METHODS IN MOLECULAR BIOLOGY

For further volumes:
http://www.springer.com/series/7651

For over 35 years, biological scientists have come to rely on the research protocols and methodologies in the critically acclaimed *Methods in Molecular Biology* series. The series was the first to introduce the step-by-step protocols approach that has become the standard in all biomedical protocol publishing. Each protocol is provided in readily-reproducible step-bystep fashion, opening with an introductory overview, a list of the materials and reagents needed to complete the experiment, and followed by a detailed procedure that is supported with a helpful notes section offering tips and tricks of the trade as well as troubleshooting advice. These hallmark features were introduced by series editor Dr. John Walker and constitute the key ingredient in each and every volume of the *Methods in Molecular Biology* series. Tested and trusted, comprehensive and reliable, all protocols from the series are indexed in Pub Med.

Allergy

Methods and Protocols

Second Edition

Edited by

Penny Lympany

Core Facilities, St. George's University of London, London, UK

Meinir G. Jones

Department of Occupational and Environmental Medicine, Imperial College London, London, UK

Humana Press

Editors
Penny Lympany
Core Facilities
St. George's University of London
London, UK

Meinir G. Jones
Department of Occupational
and Environmental Medicine
Imperial College London
London, UK

ISSN 1064-3745 ISSN 1940-6029 (electronic)
Methods in Molecular Biology
ISBN 978-1-4939-9589-9 ISBN 978-1-4939-9591-2 (eBook)
https://doi.org/10.1007/978-1-4939-9591-2

This Humana imprint is published by the registered company Springer Science+Business Media, LLC, part of Springer Nature.
The registered company address is: 233 Spring Street, New York, NY 10013, U.S.A.

Preface

Allergy is a major problem in "westernized" countries, and its prevalence continues to rise. It is therefore important to try and understand the reasons for the increase in allergy. Research, in recent years, has focused on the causes and mechanisms of allergy. In parallel, there is also an impetus to try to understand the mechanisms of natural tolerance and immunotherapy where allergy is being dampened.

This volume, *Allergy: Methods and Protocols, Second Edition, in the Methods in Molecular Biology* series, aims to assist the researcher in gaining an insight into the molecular mechanisms involved in allergy by featuring an array of protocols. These cover a range of disciplines including allergy, immunology, cell biology, and histology and include methods to investigate the cellular response to allergens, cytokine, and chemokine profile and characterization of allergens. The book is intended to be a useful bench tool for anyone embarking or continuing with their research in allergy. The techniques discussed include characterization of allergens using Western blotting and mass spectrometry, collection and sampling of airborne allergens, IgG antibodies and facilitated antigen-blocking assays, identification and characterization of allergen-specific T cells, role of antigen-presenting cells in T-cell proliferation, and measurement of allergen-specific antibodies. We thank all the authors who have shared their protocols with us and made this book possible.

London, UK *Penny Lympany*
Meinir G. Jones

Contents

Contributors

DANIEL ÁLVAREZ-SIMÓN • *Laboratori de Pneumologia, Institut de Recerca Vall d'Hebron, Universitat Autònoma de Barcelona, Barcelona, Spain*
ALLAN B. BECKER • *Department of Immunology, University of Manitoba, Winnipeg, MB, Canada; Department of Pediatrics and Child Health, University of Manitoba, Winnipeg, MB, Canada*
MARY BRIAN • *Department of Occupational and Environmental Medicine, NHLI @ Imperial College, London, UK*
JENNIFER CANIZALES • *Department of Population Health and Occupational Disease, NHLI at Imperial College, London, UK*
RISHMA CHOONIEDASS • *Department of Pediatrics and Child Health, University of Manitoba, Winnipeg, MB, Canada*
STEN DREBORG • *Department of Women's and Children's Health, Uppsala University and Academic Hospital, Uppsala, Sweden*
CECILIA DUNSTERVILLE • *King's College London, School of Immunology and Microbial Sciences and School of Life Course Sciences, Guy's Hospital, London, UK*
NATASCHA FITCH • *Department of Immunology, University of Manitoba, Winnipeg, MB, Canada*
JAMES N. FRANCIS • *Immune Targeting Systems (ITS) Ltd., London, UK*
SUSANA GÓMEZ-OLLÉS • *Laboratori de Pneumologia, Institut de Recerca Vall d'Hebron, Universitat Autònoma de Barcelona, Barcelona, Spain; Ciber Enfermedades Respiratorias (Ciberes), Madrid, Spain*
CAROLINE GRAHAM • *Department of Immunology, University of Manitoba, Winnipeg, MB, Canada*
GITTE NORDSKOV HANSEN • *ALK A/S, Hørsholm, Denmark*
THOMAS S. HAYDAY • *Cell Motility and Cytoskeleton, Randall Division of Cell and Molecular Biophysics, King's College London, London, UK*
KENT T. HAYGLASS • *Department of Immunology, University of Manitoba, Winnipeg, MB, Canada; Department of Pediatrics and Child Health, University of Manitoba, Winnipeg, MB, Canada*
LOUISA K. JAMES • *Blizard Institute, Barts and The London School of Medicine, Queen Mary University of London, London, UK*
MEINIR G. JONES • *Department of Occupational and Environmental Medicine, Imperial College London, NHLI at Imperial College, London, UK*
GIDEON LACK • *King's College London, School of Immunology and Microbial Sciences and School of Life Course Sciences, Guy's Hospital, London, UK*
JØRGEN NEDERGAARD LARSEN • *ALK A/S, Hørsholm, Denmark*
LARISA LOTOSKI • *Department of Community Health and Epidemiology, Health Science Building, University of Saskatchewan, Saskatoon, SK, Canada*
STEPHANIE J. MARSHALL • *Department of Immunology, University of Manitoba, Winnipeg, MB, Canada; Orillia Soldiers Memorial Hospital, Orillia, ON, Canada*

MONIKA RAULF • *Institute for Prevention and Occupational Medicine of the German Social Accident Insurance, Institute of the Ruhr-Universität Bochum (IPA) Center of Allergology/Immunology, Bochum, Germany;*

CLIVE ROBINSON • *Institute for Infection and Immunity, St. George's University of London, London, UK*

MOHAMED H. SHAMJI • *Immunomodulation and Tolerance Group, Allergy and Clinical Immunology, Inflammation, Repair and Develpment, National Heart and Lung Institute, Imperial College London, London, UK; Asthma UK Centre in Allergic Mechanisms of Asthma, London, UK*

WILLIAM P. STEFURA • *Department of Immunology, University of Manitoba, Winnipeg, MB, Canada*

ALICK C. STEPHENS • *King's College London, School of Immunology and Microbial Sciences and School of Life Course Sciences, Guy's Hospital, London, UK*

SUN-SANG J. SUNG • *Department of Medicine, Center for Immunity, Inflammation, and Regenerative Medicine, University of Virginia Health Sciences Center, Charlottesville, VA, USA*

VICTOR TURCANU • *King's College London, School of Immunology and Microbial Science and School of Life Course Sciences, Guy's Hospital, London, UK*

NADINE E. G. UPTON • *Asthma and Allergy, Randall Division of Cell and Molecular Biophysics, King's College London, London, UK; MRC and Asthma UK Centre for Allergic Mechanisms of Asthma, King's College London, Guy's Campus, London, UK*

ERIK WAMBRE • *Benaroya Research Institute at Virginia Mason, Seattle, WA, USA*

EVA ZAHRADNIK • *Institute for Prevention and Occupational Medicine of the German Social Accident Insurance, Institute of the Ruhr-Universitat Bochum (IPA), Center of Allergology/Immunology, Bochum, Germany*

JIHUI ZHANG • *State Key Laboratory of Microbial Resources, Institute of Microbiology, Chinese Academy of Sciences, Beijing, People's Republic of China; Institute for Infection and Immunity, St. George's University of London, London, UK*

Chapter 1

Understanding of the Molecular Mechanisms of Allergy

Meinir G. Jones

Abstract

The prevalence of allergic disease has dramatically increased over the past 30 years in Westernized countries. It is unlikely that the rapid increase in the prevalence of allergic disease is the result of genetic changes, which highlights the importance of environmental factors in the development of allergic disease. The "hygiene hypothesis" was put forward in 1989 and focused attention on the notion that exposure to microbes and their products in early life can modify the risk for development of allergic disease. Infections were thought to polarize the immunological response toward a Th2-mediated immune response causing allergic disease. However, it is likely that the Th1/Th2 imbalance is too simplistic to explain the increased prevalence of allergic disease. Current research is focusing on understanding the role of T-regulatory cells in inducing a state of tolerance and the resulting modified Th2 response observed in natural and induced tolerance.

Key words Allergic disease, Hygiene hypothesis, Immunoregulation, Immunotolerance

1 Introduction

The term "allergy" was introduced in 1906 by von Pirquet [1], who recognized that in both protective immunity and hypersensitivity reactions, antigens had induced changes in reactivity. Allergy is now used to describe a hypersensitivity reaction initiated by immunologic mechanism [2]. Allergic diseases include allergic rhinitis, allergic conjunctivitis, asthma, atopic eczema, and food allergy. IgE-mediated diseases are often referred to as atopy (from the Greek atopos, meaning out of place). The definition of atopy is a personal or familial tendency to produce IgE antibodies in response to low doses of allergens, usually proteins, and to develop typical symptoms such as asthma, rhinoconjunctivitis, or eczema/dermatitis [3].

Atopic individuals have a genetic predisposition to produce IgE antibodies against common environmental allergens. Atopic disorders are thought to be due to complex interactions between

Penny Lympany and Meinir G. Jones (eds.), *Allergy: Methods and Protocols*, Methods in Molecular Biology, vol. 2020,
https://doi.org/10.1007/978-1-4939-9591-2_1,

genetic and environmental factors. The prevalence of allergic disease has dramatically increased over the past 30 years [4–7], especially in Westernized countries. It is unlikely the rapid increase in the prevalence of allergic disease is the result of genetic changes, which emphasizes the importance of environmental factors in the development of allergic disease. The increased prevalence of allergy in Westernized countries highlights the potential influence of improved hygiene and better infection control on the development of allergy. An interesting observation was made after the reunification of Germany: Before reunification, allergic rhinitis and asthma were less common in East Germany compared with West Germany [8]. However since reunification, the prevalence of atopy and hay fever, but not asthma, has increased among children who spent their early childhood in East Germany [9]. Interestingly, exposure to farm animals remains a protective factor in the development of allergy [10], which is similar to that observed with hay fever at the turn of the century. These observations suggest that our Westernized lifestyle accounts for the increase in prevalence. Interestingly, hay fever was first reported back in the early nineteenth century and was thought to be essentially the disease of the upper social class and urban dwellers [3]. The rural working population was considered to have become tolerant through high-dose exposure in the fields.

2 Hygiene Hypothesis

The "hygiene" hypothesis was put forward in 1989 [11], and focused attention on the notion that exposure to microbes and their products in early life can modify the risk for development of allergic disorders. It is thought that helminth infection, mycobacteria, hepatitis A, endotoxin, and early-life infections create a milieu which protects against the development of allergic reactions. The distinction of Th1 and Th2 cells in mice (1989) [12] and in humans (1994) [13] provided a plausible immunological mechanism for the hygiene hypothesis. Th1 cells are responsible for cell-mediated immune responses against intracellular pathogens whereas Th2 cells direct immune responses against intestinal helminths [12]. Th1 cells cause autoimmune diseases, while Th2 cells cause allergic diseases and asthma. Th1 and Th2 cells cross regulate each other, and thus it was proposed that in allergic disease there were too many Th2 cells and not enough Th1 cells. Exposure to microbial products leads to a polarization toward the Th1 cells potentially suppressing the Th2 immune response involved in IgE-mediated allergy. Thus lack of exposure to microbes in early childhood may lead to a predominantly Th2 immune response causing allergic disease.

In parallel with an increase in prevalence of allergy in the last 30 years there has been a similar increase in autoimmune diseases such as type 1 diabetes, multiple sclerosis, inflammatory bowel disease, and systemic lupus erythematosus [14, 15]. An increase in the incidence of autoimmune diseases, plus the relative absence of autoimmunity in developing countries where chronic infections are endemic, has led to the theory that infection may actually inhibit the development of autoimmunity [14]. In view of increased prevalence of both Th1 autoimmune diseases and Th2 allergic disease in recent years, it is likely that the Th1/Th2 imbalance is too simplistic. It is more likely that there are other control mechanisms of T-cell regulation, which controls harmful T-cell responses.

3 Family Size and Allergy

One of the most robust findings in allergy which has stood the test of time is the epidemiological observation of the inverse association of allergic disease with family size, which was reported with hay fever, skin prick positivity, and specific IgE [16, 17]. Other factors found to be protective against sensitization are exposure to farm animals or domestic pets, day-care attendance, and large family size [10]. The protective influence of large family size has been interpreted as evidence in support of the hygiene hypothesis. However this does not preclude other mechanisms related to birth order [18].

It is possible that pregnancy may influence the atopic status of both the mother and the fetus. Pregnancy is an immunological challenge to the mother and it is possible that the immunoregulation, which takes place to avoid fetal rejection, may also influence the allergic response in both mother and fetus [19]. There is some evidence in support of this hypothesis. Mothers of higher parity have lower levels of total IgE, as do their newborn children [20]. They report higher rates of remission from allergic rhinitis [21] and lower rates of allergic conjunctivitis [22]. Cord blood mononuclear cell responses to house dust mite are reduced in higher birth order children [23] although this may be explained by maternal age.

In a cross-sectional study, it was observed that multiparous mothers are less often atopic, although this did not hold true for the fathers [24, 25]. In a prospective study, over a period of 7 years, it was observed that the loss of maternal atopy and hay fever are associated with a higher number of intervening pregnancies [26]. Expansion of regulatory T cells has been demonstrated in both mice [27] and humans [28]. In mice the cells were alloantigen independent although capable of suppressing an aggressive response against the fetus. Their deletion led to a failure of gestation due to immunological fetal rejection. This effect was true only for allogeneic pregnancies, the outcome of syngeneic pregnancies being unaffected. In humans, T-regulatory cells increase during early pregnancy, peaking during the second trimester and declining postpartum although remaining higher than prepregnancy [28]. The cells are capable of suppressing an allogeneic response. Allergic mothers and their neonates were found to have a stronger lymphoproliferation to alloantigen than nonallergic mothers and their neonates [29], suggesting the possibility of greater immunoregulation in nonallergic than in allergic mothers. It is not known whether the degree of regulation varies with a mother's parity nor whether it is transferred to her children.

4 Indoor Allergens

Atopic individuals are by definition sensitized to the common environmental allergens. The major allergens of the Westernized countries are Der p 1 and Der p 2, from the house dust mite (*Dermatophagoides pteronyssinus*); Fel d 1, from the cat (*Felis domesticus*); tree allergens including Bet v 1 from the birch tree (*Betula verrucosa*); and many grasses, such as Phl p 1 and Phl p 5 from timothy (*Phleum pratense*), and the ragweed allergens Amb a 1, 2, 3, 5, and 6 from short ragweed (*Ambrosia artemisiifolia*) [1]. Another allergen which has become common over the last 25 years is the glycyphagus dust mite *Blomia tropicalis*, in heavily populated tropical regions [3]. This allergen was uncommon; however it is now estimated that one billion individuals are currently sensitized.

At present there is a drive to target immunotherapy selectively to immunodominant allergens [3]. It is currently unknown whether the immunodominant allergens have intrinsic adjuvant properties that contribute to their potency. It will be intriguing to see whether removing or neutralizing the host response to immunodominant allergens will silence the allergy or redirect the immune response toward different specificities. The main allergens represent a diverse group of proteins; several are proteases which are thought to be important in the development of allergy. Currently there is much interest in the lipid binding property of immunodominant allergens [30].

Much focus has been given to understanding the mechanisms of the development of sensitization in recent years. It was proposed that exposure to indoor allergens early in life would increase the risk of allergic sensitization. If this were the case then it would follow that avoidance of allergen early in life would decrease the risk of allergic sensitization. Exposure-response studies with allergen and sensitization have demonstrated an apparent dose–response relationship with a bell-shaped curve, suggestive of a tolerance mechanism at high exposures. A bell-shaped curve was described with cat [31, 32] and house dust mite [32] allergens. Allergen avoidance trial demonstrated that reducing house dust mite concentration did not reduce but increased sensitization rates to house dust mite [33]. Cat ownership has been associated with a reduced prevalence of sensitization [34–36] and physician-diagnosed asthma [34].

Immunologically, it is known that low-dose antigen exposure favors Th2 priming whereas high-dose priming leads to a Th1 type of response [3].

5 Endotoxin

Animal exposure in the home or at work may also result in high exposures to microbial and associated products including endotoxin. Conceivably this co-exposure may confer protection, manifesting as an attenuation of the immune response to allergen at high doses. Regulatory T cells selectively express toll-like receptors which are activated by endotoxin. Exposure of CD4+CD25+ cells to the Toll-like receptor-4 ligand lipopolysaccharide induces upregulation of several activation markers and enhances their survival/proliferation [37].

The host response to environmental endotoxin appears to depend in part on the time and dose of exposure. Low doses of endotoxin induce a Th2 response whereas high-level endotoxin favors a Th1 response. In an experimental model of allergy, exposure of rats to endotoxin during early sensitization protects against their development of ovalbumin-specific IgE; co-exposure of endotoxin with allergen results in dose-dependent inhibition of acute- and late-phase allergic inflammation and bronchial hyperresponsiveness; and exposure to endotoxin after allergen challenge further exacerbates the allergic response [38]. Adult pig farmers have an inverse relationship between endotoxin and sensitization to common allergens and the overall prevalence of atopic sensitization in this population is low [39].

In contrast, other studies suggest that endotoxin is not protective. Homes of cat owners did not have higher endotoxin levels than homes without cats [40, 41]. Similarly in a study of laboratory animal workers, there was no significant relation between rat-related symptoms and endotoxin levels [42]. These results argue that the effects of cat and rat ownership cannot be explained by increased exposure to endotoxin.

6 Type 2 Immune Response

Allergy is driven by a hyperactive type 2 immune response at barrier tissues, e.g., airways, gut, and skin, requiring antigen presentation and is characterized by high levels of IL-4, IL-5, IL-9, and IL-13 traditionally associated with adaptive CD4 T-helper (Th) 2 cells. Many cells are involved with orchestrating the type 2 immune response including CD4 T-helper Th2 cells, epithelial cells, dendritic cells, macrophages, eosinophils, mast cells, basophils, and the recently identified group 2 innate lymphoid cells (ILC2) [43]. ILC2s constitutively express IL-5 and promote eosinophil production; however further signals can promote IL-5 signaling and induce IL-9 and IL-13 production leading to the typical allergic pathology including stimulating mucus production, smooth muscle cell contraction, and promoting epithelial cell repair. The ILC2 signals remain largely undefined as well as the relative contribution of ILC2s and adaptive Th2 cells in allergic responses; however ILC2s and Th2 cells appear to respond to similar signals.

A recent study suggested that IgE represents an early immunological host defense against xenobiotics or large parasites that threaten tissue integrity [44]. IgE is an ancient and highly conserved immunoglobulin, and epithelial tissues such as skin, lungs, and gut have IgE-binding cells present which can rapidly mobilize its effector functions by the induction of type 2 immunity. In an animal model, IgE was rapidly induced by cutaneous exposure to a carcinogen and the IgE response required the presence of $\gamma\delta TCR^+$ intraepithelial lymphocytes, indicating that IgE contributed to early tissue immunosurveillance against environmental xenobiotics or toxins.

7 Microbiome

The human body is home to trillions of microbes that play a critical role in educating the immune system. This microbiota is a complex community of microorganisms that includes bacteria, archaea, fungi, viruses (including bacteriophages), and protozoa species. It is becoming increasingly clear that the commensal microbes that colonize our gut, lung, and skin mediate strong regulatory effects on Th2 immune responses through effects on type 2 cytokines, dendritic cells, and regulatory T cells. Some of the regulatory mechanisms of microbial colonization include production of short-chain fatty acids butyrate and propionate which inhibits lung dendritic cells from promoting type 2 immune responses leading to the protection from allergic airway inflammation. Other mechanisms in the lung suggest that the microbiota are critical in promoting tolerance to allergens through induction of programmed death ligand (PD-L1)-dependent iTreg. Furthermore, microbial-induced iTreg can also express the transcription factor retinoic acid receptor-related orphan nuclear receptor γ (RORγt) and iTreg co-expressing FoxP3 and RORγt are required to control type 2 immune responses [16]. These studies are clearly important in unraveling as they may well help us to prevent and/or treat type 2 immune responses.

8 Cellular Response to Allergens

The cellular response of T cells in peripheral blood is often present in both healthy and sensitized individuals [45]. The epitopes recognized within allergens is also found to be similar between healthy and allergic individuals [46–50]. The cytokine profile from the in vitro T-cell culture is predominantly Th2 in the allergic individual. Th2 cytokines IL-4 and IL-13 stimulate the production of IgE; IL-5 and IL-9 are involved in the development of eosinophils; IL-4 and IL-9 promote the development of mast cells; IL-9 and IL-13 promote airway hyperresponsiveness and IL-4, IL9, and IL-13 promote the overproduction of mucus [1].

9 Modified Th2 Response

High-dose attenuation of risk of sensitization with cat allergen exposure is associated with high-titer IgG and IgG4 antibodies [31]. This response was described as a modified Th2 response since both IgE and IgG_4 require Th2 cytokine IL-4 for their production. The modified Th2 response is suggestive of clinical tolerance since the shift from specific IgE to IgG_4 resulted in a decrease in both sensitization and asthma [51].

We have recently established a modified Th2 response in laboratory animal workers. Within our cohort and cross-sectional studies on laboratory animal allergy we observed increasing risks of sensitization and work-related symptoms with increasing exposures to rats, except at highest exposure level where risks of both outcomes were lower [52, 53]. We established a significantly increased ratio of IgG_4:IgE in those workers most heavily exposed [52]. There was an almost twofold reduction in those who produced both specific IgG4 and IgE as compared to those producing specific IgE only. The attenuation at high exposures and the increased ratio of IgG_4:IgE in laboratory animal workers are suggestive of a natural form of immunotherapy.

The enteric mucosal immune system plays an extremely efficient and pivotal role in the development of tolerance. Repeated exposure to allergen through the gastrointestinal tract during life leads to the development of tolerance, even in highly atopic individuals [54]. It is proposed that exposure to aeroallergens through this route may promote the local (IgA) immune responses, which promote persistent systemic tolerance, preventing the emergence of pathogenic Th2-responsive memory T cells. The information regarding the role of IgA in mediating tolerance to allergens is at present very limited. Immunotherapy studies have shown increases in the levels of TGF-β following treatment [55]. TGF-β plays a suppressor role in mucosal allergens such as house dust mite or birch pollen and this cytokine is known to induce IgA, which works as a noninflammatory immunoglobulin isotype [55]. Levels of IgA antibodies have been shown to be upregulated following venom immunotherapy [56].

10 Natural Killer Cells

Mouse models of allergic asthma indicate that natural killer T cells are required for the development of allergen-induced airway hyperreactivity [57]. Natural killer T cells have a unique property of responding to glycolipid antigens, rather than peptide antigens presented by the nonpolymorphic class I MHC-like protein CD1d, expressed on antigen-presenting cells. Invariant natural killer T cells rapidly produce large quantities of both Th1 and Th2 cytokines, which enhance the function of dendritic cells, natural killer cells, and B cells, as well as the conventional CD4+ and CD8+ T cells [58]. The rapid production of cytokines by invariant natural killer T cells is a manifestation of innate-like immunity and provides invariant natural killer T cells with the capacity to link innate and adaptive immune responses and critically regulate adaptive immunity and a host of inflammatory diseases [58]. Recently it was observed that CD4+ invariant natural killer T cells are abundant in the lungs of patients with chronic asthma but are virtually absent from the lungs of controls and patients with sarcoidosis [58]. These natural killer cells express an invariant T-cell receptor that recognizes glycolipid antigens, which appear to be highly conserved in both man and mice. It will be important to identify glycolipid allergens from our major allergens to determine their role in both allergy and asthma.

11 Immunoregulation

The peripheral immune response has evolved several mechanisms to maintain a state of tolerance to innocuous antigens, which involves clonal deletion, anergy, and active suppression mediated by regulatory cells. Several subsets of regulatory T cells (Tr) with distinct phenotypes and distinct mechanisms of action have now been identified [59]. Recent studies suggest that naturally occurring T-regulatory cells and antigen-induced IL-10-producing T-regulatory cells have a physiological role in protecting against human allergic disease [58]. A rare mutation in the gene encoding FOXP3 results in a disease called immune dysregulation, polyendocrinopathy, and enteropathy, X-linked (IPEX). Individuals with IPEX syndrome suffer from a range of autoimmune endocrine pathologies as well as allergic symptoms including severe eczema, increased serum IgE levels, eosinophilia, and food allergies [60]. Within allergy, there is evidence that CD4+CD25+ T cells producing IL-10 are important in regulating a nonallergic response.

Healthy beekeepers show a substantial increase in IL-10-producing CD4+CD25+ T cells and monocytes, suggesting that these regulatory T cells induce tolerance to bee stings [61].

Recent interest has focused on the role of T-regulatory cells in allergic disease and immunotherapy. Seasonal atopic patients were found to have a diminished suppressive effect of T-regulatory cells compared with nonatopic controls and this was more pronounced during the hay fever season [62]. The degree of allergen exposure is likely to alter the suppressive effect of T-regulatory cells in allergic patients. At high grass pollen exposure, regulatory cells from nonatopic donors retained the ability to inhibit both proliferation and cytokine production while allergic donors failed to inhibit proliferation. At high allergen doses of wasp venom, T-regulatory cells from both allergic and healthy controls lose their regulatory function, whereas nonallergic donors retained their regulatory function at low allergen doses [63]. A study investigating regulatory differences before and after cat peptide immunotherapy demonstrated that antigen-specific proliferative responses of memory T cells were reduced after peptide immunotherapy compared with preimmunotherapy samples [64]. The CD4 cells isolated after peptide immunotherapy suppressed the proliferative response of baseline CD4-negative cells in the co-culture experiments, suggesting that peptide immunotherapy induces a population of CD4 T cells with suppressive/regulatory activity.

Grass pollen immunotherapy is associated with an increase in T-regulatory cells with IL-10+CD4+CD25+ phenotype [65]. Similarly bee venom immunotherapy demonstrated a significant increase in levels of IL-10 after therapy [66]. In a study of cat peptide immunotherapy they were able to demonstrate reduced antigen-specific proliferative responses in memory T cells following treatment. IL-10 is a potent suppressor of both total and allergen-specific IgE, whereas it simultaneously increases IgG4 production [67]. Specific IL-10 secreting T reg cells consistently represent the dominant subsets against common environmental allergens in healthy individuals, in contrast to the high frequency of allergen-specific IL-4 secreting T cells in allergic individuals [68].

In a recent pilot study, in which we investigated the role of CD4+CD25+ T cells in laboratory animal allergy, CD4+CD25− cells proliferated to a significantly greater degree than either PBMCs ($p < 0.01$) or CD25+ cells ($p < 0.001$) in all individuals (Hayley Jeal personal communication). Inhibition of proliferation to rat by CD4+CD25+ T cells did not differ between cases and controls. IL-5 suppression was increased in controls than cases although not significantly. Results from this pilot study indicate that the ability of CD4+CD25+ T regulatory cells to suppress proliferation in rat sensitized individuals compared with controls does not differ, but failure of these cells to suppress IL-5 production in cases could contribute to the development of their allergic disease.

12 Genetics

HLA class II antigens are involved in the presentation of epitopes of foreign proteins at the antigen-presenting cell surface and are important in the development of a hypersensitivity response. Epitope mapping of the major cat allergen Fel d 1 has revealed several T-cell epitopes [69]. One of these T-cell epitopes located in the carboxy-terminus of chain 2 of Fel d is associated with HLA-DRB1*0701 with preferential IL-10 induction. Production of IL-10 was enhanced in PBMC from DR-7-positive modified responders compared to their DR-7-negative counterparts. Expression of HLA-DR7, coupled with high-dose exposure to cat allergen, could favor optimal induction of T-regulatory cells in parallel with Th1 cells. When this occurs during the initiation phase of the immune response, it may result in imprinting of the regulatory mechanism necessary to prevent expansion of Th2 cells. A second immunodominant region within the chain, induced IL-5 and a strong T-cell proliferation, in allergic and modified Th2 responders but not in control subjects [69]. Thus the ratio between TRl and Th2 cells may determine the development of a healthy or allergic immune response. The generation of allergen-specific T reg cells and increased production of suppressive cytokines IL-10 and TGF-β are essentially early events in allergen-specific immunotherapy [67, 68].

Several studies have demonstrated HLA associations with low-molecular-weight chemical sensitizers [70–73]. It is likely to be more difficult to establish a HLA association with larger allergen as multiple T-cell epitopes are likely to be presented by different HLA molecules, diluting any single-HLA association. We have established in laboratory animal allergy that HLA-DR7 was associated with sensitization to rat allergen and respiratory symptoms at work whereas HLA-DR3 was protective against sensitization [74]. The major rat allergen, Rat n 1, is a relatively low-molecular-weight protein with just five identical T-cell epitopes.

13 Intradermal Exposure

The high-dose attenuation of risk of sensitization and symptoms demonstrated with laboratory animal allergens is similar to both natural tolerance seen with beekeepers that have been frequently stung by bees and the induced tolerance by subcutaneous injection of natural allergen in immunotherapy. One common theme with bee keepers, laboratory animal workers, and cat owners, who develop tolerance at high exposures, is that they are at high risk of being bitten and scratched. We suggest that the intradermal exposure to the allergens is responsible for the induced tolerance. In support of our hypothesis is the observation that repeated inhalation of cat peptides as an experimental method of immunotherapy was not—in contrast to an intradermal method—associated with the induction of hyporesponsiveness ("tolerance") in the skin or the lung. Other groups of workers at risk of developing occupational asthma, for example bakers and detergent workers, do not develop attenuation at high exposure—these workers are less likely to have an intradermal exposure.

14 Immunotherapy

Specific allergen injection immunotherapy is an effective treatment for IgE-mediated allergic diseases, which may confer long-term benefit for at least 3 years after discontinuation [75]. Immunotherapy is generally administered by either subcutaneous injection or sublingual administration of allergen.

The mechanisms associated with immunotherapy are thought to involve both humoral and cellular responses. Following immunotherapy there is a modest reduction in allergen-specific IgE and increases in allergen-specific IgG antibodies, particularly the IgG4 subclass. Effector cells are reduced at the site of allergic inflammation, including a reduction in the numbers of mast cells, eosinophils, and basophils and the release in mediator secretion. There is thought to be an immune deviation toward a Th1-type response or the induction of T-regulatory cells producing IL-10 and transforming growth factor beta.

More recently regulatory B cells (Breg) are thought to be important in maintaining and restoring tolerance to allergens, particularly the Breg subset $CD73^{-}$ $CD24^{+}CD71^{-}$ BR1 cells [76]. In those patients receiving immunotherapy with bee venom, the allergen-specific B cells increased two- to fivefold, reaching a level comparable to healthy beekeepers during the season. In parallel with IL-10, allergen-specific B cells also upregulated C-C chemokine receptor (CCR)5, a receptor for macrophage inflammatory protein 1a and b. Interestingly, there is a link between IL-10-producing BR1 cells and IgG4 production suggesting that BR1 cells may promote tolerance through IL-10-medicated suppressive effects and through directing the humoral response toward IgG_4.

Ratios of IgE to IgG4 have been found to change during specific immunotherapy [61] Specific serum levels of both IgE and IgG4 increase during the early phase of therapy, but the increase in specific IgG4 is more pronounced and the ratio of specific IgG4:IgE is increased 10- to 100-fold, suggesting a protective role for IgG4 [61]. IL-10 is a potent suppressor of both total and allergen-specific IgE, whereas it simultaneously increases IgG4 production [67].

Successful immunotherapy is associated with increases in allergen-specific IgG_1 and IgG_4 antibody concentrations occur that correlate with the clinical outcome [77–80]. It is not known whether allergen-specific IgG or IgG_4 antibodies associated with the modified Th2 response exhibit functional activity. It is possible that IgG antibodies may play a protective role by blocking leukocyte histamine release, inhibiting signal transduction and mediator release through the high-affinity IgE receptor (FcεRl) and IgG (FcγRIIB) receptors [81–84] and blocking allergen-induced IgE-dependent histamine release by basophils [85]. IgG antibodies may exert their effect by competitive inhibition of allergen-IgE complexes, which prevents complexes binding to the low-affinity IgE receptor, CD23, and subsequent antigen presentation. Others have suggested that not only quantitative changes occur with the IgG antibody but also the spectrum of the specificity of the IgG is altered [86]. One grass pollen immunotherapy study demonstrated a blunting of seasonal increases in serum allergen-specific IgG and IgG_4. Further examination showed the postimmunotherapy serum to exhibit inhibitory activity, which co-eluted with IgG_4 and blocked IgE-facilitated binding of allergen-IgE complexes to B cells. Increases in IgG and IgG blocking activity correlated with the patients' overall assessment of improvement [79].

References

1. Kay AB (2001) Allergy and allergic diseases. N Engl J Med 344:30–37
2. Johansson SGO, Hourihane JO, Bousquet J, Bruijnzeel-Koomen C, Dreborg S, Haahtela T et al (2001) A revised nomenclature for allergy. Allergy 56:813–824
3. Holt PG, Thomas WR (2005) Sensitization to airborne environmental allergens: unresolved issues. Nat Immunol 6:957–960
4. The International Study of Asthma and Allergies in Childhood (ISAAC) Steering Committee (1998) Worldwide variation in prevalence of asthma, allergic rhinoconjunctivitis, and atopic eczema: ISAAC. Lancet 351:1225–1232
5. Aberg N, Hesselmar B, Aberg B, Eriksson B (1995) Increase of asthma, allergic rhinitis and eczema in Swedish schoolchildren between 1979 and 1991. Clin Exp Allergy 25:815–819
6. Celedon JC, Soto-Quiros ME, Hanson LA, Weiss ST (2002) The relationship among markers of allergy, asthma, allergic rhinitis, and eczema in Costa Rica. Pediatr Allergy Immunol 13:91–97
7. Ninan TK, Russell G (1992) Respiratory symptoms and atopy in Aberdeen school-children: evidence from two surveys 25 years apart. BMJ 304:873–875
8. von Mutius E, Martinez FD, Fritzch C, Nicolai T, Roell G, Thiemann HH (1994) Prevalence of asthma and atopy in two areas of east and West Germany. Am J Respir Crit Care Med 149:358–364
9. von Mutius E, Weiland SK, Fritasch C, Duhme H, Keil U (1998) Increasing prevalence of hay fever and atopy among children in Leipzig, East Germany. Lancet 351:862–866
10. Upham JW, Holt PG (2005) Environment and development of atopy. Curr Opin Allergy Clin Immunol 5:67–172
11. Strachan DP (1989) Hay fever, hygiene and household size. BMJ 299:1259–1260
12. Mosmann TR, Coffman RL (1989) Thl and Th2 cells: differential patterns of lymphokine secretion lead to different functional properties. Annu Rev Immunol 7:145–173
13. Romagnani S (1994) Lymphokine production by human T cells in disease states. Annu Rev Immunol 12:27–257
14. Cooke A, Zaccone P, Raine T, Phillips JM, Dunne DW (2004) Infection and autoimmunity: are we winning the war, only to lose the peace? Trends Parasitol 20:316–321
15. Bach JF (2002) The effect of infections on susceptibility to autoimmune and allergic diseases. N Engl J Med 347:911–920

16. Strachan DP (1997) Allergy and family size, a riddle worth solving. Clin Exp Allergy 27:235–236
17. Karmaus W, Botezan C (2002) Does a higher number of siblings protect against the development of allergy and asthma? A review. J Epidemiol Community Health 56:209–217
18. Cullinan P (2006) Childhood allergies, birth order and family size. Thorax 61:3–5
19. Sacks G, Sargent I, Redman C (1999) An innate view of human pregnancy. Immunol Today 20:114–118
20. Karmaus W, Arshad SH, Sadeghnejad A, Twiselton R (2004) Does maternal immunoglobulin E decrease with increasing order of live offspring? Investigation into maternal immune tolerance. Clin Exp Allergy 34:853–859
21. Westergaard T, Begtrup K, Rostgaard K, Krause TG, Benn CS, Melbye M (2003) Reproductive history and allergic rhinitis among 31145 Danish women. Clin Exp Allergy 33:301–305
22. Forastiere F, Sunyer J, Farchi S, Corbo G, Pistelli R, Baldacci S et al (2005) Number of offspring and maternal allergy. Allergy 60:510–514
23. Devereux G, Barker RN, Seaton A (2002) Antenatal determinants of neonatal immune responses to allergens. Clin Exp Allergy 32:43–50
24. Sunyer J, Anto JM, Harris J, Torrent M, Vall O, Cullinan P et al (2001) Maternal atopy and parity. Clin Exp Allergy 31:1352–1355
25. Karmaus W, Eneli I (2003) Maternal atopy and the number of offspring, is there an association? Pediatr Allergy Immunol 14:470–474
26. Harris JM, White C, Moffat S, Mills P, Newman Taylor AJ, Cullinan P (2004) New pregnancies and loss of allergy. Clin Exp Allergy 34:369–372
27. Aluvihare VR, Kallikourdis M, Betz AG (2004) Regulatory T cells mediate maternal tolerance to the fetus. Nat Immunol 5:266–271
28. Somerset DA, Zheng Y, Kilby MD, Sansom DM, Drayson MT (2004) Normal human pregnancy is associated with an elevation in the immune suppressive CD25+CD4+ regulatory T-cell subset. Immunology 112:38–43
29. Prescott SL, Taylor A, Roper J, Wahdan A, Noakes P et al (2005) Maternal reactivity to fetal alloantigens is related to newborn immune responses and subsequent allergic disease. Clin Exp Allergy 35:417–425
30. Thomas W, Hales B, Smith W (2005) Genetically engineered vaccines. Curr Allergy Asthma Rep 5:388–393
31. Platts-Mills T, Vaughan J, Squillace S, Woodfolk J, Sporik R (2001) Sensitisation, asthma, and a modified Th2 response in children exposed to cat allergen, a population-based cross-sectional study. Lancet 357:752–756
32. Cullinan P, MacNeill SJ, Harris J, Moffat S, White C, Mills P et al (2004) Early allergen exposure, skin prick responses, and atopic wheeze at age 5 in English children, a cohort study. Thorax 59:855–861
33. Woodcock A, Lowe LA, Murray CS, Simpson BM, Pipis SD, Kissen P et al (2004) National Asthma Campaign Manchester Asthma and Allergy Study Group. Early life environmental control, effect on symptoms, sensitization, and lung function at age 3 years. Am J Respir Crit Care Med 170:433–439
34. Perzanowski MS, Ronmark E, Platts-Mills TA, Lundback B (2002) Effect of cat and dog ownership on sensitization and development of asthma among pre-teenage children. Am J Respir Crit Care Med 166:696–702
35. Ownby DR, Johnson CC, Peterson EL (2002) Exposure to dogs and cats in the first year of life and risk of allergic sensitization at 6 to 7 years of age. JAMA 288:963–972
36. Custovic A, Simpson BM, Simpson A, Hallam CL, Marolia H, Walsh D et al (2003) National Asthma Campaign Manchester Asthma and Allergy Study Group. Current mite, cat, and dog allergen exposure, pet ownership, and sensitization to inhalant allergens in adults. J Allergy Clin Immunol 111:402–407
37. Caramalho I, Lopes-Carvalho T, Ostler D, Zelenay S, Haury M, Demengeot J (2003) Regulatory T cells selectively express toll-like receptors and are activated by lipopolysaccharide. J Exp Med 197:403–411
38. Tulic MK, Holt PG, Sly PD (2002) Modification of acute and late-phase allergic responses to ovalbumin with lipopolysaccharide. Int Arch Allergy Immunol 129:119–128
39. Portengen L, Preller L, Tielen M, Doekes G, Heederik D (2005) Endotoxin exposure and atopic sensitization in adult pig farmers. J Allergy Clin Immunol 115:797–802
40. Lau S, Illi S, Platts-Mills TA, Riposo D, Nickel R, Gruber C, Niggemann B et al (2005) Multicentre Allergy Study Group. Longitudinal study on the relationship between cat allergen and endotoxin exposure, sensitization, cat-specific IgG and development of asthma in childhood--report of the German Multicentre Allergy Study (MAS 90). Allergy 60:766–773
41. Platts-Mills JA, Custis NJ, Woodfolk JA, Platts-Mills TA (2005) Airborne endotoxin in homes with domestic animals, implications for cat-specific tolerance. J Allergy Clin Immunol 116:384–389
42. Lieutier-Colas F, Meyer P, Pons F, Edelin G, Larsson P, Malmberg P et al (2002) Prevalence

of symptoms, sensitization to rats, and airborne exposure to major rat allergen (Rat n 1) and to endotoxin in rat-exposed workers, a cross-sectional study. Clin Exp Allergy 32:1424–1429

43. Dahlgren MW, Molofsky AB (2018) All along the watchtower: group 2 innate lymphoid cells in allergic responses. Curr Opin Immunol 54:13–19
44. Crawford G, Hayes MD, Seoane RC et al (2018) Epithelial damage and tissue γδ T cells promote a unique tumor-protective IgE response. Nat Immunol 19:859–870
45. Jeal H, Draper A, Harris J, Newman Taylor A, Cullinan P, Jones M (2004) Determination of the T cell epitopes of the lipocalin allergen, rat n 1. Clin Exp Allergy 34:1919–1925
46. Ebner C, Schenk S, Najafian N, Siemann U, Steiner R, Fischer GW et al (1995) Nonallergic individuals recognize the same T cell epitopes of Bet v 1, the major birch pollen allergen, as atopic patients. J Immunol 154:1932–1940
47. O'Hehir RE, Verhoef A, Panagiotopoulou E, Keswani S, Hayball JD, Thomas WR et al (1993) Analysis of human T cell responses to the group II allergen of Dermatophagoides species, localization of major antigenic sites. J Allergy Clin Immunol 92:105–113
48. Verhoef A, Higgins JA, Thorpe CJ, Marsh SG, Hayball JD, Lamb JR et al (1993) Clonal analysis of the atopic immune response to the group 2 allergen of Dermatophagoides spp, identification of HLA-DR and -DQ restricted T cell epitopes. Int Immunol 5:1589–1597
49. Van Neerven RJ, Van de Pol MM, Van Milligen FJ, Jansen HM, Aalberse RC, Kapsenberg ML (1994) Characterisation of cat ander-specific T lymphocytes from atopic patients. J Immunol 152:4203–4210
50. Carballido JM, Carballido-Perrig N, Kagi MK, Meloen RH, Wuthrich B, Heusser CH et al (1993) T cell epitope specificity in human allergic and nonallergic subjects to bee venom phospholipase A2. J Immunol 150:3582–3591
51. Hesselmar B, Aberg B, Eriksson B, Bjorksten B, Aberg N (2003) High-dose exposure to cat is associated with clinical tolerance--a modified Th2 immune response? Clin Exp Allergy 33:1681–1685
52. Jeal H, Draper A, Harris J, Newman Taylor AJ, Cullinan P, Jones M (2006) Modified TH2 responses at high dose exposures to allergen. Using an occupational model. Am J Respir Crit Care Med 174(1):21–25
53. Cullinan P, Cook A, Gordon S, Nieuwenhuijsen MJ, Tee RD, Venables KM et al (1999) Allergen exposure, atopy and smoking as determinants of allergy to rats in a cohort of laboratory employees. Eur Respir J 13:1139–1143
54. Holt PG (1994) A potential vaccine strategy for asthma and allied atopic diseases during early childhood. Lancet 344:456–458
55. Jutel M, Akdis M, Budak F, Aebischer-Casaulta C, Wrzyszcz M, Blaser K et al (2003) IL-10 and TGF-Beta cooperate in the regulatory cell response to mucosal allergens in normal immunity and specific immunotherapy. Eur J Immunol 33:1205–1214
56. Jutel M, Akdis M, Blaser K, Akdis CA (2005) Are regulatory T cells the target of venom immunotherapy? Curr Opin Allergy Clin Immunol 116:608–613
57. Dombrowicz D (2005) Exploiting the innate immune system to control allergic asthma. Eur J Immunol 35:2786–2788
58. Akbari O, Faul JL, Hoyte EG, Berry GJ, Wahlstrom J, Kronenberg M et al (2006) CD4+ invariant T-cell-receptor+ natural killer T cells in bronchial asthma. N Engl J Med 354:1117–1129
59. Akbari O, DeKruyff RH, Umetsu DT (2001) Pulmonary dendritic cells producing IL-10 mediate tolerance induced by respiratory exposure to antigen. Nat Immunol 2:725–731
60. Hawrylowicz CM (2005) Regulatory T cells and IL-10 in allergic inflammation. J Exp Med 202:1459–1463
61. Akdis CA, Blaser K (1999) IL-10 induced anergy in peripheral T cell and reactivation by microenvironmental cytokines, two key steps in specific immunotherapy. FASEB J 13:603–609
62. Ling EM, Robinson DS (2004) Relation of CD4+CD25+ regulatory T-cell suppression of allergen-driven T-cell activation to atopic status and expression of allergic disease. Lancet 363:608–615
63. Bellinghausen I, Konig B, Bottcher I, Knop J, Saloga J (2005) Regulatory activity of human $CD4^+CD25^+$ T cells depends on allergen concentration, type of allergen and atopy status of the donor. Immunology 116:103–111
64. Verhoef A, Alexander C, Kay AB, Larche M (2005) T cell epitope immunotherapy induces a CD4+ T cell population with regulatory activity. PLoS Med 2(3):e78
65. Francis JN, Till SJ, Durham SR (2003) Induction of IL-10+CD4+CD25+ T cells by grass pollen immunotherapy. J Allergy Clin Immunol 111:1255–1261
66. Tarzi M, Klunker S, Texier C, Verhoef A, Stapel SO, Akdis CA et al (2006) Induction of interleukin-10 and suppressor of cytokine signalling-3 gene expression following peptide immunotherapy. Clin Exp Allergy 36:465–474

67. Akdis CA, Blesken T, Akdis M, Wuthrich B, Blaser K (1998) Role of interleukin 10 in specific immunotherapy. J Clin Invest 102:98–106
68. Akdis M, Blaser K, Akdis CA (2005) T regulatory cells in allergy, novel concepts in the pathogenesis, prevention, and treatment of allergic diseases. J Allergy Clin Immunol 116:961–968
69. Woodfolk JA (2005) High-dose allergen exposure leads to tolerance. Clin Rev Allergy Immunol 28:43–58
70. Jones MG, Nielsen J, Welch J, Harris J, Welinder H, Bensryd I et al (2004) Association of HLA-DQ5 and HLA-DR1 with sensitization to organic acid anhydrides. Clin Exp Allergy 34:812–816
71. Map CE, Balboni A, Baricordi R, Fabbri LM (1997) Human leukocyte antigen associations in occupational asthma induced by isocyanates. Am J Respir Crit Care Med 156:S139–S143
72. Newman Taylor AJ, Cullinan P, Lympany PA, Harris JM, Dowdeswell RJ, du Bois RM (1999) Interaction of HLA phenotype and exposure intensity in sensitization to complex platinum salts. Am J Respir Crit Care Med 160:435–438
73. Young RP, Barker RD, Pile KD, Cookson WO, Newman Taylor AJ (1995) The association of HLA-DR3 with specific IgE to inhaled acid anhydrides. Am J Respir Crit Care Med 151:219–221
74. Jeal H, Draper A, Jones M, Harris J, Welsh K, Newman Taylor A, Cullinan P (2003) HLA associations with occupational sensitisation to rat lipocalin allergens, a model for other animal allergies? J Allergy Clin Immunol 111:759–759
75. Francis J, Larche M (2005) Peptide-based vaccination, where do we stand? Curr Opin Allergy Clin Immunol 5:537–543
76. van de Veen W, Stanic B, Wirz OF et al (2016) Role of regulatory B cells in immune tolerance to allergens and beyond. J Allergy Clin Immunol 138:654–665
77. Gehlhar K, Schlaak M, Becker W, Bufe A (1999) Monitoring allergen immunotherapy of pollen-allergic patients, the ratio of allergen-specific IgG4 to IgG1 correlates with clinical outcome. Clin Exp Allergy 29:497–506
78. Jutel M, Akdis M, Budak F, Aebischer-Casaulta C, Wrzyszcz MA, Blaser K (2003) IL-10 and TGF-beta cooperate in the regulatory T cell response to mucosal allergens in normal immunity and specific immunotherapy. Eur J Immunol 33:1205–1214
79. Nouri-Aria KT, Wachholz PA, Francis JN, Jabobson MR, Walker SM, Wilcock LK et al (2004) Grass pollen immunotherapy induces mucosal and peripheral IL-10 responses and blocking IgG activity. J Immunol 172:3252–3259
80. Djurup R, Osterballe O (1984) IgG subclass antibody response in grass pollen-allergic patients undergoing specific immunotherapy. Prognostic value of serum IgG subclass antibody levels early in immunotherapy. Allergy 39:433–441
81. Golden DB, Meyers DA, Kagey-Sobotka A, Valentine MD, Lichtenstein LM (1982) Clinical relevance of the venom-specific immunoglobulin G antibody level during immunotherapy. J Allergy Clin Immunol 69:489–493
82. Daeron M, Malbec O, Latour S, Arock M, Fridman WH (1995) Regulation of high affinity IgE receptor-mediated mast cell activation by murine low-affinity IgG receptors. J Clin Invest 95:577–585
83. Daeron M (1997) Negative regulation of mast cell activation by receptors for IgG. Int Arch Allergy Immunol 113:138–141
84. Zhu D, Kepley CL, Zhang M, Zhang K, Saxon A (2002) A novel human immunoglobulin Fc gamma Fc epsilon bifunctional fusion protein inhibits Fc epsilon R1-mediated degranulation. Nat Med 8:518–521
85. Ball T, Sperr WR, Valent P, Lidholm J, Spitzauer S, Ebner C et al (1999) Induction of antibody responses to new B cell epitopes indicates vaccination character of allergen immunotherapy. Eur J Immunol 29:2026–2036
86. Wachholz PA, Durham SR (2003) Induction of 'blocking' IgG antibodies during immunotherapy. Clin Exp Allergy 33:1171–1174

Chapter 2

T Cell: Primary Culture from Peripheral Blood

Monika Raulf

Abstract

Peripheral blood mononuclear cells (PBMCs) can be used to assess cell-mediated immunity in general or via antigen-specific stimulation to detect previous exposure to a variety of antigens/allergens and to monitor the response to immunotherapies. Peripheral blood is the most common source of mononuclear cells for in vitro cultures, although mononuclear cells can be obtained from other sources involved in the allergic reaction. PBMCs from individuals previously exposed to an antigen proliferate in vitro when stimulated with the specific antigen. Proliferation is measured by the incorporation of (^{3}H)-thymidine into newly synthesized DNA. This parameter is often used as an endpoint of lymphocyte stimulation induced by antigen or antigen fragments (e.g., synthetic peptides), mitogens, or anti-CD3/anti-CD28 combinations. The aim of this chapter is to describe the culture of T cells obtained from peripheral blood and the collection of cell supernatants for cytokine measurement.

Key words Peripheral blood mononuclear cells, T-cell culture, Proliferation, Cytokines

1 Introduction

The investigation of the human immune system is a key element in understanding allergic reactions. Peripheral blood mononuclear cells (PBMCs) can be used to assess cell-mediated immunity in general or, via antigen-specific stimulation, to detect previous exposure to a variety of antigens/allergens and to monitor the response to immunotherapies.

Peripheral blood is the most common source of mononuclear cells (lymphocytes and monocytes; PBMC) for in vitro cultures, although mononuclear cells can be obtained from other sources involved in the allergic reaction (lung, skin, etc.). PBMCs from individuals previously exposed to an antigen proliferate in vitro when stimulated with the specific antigen. Proliferation is measured by the incorporation of (^{3}H)-thymidine into newly synthesized DNA. This parameter is often used as an endpoint of lymphocyte stimulation induced by antigen or antigen fragments (e.g., synthetic peptides), mitogens, or anti-CD3/anti-CD28 combinations.

Penny Lympany and Meinir G. Jones (eds.), *Allergy: Methods and Protocols*, Methods in Molecular Biology, vol. 2020,
https://doi.org/10.1007/978-1-4939-9591-2_2,

Measurable amounts of cytokines can be detected in such cultures. In some cases, an enhanced expression of cytokine receptors and activation markers can be detected on lymphocyte surfaces by flow cytometry.

In addition to basic nutrients, in vitro cultures of PBMC require a serum supplement, usually of human or fetal calf origin.

It is frequently difficult to perform studies on PBMCs the same day they are obtained. However, it is feasible to freeze and thaw the separated PBMC without significant loss of function.

2 Materials

2.1 General Comments on Sterile Working and Biosafety Practice

All solutions and equipment coming into contact with cells must be sterile and a proper sterile technique should be used accordingly. Usually as a minimum, a lamina flow hood filtering the air to remove airborne bacteria and fungi is necessary. However, laminar flow cabinets are normally produced to protect the working area and not the operator and are therefore not suitable for working with potential biohazards. Immunological studies of the human immune system pose special safety problems associated with the risk for infection with human disease agents. Invariably, blood samples should be treated as though they were a potential source of hepatitis or HIV infection. If your risk assessment suggests that your sample may present such a hazard, then a Class I or II microbiological safety cabinet and appropriate personal protective equipment should be used, i.e., wearing laboratory suits, latex gloves, and eye protectors. Disinfection of all equipment after use is recommended (e.g., with alcohol or Barrycidal).

Work in the laboratory environment is closely regulated by legislation, usually reinforced and exemplified by institutional and local codes of practice. Many of the requirements for "good laboratory practice" rely on common sense or are based on a thorough knowledge of the likely risks and their avoidance (e.g., hazardous procedures or chemicals). Eating, drinking, smoking, or application of cosmetics in laboratory areas should be prohibited. A large number of commonly used laboratory chemicals are potentially carcinogenic or mutagenic, for example phorbol esters (PMA) or propidium iodide, and handling them with care is necessary [1, 2].

In addition, there are defined legal requirements for the handling of radioisotopes (*see* (^{3}H)-thymidine labeling). The work area should be especially designed for their use. The design of apparatus and experimental procedures should minimize the handling of radioactive material and avoid exposure to radiation. Appropriate shielding and distance reduce the radioactive dose received.

2.2 Culture Media, Supplements, Reagents, and Equipment

Many different culture media are available. RPMI 1640 was specifically designed for the culture of human cells. It is a double-buffering system containing bicarbonate (24 mM) and HEPES (50 mM) (*N*-2-hydroxyethyl-piperazine *N*-2-ethanesulfonic acid) buffered by CO_2 in the air, as this approximates physiological conditions in closed culture conditions (5% CO_2 in air in a gassed incubator). Although 20 mM HEPES alone can control the pH of the culture medium within physiological limits, cells grow better in the presence of CO_2 and HCO_3^-. Oxygen tension is also important for the growth of cells. In static cultures, the depth of the medium should be greater than about 5 mm. Most cells grow well at pH 7.4. At this pH phenol red, the most commonly used indicator is salmon. It is orange at pH 7.0, yellow at pH 6.5, and blue ("livid") under alkaline conditions.

For the prevention of bacterial contamination in cell cultures, an antibiotic cocktail of penicillin (100 U/mL) and streptomycin sulfate (100 μg/mL) or gentamycin (30 μg/mL; more stable but more expensive) is recommended. Protection from yeast contamination is possible by adding fungizone (amphotericin B) up to a final concentration of 10 μg/mL.

The growth of cells in cultures requires a complex mixture of nutrients and other essential components. Theoretically, it should consist of a totally defined set of media additives that result in vigorous cell growth without causing extraneous cell stimulation. Such media additives have been devised but they are usually not as satisfactory as fetal calf serum (FCS), an easily obtained and relatively cheap material that normally contains all components necessary for the growth of human cells (heat inactivation for 30 min at 56 °C reduces the number of viral and other adventitious contaminants and inactivate complements; filter-sterilized (0.45 μm filter)).

Alternatively, cell cultures can grow in serum-free medium (e.g., Ultraculture; Yssel's medium which is based on a modification of Iscove's modified Dulbecco's medium) [3]. In some cases stimulation experiments will be performed in serum-free ultraculture medium (Bioproducts, Heidelberg, Germany) supplemented with 2 mM GlutaMAX™ 1 (Life Style Technology), antibiotic/antimycotic solution (Sigma, Deisenhofen, Germany), and 20 mM β-mercaptoethanol (Life Style Technology) [4].

In some experiments involving the culture of human lymphocytes, it is preferable to replace FCS with human AB serum because FCS can be mitogenic for human cells. Since the capacity of human AB serum to support lymphocyte cultures can vary, the screening of various batches is recommended. In addition, human AB serum should be heat inactivated for 30 min at 56 °C.

Nonessential amino acids may be required for some applications. Glutamine is a nonessential amino acid that serves not only as a primary respiratory fuel, but also as a necessary substrate for nucleotide synthesis in rapidly proliferating cells such as lymphocytes. Glutamine can be produced in sufficient quantities under stable conditions, but it becomes a limiting substrate during metabolic stress. Optimal lymphocyte functions have been demonstrated when the glutamine concentration is set around 0.6–2.0 mM [5, 6].

Although the precise mode(s) of action of 2-mercaptoethanol (2-ME) has not been defined it must be included in media (final concentration 50 μM) used for procedures with primary cultures. 2-ME (50 mM in PBS diluted solution; stored at 4 °C) must be added to media immediately before use, because its activity rapidly declines if diluted.

A variety of ingredients and reagents are supplemented to media shortly before use; they are typically made in large batches at 100× or 200× concentrations and stored in small aliquots of convenient size until use at −20 °C and pre-warmed at 37 °C before use.

It is possible to purchase sterile media in solution. Alternatively, packaged, premixed powders can be purchased and reconstituted in 10–20 L batches, which must then be filter-sterilized (0.45 μm filter). The media can be stored at 4 °C (*see* the manufacturer's recommendations).

1. Complete RPMI (*R*oswell *P*ark *M*emorial *I*nstitute) medium (500 mL) containing 439.5 mL RPMI1640 cell culture medium with GlutaMAX™ I-supplement and 25 mM HEPES (Gibco, BRL; Life Technologies GmbH Paisley; UK), 5 mL penicillin/streptomycin (10,000 U/mL penicillin and 10,000 μg/mL streptomycin; Gibco, BRL), 5 mL sodium pyruvate MEM (100 mM; Gibco, BRL), 0.5 mL 2-mercaptoethanol (1000×, Gibco, BRL), 50 mL FCS (Biochrom, Berlin), or human AB-serum (both heat inactivated).
2. Hanks' balanced salt solution (HBSS) without calcium and magnesium: D-Glucose (1.0 g/L), KCl (0.4 g/L), KH_2PO_4 (0.06 g/L), NaCl (8.0 g/L), $NaHCO_3$ (0.35 g/L), Na_2HPO_4 (0.048 g/L).
3. Phosphate-buffered saline (PBS; Dulbecco's) (10×): 80 g NaCl, 23 g $Na_2H\ PO_4\ 2\ H_2O$, 2 g $KH_2\ PO_4$, 2 g KCl. Make up to 1000 mL with H_2O. For the ready-to-use PBS buffer (1×), mix 100 mL PBS (10×) with 800 mL H_2O; adjust to desired pH (7.2–7.4) with NaOH. Make up to 1000 mL with H_2O.

For cell cultures and experiments, special equipment and utensils are necessary including CO_2 humidified incubator, biosafety cabinet (laminar flow hood; Kendro Laboratory Products), autoclave, centrifuges (e.g., Beckman Instruments, Munich), multiwell harvester or cell harvester (PHD, Cambridge Technologies, or 1450 Microbeta Trilux, Perkin Elmer Wallac GmbH, Freiburg), etc.

1. *Thymidine*: (^{3}H)-labeled thymidine-methyl is added to each cell-containing well for determination of the proliferation response. Purchased from Dupont, Germany, NEN Division, Dreieich, Germany.
2. *Ficoll-Paque* (or Ficoll-Paque plus; Amersham Biosciences Europe GmbH, Freiburg Germany, or Pharmacia LKB, Uppsala, Sweden) for in vitro isolation of lymphocytes; should be stored between 4 and 25 °C and protected from direct light. Cold storage will increase the shelf life. Ficoll-Paque plus provides a sterile, ready-to-use Ficoll-sodium diatrizoate solution (contains nonionic saccharose polymer, sodium-diatrizoate, and ethylenediaminetetraacetic acid-disodium) of the appropriate density, viscosity, and osmotic pressure for use in a simple and rapid lymphocyte isolation procedure.
3. *PBS, BSA, EDTA*: Buffer used for the pan T-cell isolation kit; PBS with 0.5% bovine serum albumin (BSA) and 2 mM EDTA; should be degassed by applying vacuum or sonification.
4. *Eosin B* for microscopy (Merck Eurolab, Darmstadt, Germany): Prepare the 1% eosin stock solution by dissolving 100 mg eosin in 10 mL complete medium and sterile filtration; storage at +4 °C for 1 month is possible; dilute the stock solution 1:10 with complete medium for use.
5. *Freezing medium*: A mixture prepared of 440 mL RPMI 1640 with Glutamax I, 5 mL penicillin/streptomycin, 5 mL sodium pyruvate, 100 mL FCS medium, and 50 mL DMSO. Aliquoted in 50 mL and stored at −20 °C.
6. *PHA* (phytohemagglutinin; lectin from *Phaseolus vulgaris*; Sigma, Deisenhofen, Germany): 5 mg Lyophilisate should be dissolved in 1 mL sterile HBSS (allowed to stand for 10 min for complete dissolution); carefully mixed, aliquoted in 10 μL portion (50 μg), and stored at −20 °C.
7. Hapten-antibody cocktail of antibodies for pan T-cell isolation kit: A cocktail of CD11b, CD16, CD19, CD36, and CD56 antibodies is used for the depletion of non-T cells. These antibodies are hapten conjugated.
8. Reagents for polyclonal cell stimulation: Use combinations of PMA (1 ng/mL) and calcium ionophore A23187 (500 ng/mL) both from "Sigma Chemicals"; PMA and soluble anti-CD3 mAb (1 μg/mL) (anti-CD3 were purchased from Ortho Pharmaceuticals USA); and anti-CD28 mAb (1 μg/mL) and coated anti-CD3 mAb to plates.

3 Methods

3.1 Obtaining Peripheral Blood

Blood should be taken by trained staff in designated areas, and biosafety practices must be followed. Collect blood in heparinized tubes (20 mL heparinized blood for 2 –3 × 10^7 cells).

3.2 Preparation of Human Mononuclear Cell Population (PBMC)

The use of human peripheral blood as a source of lymphoid cells is facilitated by Ficoll-Hypaque density gradient centrifugation [7]. This simple and rapid method of purifying peripheral blood mononuclear cells (PBMCs) takes advantage of the density differences between mononuclear cells and other blood materials. Mononuclear cells and platelets collect on top of the Ficoll-Hypaque layer because they have a lower density: in contrast, erythrocytes and granulocytes (neutrophils and eosinophils) have a higher density than Ficoll-Hypaque and collect themselves at the bottom of the gradient. Platelets are separated from the mononuclear cells by subsequent washing. Removal of immature cells (contaminants of cord blood and peripheral blood from infants) requires additional steps. All procedure steps have to be done under sterile conditions using a laminar flow cabinet.

1. Transfer the fresh heparinized blood into a 15 or 50 mL conical centrifuge tube, add an equal volume of HBSS (room temperature) or PBS, and mix it well. (Using blood from a leukophoresis donor, blood dilution with buffer of 1:3 or 1:4 (blood:buffer) is recommended.) (Alternatively, instead of 50 mL conical centrifuge tubes use LeucoSep tubes (Greiner, Frickenhausen, Germany) which have a special permeable disk membrane in their lower part.)
2. Place Ficoll-Paque plus solution (Pharmacia LKB, Uppsala, Sweden; density 1.077 g/L) in a 15 or 50 mL conical centrifuge tube. Use 3 mL Ficoll-Paque solution per 10 mL blood/buffer mixture.
3. Slowly layer the blood/buffer mixture over the Ficoll-Paque solution by placing the tip of the pipette containing the blood/buffer mixture at the surface of the Ficoll-Paque solution. (Alternatively, slowly layer the Ficoll-Paque solution underneath the blood/buffer mixture by placing the tip of the pipette containing the Ficoll-Paque solution at the bottom of the tube.)
4. Centrifuge the capped tube for 30 min at 900 × *g* (room temperature) using no brake.
5. Use a sterile pipette and remove the upper layer containing the plasma and most of the platelets. Change the pipette and transfer the next layer containing the mononuclear cells (lymphocytes, monocytes, and basophils) to another centrifuge tube.

6. Wash the PBMC by adding excess HBSS (more than three times the volume of the cell layer) and centrifuge them for 10 min at 400 × *g* at room temperature. Discard the supernatant into an appropriate disinfectant solution, resuspend the cell pellet carefully in HBSS (step by step; first in a small volume, mixing gently, adding HBSS to a final volume of 10 mL into the tube) and repeat the washing procedure once again.
7. Resuspend the PBMC in complete RPMI medium. Count cells and determine viability (*see* Subheading 3.4).

3.3 Isolation of T Cells (Immunomagnetic Purification of T Cells)

For some research applications isolation of purified T cells is necessary (e.g., studies on signal transduction, regulation of T-cell cytokine expression, induction of T-cell anergy). We used the magnetic activated cell sorter (MACS®) T-cell isolation kit for indirect isolation of untouched $CD3^+$ T cells from human peripheral blood mononuclear cells (MACS®, Miltenyi Biotec, Bergisch-Gladbach, Germany). This T-cell isolation kit is based upon an indirect magnetic labeling system with depletion of B cells, monocytes, NK cells, dendritic cells, erythroid cells, platelets, and basophils. For this purpose, a cocktail of CD11b, CD16, CD19, CD36, and CD56 antibodies is useful for the depletion of non-T cells. The T cells are isolated following the manufacturer's instructions.

In brief, a MACS® column-type LS^+/VS^+ is used. It is a prerequisite to isolate PBMC cells without any clumps as the cells pass through a 30 mm nylon mesh or filter.

1. Count the isolated PBMC cells (*see* Subheading 3.4) and wash them with PBS buffer with 2 mM EDTA and 0.5% BSA (*see* **Note 1**) by centrifugation of the cell suspension for 10 min at 400 × *g* at room temperature.
2. Remove supernatant completely and resuspend cell pellet in PBS buffer with 2 mM EDTA and 0.5% BSA to a total volume of 80 μL/1 × 10^7 total cells.
3. Add 20 μL hapten antibody cocktail to 1 × 10^7 total cells, mix well, and incubate for 10 min at 6–12 °C.
4. Wash the cells carefully with PBS buffer with 2 mM EDTA and 0.5% BSA by adding 10–20 times the labeling volume.
5. Centrifuge for 10 min at 400 × *g* at room temperature and remove the supernatant.
6. Repeat the washing step. Resuspend the cells carefully in 80 μL of PBS buffer with 2 mM EDTA and 0.5% BSA for 1 × 10^7 total cells.
7. Add 20 μL MACS® anti-hapten microbeads to 1 × 10^7 total cells, to label the cells magnetically.
8. Mix the cell suspension well and incubate them for 15 min at 6–12 °C.

9. Wash the cells carefully with PBS buffer with 2 mM EDTA and 0.5% BSA by adding 10–20 times volume (approx. 15 mL) and centrifuging at 400 × *g* for 10 min.
10. Place the column in the magnetic field of an appropriate MACS® separator.
11. Prepare the LS^+/VS^+ column by washing with 3 mL PBS buffer with 2 mM EDTA and 0.5% BSA.
12. Apply cell suspension onto the column; the unlabeled cells will not be retained on the column, and will come out in the effluent.
13. Collect the effluent as negative fraction, representing the enriched T-cell fraction.
14. Rinse with 3–4 mL of PBS buffer with 2 mM EDTA and 0.5% BSA and collect the effluent (enriched T-cell fraction).
15. Remove column from the separator and elute outside of the magnetic field all positive non-T cells.
16. Check the purity of the untouched T cells by staining an aliquot of the T-cell fraction with the fluorochrome conjugate antibody against T cells (e.g., CD3-PE) and analyze by flow cytometry. To determine if any remaining non-T cells in the T-cell fraction are leukocytes or rather erythroid cells, counterstain an aliquot of the cell fractions with an antibody against CD45 coupled to another fluorochrome (e.g., CD45-FITC). In this case, T cells are double-positive stained.

3.4 Determination of Cell Count and Cell Viability

Cells can be counted using Coulter counter or a hemocytometer. A Coulter counter is an electronic particle counter. It is based on the principle that particles (cells suspended in an electrolyte) passing through an aperture in which an electronic current is flowing will alter the electrical resistance of the electrolyte and give rise to changes in the current flow and voltage. A hemocytometer (improved by Neubauer ruling; Brand, Wertheim, Germany) is a special type of microscope slide (cell counting chamber), which is divided into squares of a defined area over which a defined volume of cell suspension is distributed. Counting the number of cells in a defined volume can give us the number of cells/mL in a cell suspension. The hemocytometer can be used to count all cells, or determine the number of viable cells in a culture. Viability is determined by either trypan blue or eosin dye exclusion test (*see* **Note 2**). Determination of cell viability is recommended when using thawed PBMC.

The following procedure can be used for the determination of viable cells with eosin dye exclusion test.

1. Centrifuge the cell suspension (10 min at 400 × *g* at room temperature), remove the supernatant completely, and resus-

pend in a defined volume (e.g., 1 mL) in complete medium RPMI. The cells need to be well mixed and uniformly suspended in the suspension.

2. Ensuring that both are clean and free from any grease, place coverslip on hemocytometer.
3. Gently mix 50 μL cell suspension with 450 μL eosin ready-to-use solution in a small plastic tube.
4. Dip a 0.1 or 1 mL pipette into the cell-eosin suspension to form a small drop on the end of the pipette and transfer gently to the surface of slide at the periphery of the coverslip.
5. Place hemocytometer on the stage of the microscope and focus on the cells.
6. Count the number of viable cells (unstained, in contrast to the red dead cells) at each of the four corner squares (the total volume of each corner square is 0.1 mm^3) (*see* **Note 3**). Cells falling across the top and left border lines of a square are considered to be in that square, whereas those that lie on the bottom and right borders are excluded. Count any clumps of cells as one cell.
7. Calculate the viable number of cells per mL of cell suspension as follows:

viable cell number/mL = (total number of cells in four corner squares/4) × 10^5 (the factor 10^5 includes the cell dilution of 1:10 in the eosin).

3.5 Cryopreservation of Cells (Freezing and Thawing of Cells)

Freshly isolated PBMC or cell lines should be used for culturing and stimulation experiments. However, they can be stored in culture medium at 4 °C for at least 2 days prior to use, or frozen as soon as possible. Cell concentrations up to 10^7 cells/mL can be successfully frozen in special cryovial tubes (sterile; volume 1.8 mL). A stepwise freezing process is recommended (1–2 °C/min for the first 30 °C). Dimethyl sulfoxide (DMSO) (or alternatively, glycerol) as an additive in the culture medium (cryoprotection solution) avoids the development of ice crystals during the freezing process. DMSO must be handled with care (avoid skin contact) and avoid the accumulation of toxic peroxide in the DMSO solution by using a fresh bottle every 3 months.

1. Prepare freezing medium with dimethyl sulfoxide (DMSO) (RPMI with GlutaMAX™ with 20% FCS, 10% DMSO, 1% penicillin/streptomycin, 1% sodium pyruvate) and store at −20 °C (add DMSO to medium and not vice versa).
2. Centrifuge the PBMC at 500 × *g* (room temperature) using a 50 mL conical centrifuge tube, discard the supernatant, and save the cell pellet. Place the cells in the tube in an ice bath.

3. Add the pre-cooled freezing medium (+4 °C) to the cell pellet to achieve a final cell concentration of 2×10^6 cells/mL and resuspend cells gently (avoid cell sedimentation).
4. Transfer 1 mL of the resuspended cells to each labeled cryovial (use an indelible marker). Cap the vial and immediately place it for 1 h in a freezer storage box in −20 °C freezer. Then, place the cryovials overnight into a −70 °C freezer. For long-term storage (several years for human freshly isolated PBMC), transfer cells to a liquid nitrogen container (−196 °C).
5. Thawing the frozen PBMC begins with pre-cooling the cells (+4 °C). Retrieve the cryovial containing the cells from the "liquid nitrogen freezing container."
6. Take the cryovial to the laminar flow and disinfect the outside of the vial with alcohol (70%).
7. Swirl cryovial gently in glove-protected and disinfected hands until PBMCs are thawed or alternatively thaw vial quickly in 37 °C water bath.
8. Open the cryovial gently and transfer the cells into a sterile 15 mL Falcon tube containing 12 mL of the pre-cooled media. (Alternatively, resuspend the cells gently using a sterile 1 mL pipette, transfer them into a sterile 15 mL Falcon tube, and add dropwise 9 mL complete RPMI media with gentle shaking over a time period of about 2–3 min.)
9. Cap the tube, centrifuge for 5 min at 500 × *g* at room temperature, discard the supernatant (under sterile conditions in the laminar flow), resuspend the cells in complete RPMI, and repeat the washing procedure as above twice. Examine the cell viability and determine cell count. The cells are ready for use at this stage and should be transferred to tissue culture plates or flasks.
10. In some cases, it is necessary to remove the dead cells. For this purpose, centrifuge the cells (10 min at 400 × *g* at room temperature), resuspend in 2 mL sterile PBS, by using a 2 mL pipette place 2 mL of FCS under the cell suspension, centrifuge the suspension for 5 min at 500 × *g*, and remove the supernatant. Wash the cells once with complete RPMI and determine the number of viable cells.

3.6 Culturing and Stimulation of PBMC

A number of agents can specifically or nonspecifically induce T-cell activation resulting in cytokine production, cytokine receptor expression, and ultimately proliferation of the activated T cells. Some agents are capable of nonspecific activation of unprimed T cells in culture. Calcium ionophore and phorbol ester stimulation can directly cross-link the T-cell receptor (TCR) on a large percentage of responder cells. Lectins, such as phytohemagglutinin (PHA), indirectly cross-link the TCR, and accessory cells are necessary with concentrations of 1–5 μg/mL. The use of anti-CD3 or anti-TCR antibodies in soluble forms (rather than plate bound) also requires accessory cells. When using superantigens, such as staphylococcus enterotoxin, accessory cells must express the appropriate MHC class II molecules.

For antigen-specific stimulation of PBMC, peripheral blood cells from donors previously exposed to antigen can be used successfully. In the case of tetanus toxoid, donors should ideally have received a booster injection about 1 month to 1 year prior to the use of their PBMCs. To study PBMC reaction induced by allergens, peripheral blood from atopic donors can be stimulated specifically with allergens, which induces the IgE response in this subject (for example house dust mite allergen (Der p 1), grass pollen (Phl p 1–5), latex allergen (e.g., Hev b 1–10), and so on). Patients should be tested for allergen-specific serum IgE levels. Although there is not always a positive correlation between RAST score and success rate in the induction of allergen-specific PBMC response, in some cases (e.g., for the generation of Th2 clones) donors with a RAST class >3 should be chosen preferentially.

The antigen concentration used for T-cell proliferation assay needs to be optimized. It is common for Th2 responses to be induced preferentially with low allergen concentrations, whereas Th1 responses are more frequently induced by higher allergen concentration. The sensitization is not important for stimulation of PBMCs, as cells from nonallergic but exposed subjects also demonstrate proliferation response in the presence of allergen [8]. This is not surprising, as cells from nonallergic but exposed subjects, recognize the antigen and show strong IgG binding to the antigen, and immunocompetent cells are stimulated in this polyclonal system. The observation that nonallergic subjects show a proliferative response to allergen is in accordance with the observation of other authors, although there is some controversy as to whether the proliferation of PBMC from allergic and nonallergic subjects is similar or lower for the latter [3, 8].

3.7 Measurement of Proliferative Responses of Cultured Lymphocytes (Mitogen and Antigen Induced)

Although proliferation is not a specific effector function of T lymphocytes, in contrast to helper function for B lymphocytes or cytotoxicity, proliferation assays are reliable and simple and easy to perform and have been widely used to assess the overall immunocompetence of the T cells.

1. For the proliferation assay PBMCs were “seeded” at a concentration of 2 × 10^4 cells/well in a 96-well culture plate (U-bottom; total volume 200 μL) in triplicate or increased number of replicates (hexaplicates) and stimulated with the antigen (*see* **Note 3**). Appropriate dilution of various antigen diluted (10–0.01 μg/mL) in complete medium was then added in 0.1 mL aliquots. As a positive control, stimulation

with the mitogen PHA (5 μg/mL; phytohemagglutinin) is used. Cells incubated with no antigen provide a medium control, to give a baseline level of T-cell proliferation.

In the case of mitogen-specific stimulation an incubation time of 3 days is performed. In the case of allergens, 5 or 6 days is a good time, although this needs to be optimized for each allergen. For (^{3}H)-thymidine incorporation with allergens we performed a 5-day incubation in a humidified atmosphere at 37 °C and 5% CO_2 (*see* **Notes 4–8**).

2. For the final 12 h of incubation, 37.4 kBq (1 μCi) of (^{3}H)-thymidine-methyl (Dupont, Germany, NEN Division, Dreieich, Germany) was added to each well (20 μL) and the incorporated radioactivity was assessed.
3. A semiautomated cell-harvesting apparatus is used to lyse the cells with water and precipitate the tritium-labeled DNA onto glass fiber filters. The dried filter pads were counted by liquid scintillation spectroscopy.
4. Results were calculated as stimulation indices (SI value). The SI value is the ratio of the mean counts per minute obtained in three (or more) similar cultures with allergen or antigen to that obtained in the antigen-free culture (the medium control).
5. In the case of allergen-specific stimulation, it is important to set a cutoff point for determination of a positive response. An SI value of 1.0 indicates that there is no antigen-specific response. An SI value of 2 or 3 is often considered as a positive stimulation index.

3.8 Measurement of Receptors and Activation Markers on Lymphocyte Surfaces by Flow Cytometry

T-cell activation can be determined by measuring activation markers expressed on the cell surface of stimulated cells. For example, markers like CD25 (IL-2 receptor) and/or CD71 (transferrin receptor) are expressed on proliferated cells. The expression of these special markers is time dependent, e.g., CD69 is an early proliferation marker. In addition, expression of T-cell receptors or intracellular cytokines for further characterization of T cells can also be determined in PBMC cultures by flow cytometry.

1. Using sterile technique, 2×10^6 PBMC/mL is incubated in a 24-well culture plate in the presence or absence of antigen/allergen at different concentrations and for different times at 37 °C in 5% CO_2.
2. After incubation, the cells are harvested and transferred to tubes and centrifuged for 10 min at $500 \times g$. Discard the supernatant.
3. Resuspend the cells in medium and count. Adjust cell count to 2×10^6/mL.

4. Pipette 50 μL PBMC cell suspension in a polypropylene tube and incubate with 8–10 μL of the chosen fluorochrome-labeled antibody to determine its expression.
5. Incubate in the dark for 30 min at 4 °C.
6. Add 2 mL PBS and centrifuge the labeled cell suspension for 5 min at 500 × *g*. Discard the supernatant.
7. Repeat the washing step. Add 250 μL PBS with 0.2% paraformaldehyde to fix the cells.
8. Measure activation and cell surface marker expression by flow cytometry.

3.9 Collecting Supernatants for Further Cytokine Determination

The concentrations of soluble cytokines (like IL-4, IL-5, IL-10, IL-13, and interferon-gamma (IFNγ)) in culture supernatants could be measured with commercially available sandwich ELISAs (technique using combinations of unlabeled and biotin-coupled mAb of different epitopes of each cytokine).

1. Incubate 10^6 PBMCs/mL in the presence or absence of antigen/allergen in either 24- (final volume 1 mL), 48- (500 μL), or 96-well (200 μL) plate.
2. For polyclonal stimulation, use combinations of PMA (1 ng/mL) and calcium ionophore A23187 (500 ng/mL) both from "Sigma Chemicals"; PMA and soluble anti-CD3 mAb (1 μg/mL); and anti-CD28 mAb (1 μg/mL and coated anti-CD3 mAb) to coat plates with anti-CD3 mAb; incubate a 96-well flat-bottom plate with 10 μg/mL anti-CD3 mAb diluted in PBS; and wash twice with 100 μL of RPMI.
3. Incubate the cells at 37 °C, 5% CO_2, for 16 h/24 h (for IL-4 and IL-2) and 48 h or longer for IFNγ-, IL-5-, IL-13-, etc. and harvest the supernatant which can be frozen (−20 °C or better −70 °C) prior to cytokine analysis.
4. Determine cytokine production levels by specific cytokine ELISAs. Be sure that the supernatant is cell free (supernatant should be used after centrifugation).

4 Notes

1. Buffer is degassed by vacuum pump or sonification. Excess gas in buffer can form bubbles in the matrix of the column during separation, which may lead to clogging of the column and decrease the quality of separation.
2. Dye exclusion test is based on the principle that nonelectrolyte dyes penetrate into dead cells, whereas live cells with intact plasma membranes do not allow the entry of such substances. Exclusion dyes will eventually penetrate live cells, so quantifi-

cation should be performed within 30 min of adding dye to cell suspension. Antigen preparations can lead to nonspecific activation of T cells, e.g., casein which if contaminated with lipopolysaccharide (LPS) can result in unspecific T-cell stimulation [9]. LPS can be removed from the protein fractions by polymyxin B coupled to a solid phase as described [10].

3. As an alternative to (^{3}H)-thymidine incorporation, cell growing (proliferation) can be monitored using nonradioactive methods. Proliferation can be determined by photometric method using MTT (3-(4,5 dimethythiazol-2-yl)-2,5-diphenyl tetrazolium bromide) or else by flow cytometry using a combination of ethidium bromide and bromodeoxyuridine (BrdU).
4. The level of (^{3}H)-thymidine incorporation should not be regarded only as a reflection of cellular proliferation: some nondividing cells will synthesize DNA and "cold" thymidine released by disintegrating cells will compete with incorporation of labeled thymidine. Therefore, measurements of DNA synthesis should be accompanied by counting viable cells over the length of the culture period if a true estimate of cellular proliferation is to be obtained. Of course, cell death of nonactivated cells will also interfere with the accuracy of this last parameter.
5. The sensitivity of proliferation assays is such that small errors in cell numbers will result in large differences in (^{3}H)-thymidine incorporation. When values obtained in triplicate cultures correspond poorly (for example >5% differences in CPM values >1000), technical problems such as cell clumping, dilution, and pipetting should be considered.
6. Excessively high values may be obtained from contaminated wells, as thymidine will be incorporated into replicating bacteria; therefore, it is a good practice to check the wells from microtiter plates under inverted microscope for contamination. Contamination may also interfere with proliferation of the activated lymphocytes. It is also useful to check the blast formation by microscopic examination of the cultures. Activating lymphocytes will tend to enlarge and detection of blast will give a general indication of successful activation [2].
7. The main problem that may occur with proliferative response assays is high levels of background (^{3}H)-thymidine incorporation in control cultures without antigen. This problem is frequently due to the FCS used to supplement the cultures which may be mitogenic for B cells. Different lots of FCS should be screened to select those that are nonstimulatory or only weakly stimulatory in the absence of any stimuli.

8. The culture period required for stimulation—after which the cells are to be labeled—varies for different laboratories, media, and types of responding and stimulator cells. Conditions eliciting weak responses such as most allergens will require a longer period of time (5–6 days) than those eliciting a higher frequency of responding T cells (3–4 days). Because laboratory conditions vary, it will be necessary to run a kinetic assay to determine the optimal time of T-cell proliferation. Addition of thymidine on days 2, 3, 4, 5, and 6 will provide a useful test. Further extension of culture periods will not yield any improvements, due to exhaustion of nutrients in the medium (yellow color indicating acidic condition).

References

1. Hudson L, Hay FC (1989) Practical immunology. Blackwell Scientific Publications, Oxford
2. Coligan JE, Kruisbeek AM, Margulies DH, Shevach EM, Strober W (eds) (1996) Current protocol immunology. John Wiley & Sons, Inc., New York
3. Kahlert H, Stüwe H-T, Cromwell O, Fiebig H (1999) Reactivity of T cells with grass pollen allergen extract and allergoid. Int Arch Allergy Immunol 120:146–157
4. Yssel H, De Vries JE, Koken M, Blitterswijk WV, Spits H (1984) Serum-free medium for generation and propagation of functional human cytotoxic and helper T cell clones. J Immunol Methods 72:219–227
5. Rohde T, Maclean DA, Pedersen BK (1996) Glutamine, lymphocyte proliferation and cytokine production. Scand J Immunol 44:648–650
6. Horig H, Spagnoli GC, Filguerira L, Babst R, Gallati H, Harder F, Juretic A, Heberer M (1993) Exogenous glutamine requirement is confined to late events of T cell activation. J Cell Biochem 53:343–351
7. Böyum A (1968) Isolation of mononuclear cells and granulocytes from human blood. Isolation of mononuclear cells by one centrifugation, and of granulocytes by combining centrifugation and sedimentation at 1 g. Scand J Clin Lab Invest 97:77–89
8. Raulf-Heimsoth M, Chen Z, Liebers V, Allmers H, Baur X (1996) Lymphocyte response to extracts from different latex materials and to the purified latex allergen Hev b 1 (rubber elongation factor). J Allergy Clin Immunol 98:640–651
9. Werfel T, Ahlers G, Schmidt P, Boeker M, Kapp A (1996) Detection of a κ-casein-specific lymphocyte response in milk-responsive atopic dermatitis. Clin Exp Allergy 26:1380–1386
10. Karplus TE, Ulevitch RJ, Wilson CB (1987) A new method for reduction of endotoxin contamination from protein solutions. J Immunol Methods 105:211–220

Chapter 3

Measurement of Allergen-Specific Inhibitory Antibody Activity

Mohamed H. Shamji and James N. Francis

Abstract

Specific allergen immunotherapy (AIT) is an effective treatment for IgE-mediated allergic diseases and involves T- and B-cell-mediated events. IgE receptors on the surface of antigen-presenting cells facilitate the presentation of allergens in the presence of specific IgE antibody resulting in T-cell activation. Interference with these IgE-dependent mechanisms by "blocking" IgG antibodies suppresses pro-inflammatory Th2 cell responses and manifests as a reduction in allergic responses in vivo.

In vitro assays used to measure the inhibition of binding of allergen-IgE complexes have previously utilized proliferation of antigen-specific T-cell clones as an assay readout. Here we describe two simplified assays to measure allergen binding without the complexity of generating T-cell clones. The IgE-facilitated allergen binding assay (IgE-FAB) utilizes flow cytometry to measure the binding of allergen-IgE complexes to EBV-transformed B cells. The enzyme-linked immunosorbent-facilitated antigen binding (ELIFAB) assay uses standard ELISA-based techniques to measure allergen-IgE binding to plate-bound CD23, the low-affinity IgE receptor expressed on B cells.

Key words Allergen immunotherapy, Inhibitory antibodies, IgG, Facilitated-allergen binding assay, ELIFAB, Allergy

1 Introduction

Allergen immunotherapy (AIT) administered either subcutaneously (SCIT) or sublingually (SLIT) is an effective treatment for IgE-mediated diseases. Several well-controlled studies have confirmed that AIT is clinically effective and induces allergen-specific clinical and immunological tolerance [1–3]. The immunologic tolerant state induced following AIT has been shown to be associated with both T-cell mechanisms [4–7] and B-cell responses, in particular induction of IgG4 antibodies [8, 9]. These allergen-specific antibodies are thought to function by competing with IgE to bind to allergen and thereby reducing binding of allergen-IgE complexes to mast cells, basophils, and other IgE receptor-expressing cells [10]. Receptors for IgE expressed on the surface of

Penny Lympany and Meinir G. Jones (eds.), *Allergy: Methods and Protocols*, Methods in Molecular Biology, vol. 2020, https://doi.org/10.1007/978-1-4939-9591-2_3,

antigen-presenting cells have been shown to facilitate the presentation of allergens in the presence of specific IgE antibody resulting in effective T-cell activation at low concentrations of allergen [11]. Interference with these IgE-dependent mechanisms by "blocking" IgG antibodies may downregulate T-cell responses and manifest as a reduction in allergic responses in vivo.

Previous studies have shown that serum obtained from subjects receiving birch pollen immunotherapy inhibits IgE-facilitated presentation of allergen by B cells to an allergen-specific T-cell clone [12, 13]. Another study demonstrated that serum obtained from a clinical trial of grass pollen immunotherapy could inhibit IgE-facilitated allergen presentation to a grass-specific T-cell clone [14]. The vigor of proliferative responses by T-cell clones was shown to be representative of the binding of allergen-IgE complexes to B cells. This chapter describes two simplified serum-based assays that can be employed to measure the binding of allergen-IgE complexes to B cells—substituting more complex assays involving use of antigen-specific T-cell clones.

The IgE-FAB assay involves incubation of serum, known to contain high levels of allergen-specific IgE (>100 kU/mL; indicator serum), with low concentrations of allergen extract in the presence or absence of "test serum" with potential inhibitory activity [15, 16]. The resulting allergen-IgE complexes are subsequently incubated with an EBV-transformed human B-cell line. These cells express high levels of the low-affinity IgE receptor (CD23, FcεRII) which binds allergen-IgE complexes. Detection of allergen-IgE complexes on the surface of B cell can be achieved using either a biotinylated allergen or a fluorescent antibody against IgE and analyzed using flow cytometry (Fig. 1). In the presence of inhibitory serum, isolated from subjects treated with AIT, the number of allergen-IgE complexes bound to B cells is decreased.

The IgE-FAB assay has been applied to the measurement of functional antibody activity from a variety of different environmental and occupational allergens including grass pollen [8, 9, 15], birch pollen [17], ragweed [18], peanut [19], bee venom [20], and rat urine [21].

Although reliable and reproducible in experienced hands, the IgE-FAB assay has a number of technical restrictions that may limit the routine application of this assay. Firstly the assay requires the generation and maintenance of viable EBV-transformed B cells and continued expression of surface FcεRII/CD23 receptors, both of which are compromised during prolonged culture. Moreover, the dependence on labile B-cell lines precludes routine standardization of the assay between different laboratories and poses challenges when analyzing large numbers of samples from clinical studies. Secondly, the detection of allergen-IgE complexes in the IgE-FAB assay requires a flow cytometer that may not be available in all labo-

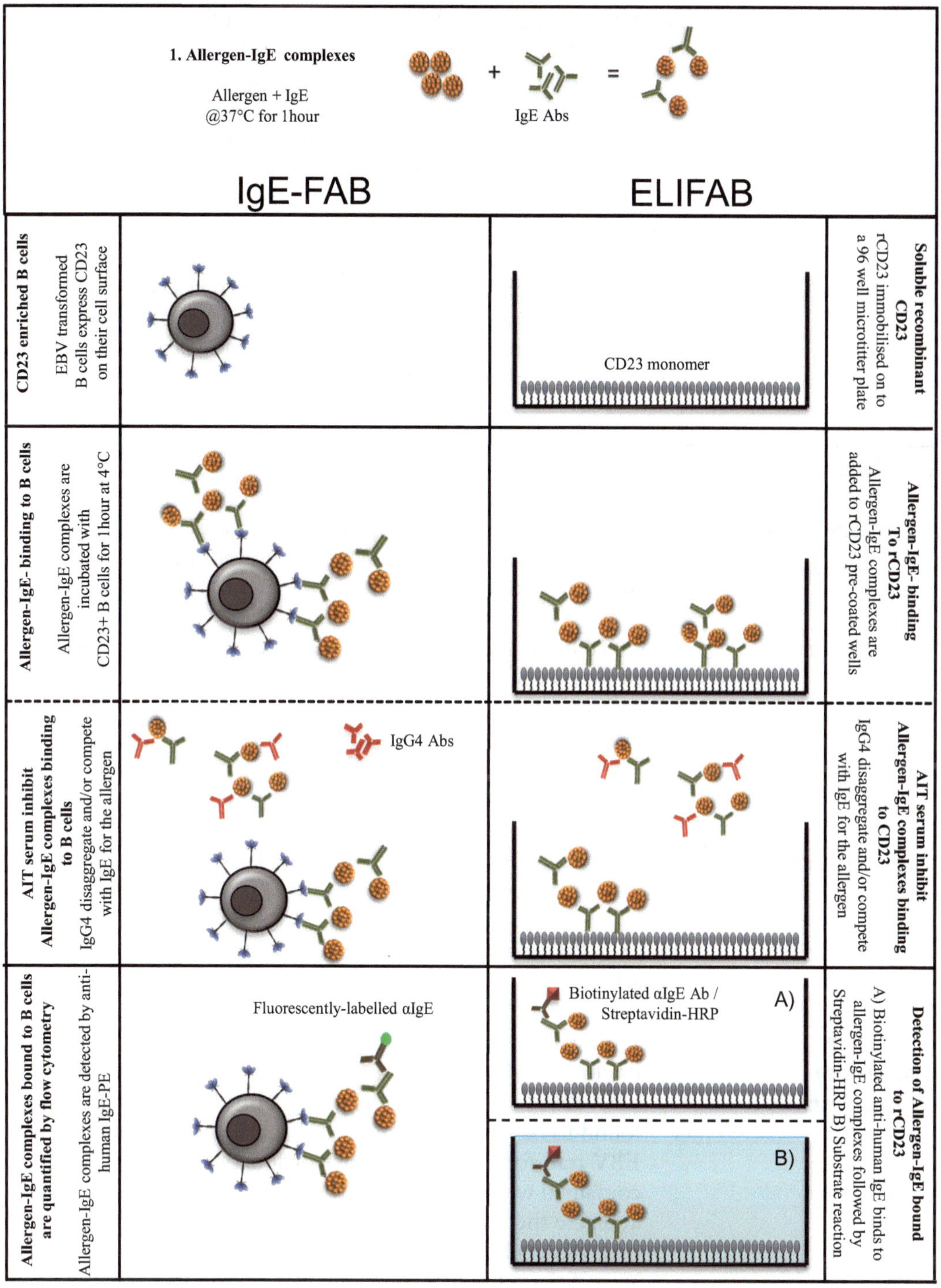

Fig. 1 Detection of allergen-IgE complexes on the surface of B cells using flow cytometry

ratories. Instead the ELIFAB procedure utilizes the more commonly available microplate absorbance reader.

The enzyme-linked immunosorbent-facilitated antigen binding (ELIFAB) assay is an alternative cell-free assay which substitutes EBV-transformed B-cell lines with soluble CD23 monomers bound to a solid surface and the assay follows the basic principles of a standard ELISA protocol using a 96-well plate [22]. Briefly, test serum is incubated with allergen and high-IgE indicator serum as per the IgE FAB assay. This mixture is added to the CD23-coated wells and IgE-allergen complexes bound to CD23 are revealed using a biotinylated anti-IgE antibody followed by peroxidase and a colorimetric substrate system. Plates can be read using standard laboratory microplate absorbance reader.

2 Materials

2.1 Assay Buffers

2.1.1 FAP Buffer (pH 7.2)

8.10 g NaCl, 0.16 g NaH2PO4, 0.98 g Na2HPO4, 1.0 g BSA (0.1%): Dissolve in 1 L of distilled H_2O, and adjust pH to 7.2. Store for up to 2 weeks at 4 °C.

2.1.2 EBV Growth Medium

RPMI 1640 supplemented with 1% (v/v) L-glutamine, 10% heat-inactivated FCS, and 1% (v/v) penicillin/streptomycin mixture. Store at 4 °C for up to 4 weeks.

2.1.3 TMB Substrate Solution

For one plate, add 11 mL of phosphate-citrate buffer at pH 5.0 to 110 μL of TMB solution and 6 μL H_2O_2 (30%).

2.1.4 ELIFAB Buffer

PBS/Tween (4 mL Tween 20, 250 mL 10 × PBS in 10 L distilled H_2O).

2.1.5 Blocking Buffer

1% BSA/PBS solution; 200 μL (5 g BSA, 500 mL PBS) to be added to each well.

2.2 Serum and Allergen Requirements

1. Indicator serum should be obtained from an atopic (allergic) donor with high allergen-specific IgE levels (as measured by CAP-RAST). Serum with levels of >100 kU/mL are generally found to be a suitable indicator serum as the level of binding to EBV-transformed B cell is proportional to the amount of IgE contained within the serum. If serum with >100 kU/mL is not available then it is worthwhile testing serum with 50–100 kU/mL. Generally, serum with <50 kU/mL does not bind in the assay. Serum (or plasma) from allergic donors is commercially available.
2. Inhibitory serum to be tested in the assay can be obtained from subjects undergoing AIT treatment or with signs of clinical remission/tolerance. Serum can be collected using standard blood tubes with clotting agent.

3. Allergen is commercially available or can be isolated by standard laboratory methods. Freeze-dried allergen should be dissolved in sterile RPMI-1640 medium at 1–5 mg/mL, aliquoted, and stored at −20 °C.

3 Methods

3.1 IgE-Facilitated Allergen Binding (IgE-FAB) Assay

3.1.1 Cultivation of EBV-Transformed B Cells

Detailed description of the generation of EBV-transformed B cells is beyond the remit of this protocol. Briefly, supernatant from an EBV-producing cell line (e.g., B-958) is cultured with peripheral blood mononuclear cells from an atopic donor. Transformed B cells are enriched for high CD23 expression by the use of magnetic bead separation and stored in liquid nitrogen for long-term storage until use.

1. EBV-transformed B cells are rapidly thawed at 37 °C, washed twice in 50 mL of RPMI-1640 medium, and cultured in vented-cap, canted-neck cell culture flask (Falcon) at 37 °C, 5% CO_2, and 95% relative humidity.
2. Subculture cells two to three times a week to maintain cell density of 1.0–2.0 × 10^6 cells/mL and viability above 95%.
3. Use cells after a minimum of 10–14 days after the start of the culture period and a maximal of 60 days.
4. Routinely check CD23 expression on B cells by flow cytometry, e.g., using anti-human CD23-PE antibody (Miltenyi Biotec). Numbers of B cells expressing CD23 should be >98% and levels of expression should lie approximately one fluorescence log higher than controls.

3.1.2 IgE-FAB Analytical Procedure

Serum Preparation

Serum stored at −80 °C should be first left for 24 h at −20 °C. Thaw serum in a water bath at 37 °C for 10 min. Serum-containing precipitants may be filtered before use in the assay.

Allergen Dilution

Allergen should be freshly prepared in RPMI-1640 medium to a working dilution 10× greater than the required final concentration; for example, if a final allergen concentration of 1 μg/mL is required, the working stock solution should be prepared at 10 μg/mL.

Complexing Allergen with Serum Antibodies

1. 20 μL of "test" serum, the inhibitory activity of which is to be tested, is added to a 96-well U-bottomed plate. Control wells should contain 20 μL of RPMI-1640 medium.
2. Add 20 μL of "high-IgE" indicator serum.
3. Add 5 μL of the diluted allergen.

4. Mix gently by tapping the side of the plate and place a lid on the plate to minimize evaporation.
5. Incubate serum/allergen for 1 h at 37 °C.

Preparation of EBV-B Cells

1. Transfer cells from culture flask into a 50 mL centrifuge tube.
2. Wash cells by centrifugation at 490 × *g* at 4 °C for 7 min.
3. Repeat wash step with 50 mL cold RPMI-1640 medium (centrifuge at 490 × *g* at 4 °C for 7 min).
4. Resuspend cells in 10 mL of RPMI-1640 medium.
5. Count cells using a standard laboratory technique incorporating a cell viability dye where possible.
6. Centrifuge the cells and resuspend to 2×10^7 cells/mL in FAB buffer; dissolve in 1 L of dH_2O; adjust pH to 7.2; store for up to 2 weeks at 4 °C.
7. Store cells on ice and mix thoroughly prior to use.

Incubation of EBV-B Cells with Pre-complexed Allergen

Add 5 μL of EBV-B cell solution (100,000 cells per test) to allergen–serum complexes on the 96-well plate. Mix gently and incubate for 30 min on ice.

Staining of Allergen-IgE Complexes Bound to B Cells (*See* Note 1)

1. Wash EBV-B cells from the previous step twice with 150 μL of FAB buffer by centrifugation at 490 × *g* at 4 °C for 7 min.
2. Dilute anti-human IgE-PE antibody (Miltenyi Biotec, Surrey, UK) 1:30 (e.g., 20 μL in 580 μL FAB buffer) and add 20 μL of diluted anti-human IgE-PE antibody to wells.
3. Incubate for 30 min on ice in the dark.
4. Wash cells with 150 μL FAB buffer per well (centrifuge at 490 × *g* at 4 °C for 7 min) and resuspend in 100 μL of Cell Fix (BD Biosciences) per well, diluted 1:10 as recommended.
5. Analyze surface staining by flow cytometry. If possible analysis should be conducted as soon as practicably possible but, if necessary, cells can be stored overnight without a significant loss in performance.

Flow Cytometry

Acquisition by flow cytometry should be tailored to an individual cytometer and specific settings are beyond the remit of this protocol. The following advice may be helpful:

1. Using a forward/side scatter plot identify the EBV cell population and gate the main population.
2. Set a histogram plot for PE and adjust the voltage so that the cell population appears in an appropriate position as the negative control population.

3. Acquire cells using the serum-positive control (*see* below) to ensure that an increased signal can be detected over the positive control (essentially this is the population that will be decreased by inhibitory antibodies present in test serum).
4. Acquire 5000 gated cells per sample.

The following controls should be included in each experiment where possible:

(a) Cells only (i.e., no PE stain; however, cells should be incubated with human serum as this can increase background fluorescence).

(b) Cells + isotype control for anti-human IgE-PE.

(c) Cells + anti-human IgE-PE.

(d) Indicator serum/allergen + anti-human IgE-PE (serum-positive control).

(e) Internal negative control for inhibition (e.g., serum from healthy donors).

(f) Internal positive control for inhibition (e.g., known serum from AIT-treated patient).

High-Throughput Sample Analysis

The above protocol uses standard 5 mL Falcon "FACS" tubes in the assay. For multiple samples, a 96-well U-bottomed plate (Nunc) may be used. In this case, a centrifuge equipped with microplate carriers is required and wash steps should be carried out using a multichannel pipette. In addition, wash volumes should be reduced to 250 μL (or so that the maximal volume of the well is not exceeded). For FACS analysis, contents of the wells should be mixed well and transferred to microtubes (Bioquote, UK). Microtubes can be place in a standard FACS tube and used as normal. Alternatively the plate can be used directly on an appropriately equipped flow cytometer, e.g., using a high-throughput sample (HTS; BD).

3.1.3 Optimization of the IgE-FAB Assay

It is essential to optimize the IgE-FAB assay for your allergen of choice. The following experiments should be completed before using the assay on large numbers of test samples.

1. Identification of a suitable indicator serum (containing high allergen-specific IgE levels, *see* Subheading 2.2): Potential serum to be used as indicator serum should be first tested for binding with a limited dose–response of allergen (e.g., 0.01, 1, and 100 μL/mL) without inclusion of inhibitory serum. If indicator serum is of limited availability, dilutions of serum (in RPMI-1640 medium) can be tested for binding in the assay. Also, pooled serum can be used in place of serum from a single donor.

2. Any serum showing binding of >30% (at any allergen concentration) should be further tested using a more comprehensive dose–response curve (e.g., half logarithmic doses from 1 μg/mL to 100 μg/mL). Typical optimal binding occurs at 0.1–5 μg/mL. It is desirable to achieve binding of >50% although binding in the range of 70–80% is optimal; lower binding of indicator serum may cause increased assay variability.
3. Once a suitable indicator serum is identified, the time course of allergen-IgE complex binding to B cells should be optimized (*see* Subheading "Incubation of EBV-B Cells with Pre-complexed Allergen"). Binding time between 2 and 120 min can be tested (e.g., 2, 10, 30, 60, and 120 min).
4. If serum with potential inhibitory activity is available, this should be tested in the assay before running large numbers of test samples. The assay should be run using a dose range of allergen concentrations in the presence or absence of potential inhibitory serum. As inhibition of facilitated allergen binding occurs at low allergen concentrations, an allergen concentration should be chosen that generates binding of >50% (or less, *see* above) but also allows the maximal inhibition of binding by test sera.

3.2 Enzyme-Linked Immunosorbent-Facilitated Antigen Binding (ELIFAB) Assay

3.2.1 ELIFAB Analytical Procedure

Coat Plate with sCD23

1. A stock solution of sCD23 is made by reconstituting 50 μg of lyophilized sCD23 protein (R&D) in 100 μL PBS. Prepare dilutions of stock sCD23 in PBS (approx. 10 μg/mL—optimization of this concentration is recommended—refer to Subheading 3.2.1).
2. Pipette 50 μL of diluted sCD23 to each well of a 96-well microtiter plate (Nunc MediSorp).
3. Cover plate and leave overnight at room temperature.

Prepare Allergen Complex with Serum Antibodies

1. Add 20 μL of indicator serum (*see* Subheading 2.2) into the bottom of a separate 96-well round-bottomed plate (Nunc) using a repeater or multichannel pipette, followed by 20 μL of serum of which inhibitory activity is to be tested. 20 μL of RPMI-1640 medium can be used in negative control wells.
2. Prepare allergen of interest in RPMI-1640 medium to a working dilution 10× greater than the required final concentration. Add 5 μL of the working stock into each well.
3. Cover plate and incubate allergen/serum for 1 h at 37 °C and 5% CO_2.

Block Plate with 1% BSA (Perform Immediately After Allergen Complex Preparation)

1. Wash the plate prepared in Subheading "Coat Plate with sCD23" twice with 200 μL/well of ELIFAB buffer.
2. Add 200 μL of blocking buffer to each well. Cover plate and incubate for 1 h at 37 °C. Be sure that the time lag between the BSA blocking and allergen complex incubations is minimal.

Adding Allergen Complex into sCD23-Coated Plate

1. Wash the BSA-blocked plate three times with 200 μL/well PBS/Tween20.
2. Transfer all preincubated allergen complex onto the sCD23-coated plates, and cover and leave on shaker at 650 rpm for 1 h at room temperature.

Conjugate (Antibody Detection)

1. Wash the plate four times with 200 μL/well PBS/Tween20.
2. Dilute the biotinylated IgE-specific detection antibody 1:1000 (BD bioscience) in 1% BSA/PBS and pipette 100 μL into each well.
3. Incubate covered plate on shaker at 650 rpm for 1 h at room temperature.

Streptavidin Peroxidase

1. Wash the plate five times with 200 μL/well PBS/Tween20.
2. Dilute streptavidin peroxidase 1:1000 (Sigma) in 1% BSA/PBS.
3. Pipette 100 μL into each well and incubate on a shaker at 650 rpm for 30 min at room temperature.

Chromogenic Substrate (TMB)

1. Wash the plate six times with 200 μL/well PBS/Tween20.
2. Prepare the TMB substrate solution immediately before use. Alternatively use a commercially available ready-made substrate solution.
3. Add 100 μL of TMB substrate solution into each well.
4. Leave to incubate for up to 10 min in the dark.
5. Stop reaction with 50 μL per well of 1.8 M H_2SO_4.
6. Read plate on a microplate absorbance reader at 450 nm.
7. Results are expressed as allergen-IgE binding to sCD23 (OD_{450}).

3.2.2 Optimization of the ELIFAB Assay

The ELIFAB assay needs to be optimized for your allergen of choice. In addition to the optimization recommendations in Subheading 3.1.3 for the IgE-FAB assay, the following experiment should be completed before using the assay on large numbers of test samples.

1. A range of concentrations of immobilized sCD23 (e.g., 0.01, 1, 3, and 30 μg/mL) should used to identify optimal allergen-IgE binding to sCD23.

4 Notes

1. Allergen-IgE complexes can also be detected using biotinylated allergen. In such a case optimal binding/inhibition should first be established using the biotinylated allergen. Detection of complexes is achieved using streptavidin-PE (BD Biosciences).

   Fresh preparation of reagents, buffers, and adherence to incubation times is crucial for its optimal performance and reproducibility of the ELIFAB assay. When analyzing the results, it is important to account for allergen-specific IgE present in the post-immunotherapy "test" sample, which may increase the binding of allergen-IgE complexes to sCD23 above that of the indicator serum alone. Therefore, data from the clinical trial is expressed as the percentage relative binding of allergen-IgE complexes, where binding with indicator serum alone is normalized to 100%.

Acknowledgments

The authors would like to thank Peter Würtzen, Stephen J Till, Rebecca Parkin, and Natalia Do Couto Francisco for their contributions to this protocol.

References

1. Durham SR, Walker SM, Varga EM et al (1999) Long-term clinical efficacy of grass-pollen immunotherapy. N Engl J Med 341:468–475
2. James LK, Shamji MH, Walker SM et al (2011) Long-term tolerance after allergen immunotherapy is accompanied by selective persistence of blocking antibodies. J Allergy Clin Immunol 127:509–516
3. Durham SR, Emminger W, Kapp A et al (2012) SQ-standardized sublingual grass immunotherapy: confirmation of disease modification 2 years after 3 years of treatment in a randomized trial. J Allergy Clin Immunol 129:717–725
4. Wambre E, DeLong JH, James EA et al (2012) Differentiation stage determines pathologic and protective allergen-specific CD4+ T-cell outcomes during specific immunotherapy. J Allergy Clin Immunol 129:544–551
5. Francis JN, Till SJ, Durham SR (2003) Induction of IL-10+CD4+CD25+ T cells by grass pollen immunotherapy. J Allergy Clin Immunol 111:255–261
6. O'Hehir RE, Gardner LM, de Leon MP et al (2009) House dust mite sublingual immunotherapy: the role for transforming growth factor-beta and functional regulatory T cells. Am J Respir Crit Care Med 180:936–947
7. Swamy RS, Reshamwala N, Hunter T et al (2012) Epigenetic modifications and improved regulatory T-cell function in subjects undergoing dual sublingual immunotherapy. J Allergy Clin Immunol 130:215–217
8. Nouri-Aria KT, Wachholz PA, Francis JN et al (2004) Grass pollen immunotherapy induces mucosal and peripheral IL-10 responses and blocking IgG activity. J Immunol 172:3252–3259
9. Shamji MH, Ljørring C, Francis JN et al (2012) Functional rather than immunoreactive levels of IgG4 correlate closely with clinical response to grass pollen immunotherapy. Allergy 67:217–226
10. van de Veen W, Stanic B, Yaman G et al (2013) IgG4 production is confined to human IL-10-

producing regulatory B cells that suppress antigen-specific immune responses. J Allergy Clin Immunol 131:1204–1212

11. Garcia BE, Sanz ML, Gato JJ et al (1993) IgG4 blocking effect on the release of antigen-specific histamine. J Investig Allergol Clin Immunol 3:26–33
12. van der Heijden FL, van Neerven RJ, Kapsenberg ML (1995) Relationship between facilitated allergen presentation and the presence of allergen-specific IgE in serum of atopic patients. Clin Exp Immunol 99:289–293
13. van Neerven RJ, Wikborg T, Lund G et al (1999) Blocking antibodies induced by specific allergy vaccination prevent the activation of CD4+ T cells by inhibiting serum-IgE-facilitated allergen presentation. J Immunol 163:2944–2952
14. van Neerven RJ, Arvidsson M, Ipsen H et al (2004) A double-blind, placebo-controlled birch allergy vaccination study: inhibition of CD23-mediated serum immunoglobulin E-facilitated allergen presentation. Clin Exp Allergy 34:420–428
15. Wachholz PA, Soni NK, Till SJ, Durham SR (2003) Inhibition of allergen-IgE binding to B cells by IgG antibodies after grass pollen immunotherapy. J Allergy Clin Immunol 112:915–922
16. Shamji MH, Wilcock LK, Wachholz PA et al (2006) The IgE-facilitated allergen binding (FAB) assay: validation of a novel flow-cytometric based method for the detection of inhibitory antibody responses. J Immunol Methods 317:71–79
17. Kinaciyan T, Jahn-Schmid B, Radakovics A et al (2007) Successful sublingual immunotherapy with birch pollen has limited effects on concomitant food allergy to apple and the immune response to the Bet v 1 homolog Mal d 1. J Allergy Clin Immunol 119:937–943
18. Klunker S, Saggar LR, Seyfert V et al (2007) Combination treatment with omalizumab and rush immunotherapy for ragweed allergic rhinitis: induction of inhibitory antibody responses. J Allergy Clin Immunol 120:688–695
19. Jones SM, Pons L, Roberts JL, Scurlock AM et al (2009) Clinical efficacy and immune regulation with peanut oral immunotherapy. J Allergy Clin Immunol 24:292–300
20. Varga EM, Francis JN, Zach MS et al (2009) Time course of serum inhibitory activity for facilitated allergen-IgE binding (FAB) during bee venom immunotherapy in children. Clin Exp Allergy 39:1353–1357
21. Jones M, Jeal H, Schofield S et al (2014) Rat-specific IgG and IgG4 antibodies associated with inhibition of IgE-allergen complex binding in laboratory animal workers. Occup Environ Med 71:619–623
22. Shamji MH, Francis JN, Wurtzen PA et al (2013) Cell-free detection of allergen-IgE cross-linking with immobilized phase CD23: inhibition by blocking antibody responses after immunotherapy. J Allergy Clin Immunol 132:1003–1004

Chapter 4

Immunoelectrophoresis for the Characterization of Allergen Extracts

Gitte Nordskov Hansen and Jørgen Nedergaard Larsen

Abstract

Immunoelectrophoresis can be used for analysis of individual proteins in complex mixtures. The conditions involved in immunoelectrophoresis are mild, avoiding the risk of denaturation, and it is possible to perform relative quantification of individual components. The fundamental disadvantage is the dependence on rabbit antisera as reagents. The usefulness of immunoelectrophoresis in allergy research is greatly enhanced by the possibility of identification of allergens to which the individual in question has IgE.

The common principle is characterized by two independent electrophoreses having direction of current perpendicular to each other, i.e., crossed immunoelectrophoresis (CIE). This ultimately results in the formation of characteristic bell-shaped precipitates, each precipitate representing one antigen. There is a linear relationship between the amount of antigen and size of precipitate for a given antibody concentration for each precipitate and so relative quantification can be performed. The sensitivity and resolution power of CIE are very high and there are multiple variations of the technique, some of which will be illustrated in this chapter.

Key words Immunoelectrophoresis, Crossed immunoelectrophoresis (CIE), Allergen, IgE

1 Introduction

Immunoelectrophoresis is the common name for a versatile family of electrophoretic precipitation-in-gel techniques, which can be used for analysis of individual proteins in complex mixtures [1, 2]. Compared to corresponding techniques, the major advantages of immunoelectrophoresis are firstly that experimental conditions are mild avoiding the risk of denaturation, and secondly the possibility of performing relative quantification of individual components. A disadvantage is the dependence on rabbit antisera as reagents.

The common principle is characterized by two independent electrophoreses having direction of current perpendicular to each other, i.e., crossed immunoelectrophoresis (CIE) (Fig. 1a). The first-dimension electrophoresis is performed in an agarose gel at

Penny Lympany and Meinir G. Jones (eds.), *Allergy: Methods and Protocols*, Methods in Molecular Biology, vol. 2020, https://doi.org/10.1007/978-1-4939-9591-2_4,

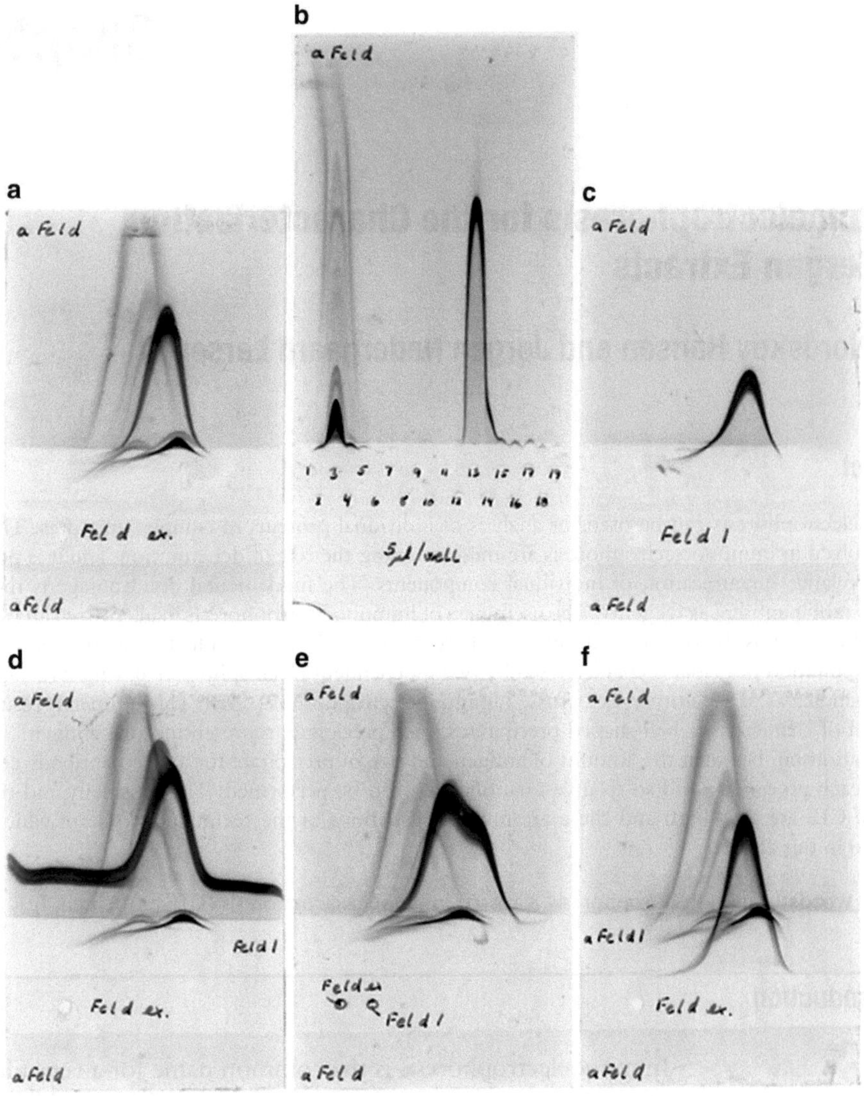

Fig. 1 Different types of immunoelectrophoresis of cat hair extract (Fel d) using a polyclonal rabbit antibody raised against the same extract (a Fel d). (**a**) CIE of Fel d extract, (**b**) FRIE following a purification (immunoabsorption) of the major allergen Fel d 1, (**c**) CIE of purified Fel d 1 against a Fel d, (**d**) CLIE with Fel d 1 in intermediate gel for identification of the allergen, (**e**) TCIE with Fel d extract and Fel d 1 showing a double peak, (**f**) CIIE with monospecific Fel d 1 in intermediate gel

pH 8.6. Protein mixtures are separated into sharp bands according to a complex relation between mass and charge. In the second-dimension electrophoresis performed perpendicular to the first, the gel on both sides of the track of proteins resulting from the first dimension electrophoresis is replaced by a gel containing polyclonal rabbit antiserum. Again, the electrophoresis is performed at pH 8.6, at which pH the average charge of the antibody molecules is zero resulting in minimal mobility of the antibody molecules during electrophoresis. Formation of antigen–antibody complexes during second-dimension electrophoresis will result in the formation of characteristic bell-shaped precipitates, each precipitate representing one antigen. The size of the precipitate will depend on the ratio between antigen and antibody as well as the average avidity of the interaction and is not a direct measure of antigen concentration. Relative quantification, however, can be performed, as there is a linear relationship between the amount of antigen and size of precipitate for a given antibody concentration for each precipitate. This is a major advantage when applied in allergen extract standardization. Furthermore, the usefulness of immunoelectrophoresis in allergy research is greatly enhanced by the possibility of incubating the electrophoretic plate with allergic patients' serum IgE for simple and reliable identification of allergens to which the individual in question has IgE.

A major advantage of immunoelectrophoresis is the providing of a range of possibilities for immunochemical analyses of individual proteins directly in a complex protein mixture. Experiments are performed under mild conditions without increased risk of protein denaturation, an important aspect when studying allergen–IgE interactions. The sensitivity and resolution power of CIE are very high; at optimal conditions about 50 antigens may be distinguished on one immunoplate, and at least 20 antigens may be quantified. Furthermore, the ease of preparation and stability of immunoglobulins make rabbit antisera useful as reference reagents for the characterization of complex allergen extracts. The dependence on antiserum, however, may also represent a drawback. When used for assessment of allergen extract complexity and for identification of allergic reactivities, it is essential to perform additional experiments to verify that all relevant allergens are precipitated by the antiserum. A limitation of the technique is that protein antigens with pI near 8.6 are difficult to analyze. The buffer pH 8.6 cannot be changed without chemical modifications of the immunoglobulins (e.g., carbamylation).

Multiple variations of immunoelectrophoresis may be designed, some of which will be illustrated in this chapter.

Crossed radio-immunoelectrophoresis (CRIE, Fig. 2a, b) is used for the identification of allergens. The cold dried CIE plate is incubated with allergic patients' IgE and developed using labeled anti-IgE and autoradiography. CRIE analyses of serum samples from several allergic patients may be used to construct an allergogram (Fig. 2d), a graphic representation of the relative importance of individual allergens.

Under carefully controlled experimental conditions the area delimited by the precipitate is proportional to the amount of antigen applied. Thus, quantitative immunoelectrophoresis (QIE, Fig. 3c) can be used for quantification of individual components in complex mixtures, for example, in batch-to-batch standardization. QIE is a method to quantify antigens without the need for monospecific antibodies.

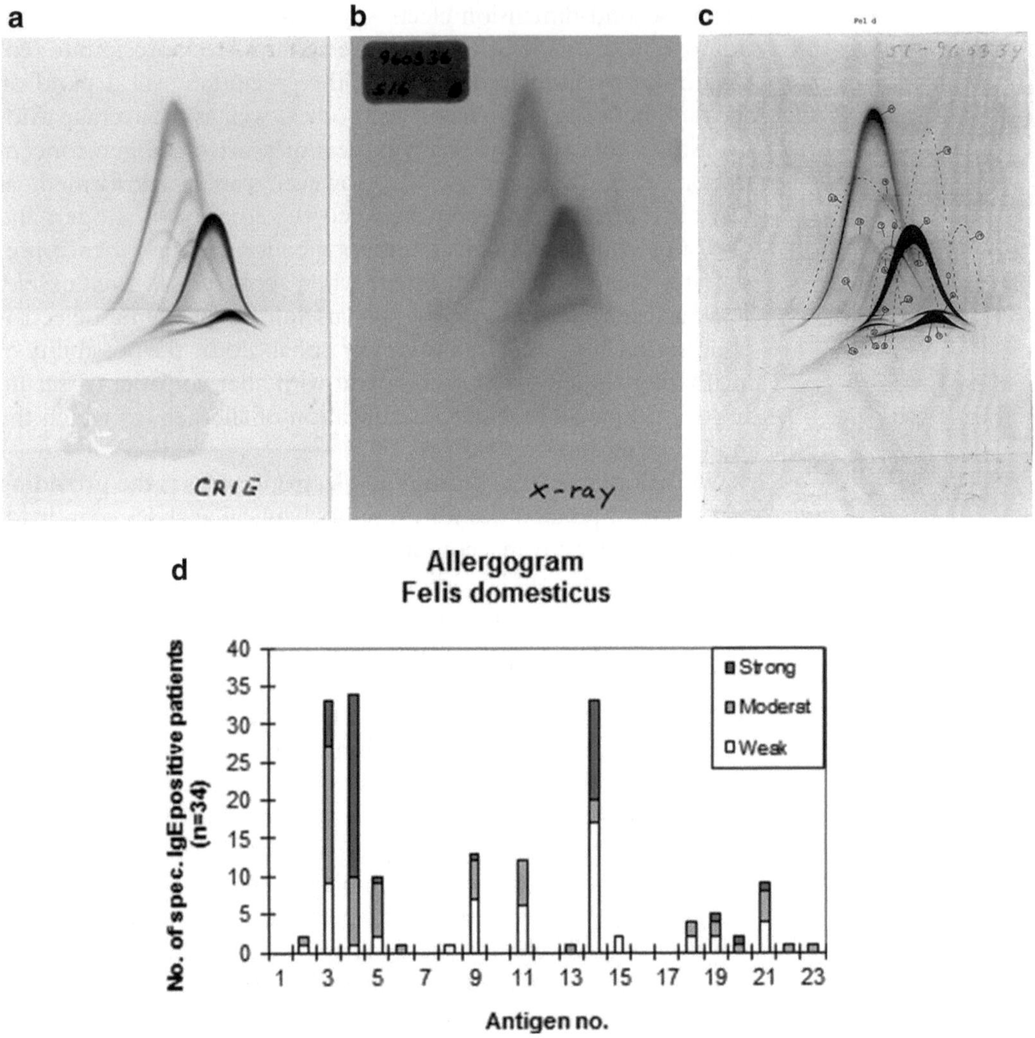

Fig. 2 CRIE and allergogram on Fel d extract. (**a**) Stained CRIE plate and (**b**) corresponding X-ray print from a cat-allergic patient, (**c**) reference picture with numbered precipitates, (**d**) allergogram from CRIE investigation of 34 cat-allergic patients' sera

A unique application is the use of fused rocket immunoelectrophoresis (FRIE, Fig. 1b) for the monitoring of a protein purification procedure. Aliquots of each fraction following a biochemical fractionation (e.g., a chromatographic step) are applied in wells in an agarose gel containing polyspecific rabbit antibody, and electrophoresis is performed in only one dimension. The wells are placed close together resulting in one large fused precipitate. Precipitates on the FRIE plate can be identified using crossed-line immunoelectrophoresis (CLIE, Fig. 1d), in which an aliquot from the relevant fraction is added to an intermediate gel in a CIE design (Fig. 1a).

If only limited amount of material is available tandem crossed immunoelectrophoresis (TCIE, Fig. 1e) can be used as an alternative for this purpose. In TCIE, two wells about 0.75 cm apart are

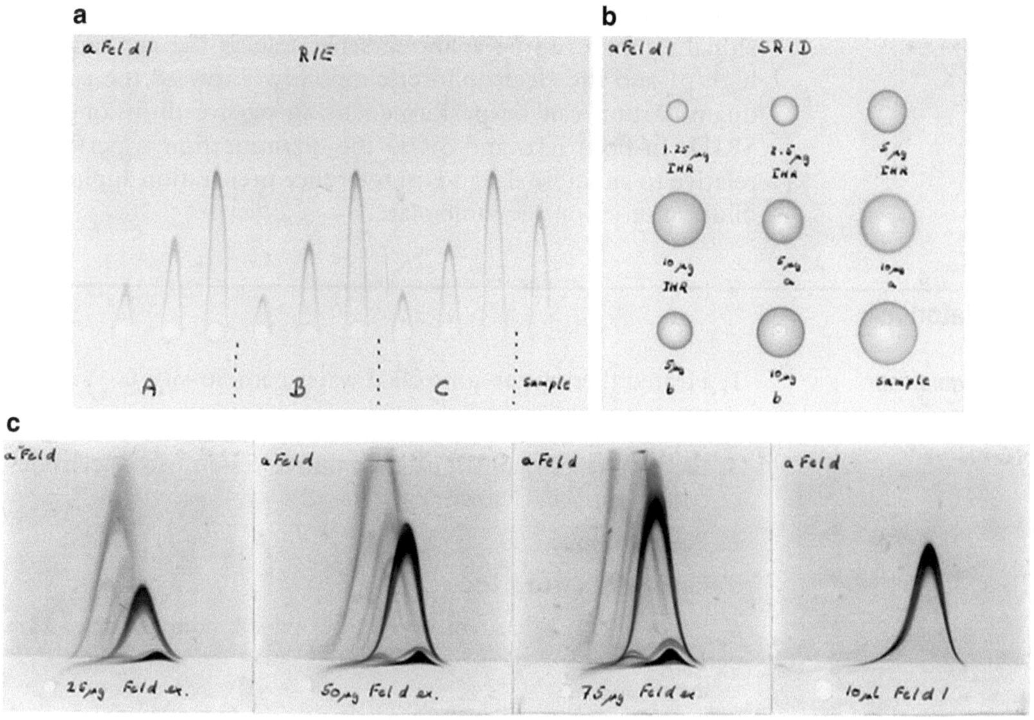

Fig. 3 Quantification methods using monospecific and polyspecific antibodies raised against Fel d 1 (**a**, **b**) and Fel d extract (**c**). (**a**) RIE of three dilutions of three Fel d batches and a sample, (**b**) SRID of four dilutions of in-house reference and different samples, (**c**) QIE of three concentrations of Fel d extract and a sample (Fel d 1)

placed alongside in the first-dimension gel; one well is filled with the reference extract and the other well with the sample to be analyzed. The precipitate formed by the antigen in the sample will make a perfect fusion with the precipitate formed by the identical antigen in the reference extract resulting in a double peak. In addition, TCIE is ideal for the study of partial cross-reactivity from which partially fused precipitates will result.

Having access to the purified protein antigen of interest, Fig. 1c, enables the production of monospecific, polyclonal rabbit antibodies by repeated immunization using the purified antigen. The specificity of the monospecific antiserum can be analyzed in crossed intermediate gel immunoelectrophoresis (CIIE, Fig. 1f) in which the monospecific antiserum is placed in an intermediate gel in a CIE design. The precipitate resulting from the monospecific antiserum will precipitate in the intermediate gel.

The monospecific antiserum can furthermore be used for identification of the antigen in an unknown mixture by CIIE or for quantification by rocket immunoelectrophoresis (RIE, Fig. 3a) or single radial immunodiffusion (SRID, Fig. 3b). In RIE multiple samples can be quantified on the same plate, as only one dimension is performed, as mentioned for FRIE.

In RIE, however, the wells are placed further apart so that individual samples can be analyzed separately. If the antigen has a high pI and the electrophoretic mobility is toward the cathode quantification can be performed using passive diffusion, as in SRID. In both RIE and SRID the quantification is performed relative to an internal standard reference preparation applied as a dilution series on the same plate.

2 Materials

2.1 Equipment

1. Heated thermostat-controlled water bath 56–60 °C.
2. Cooled thermostat-controlled water bath 15 °C.
3. Electrophoresis apparatus (two buffer vessels, two electrodes, cooled surface, chamber).
4. Power supply.
5. Glass plates (std sizes, e.g., 5 × 5, 5 × 7, 10 × 7 cm).
6. Paper wicks: Whatman no. 1 filter paper, standard size: 21 × 10 cm.

2.2 Buffers and Solutions

2.2.1 Buffer for Electrode Vessels and Agarose Gel

1. 5,5-Diethylbarbituric acid (Veronal) Mw 184.20 112.1 g.
2. Tris (Sigma 7–9) Mw 121.14 221.5 g.
3. Calcium lactate (purum) Mw 308.30 2.7 g.
4. Milli-Q H_2O to 5 L.
5. Dissolve overnight by stirring. Store at +5 °C.
6. Dilute 1 + 4 before use to obtain ionic strength of 0.02, pH 8.6.

2.2.2 Agarose Gel

1. 1% (w/v) Litex agarose-type HSA (M_r = −0.13) in the above-mentioned buffer.
2. The agarose is heated under stirring, boiled for 2 min, and kept fluid in a water bath at +56 °C.

2.2.3 Staining Solution

1. Coomassie Brilliant Blue R-250 5 g.
2. Ethanol 96% 450 mL.
3. Milli-Q water 500 mL.
4. Glacial acidic acid 50 mL.
5. Dissolve overnight by stirring. After filtration the solution is ready for use.

2.2.4 Destaining Solution

1. Ethanol 96% 450 mL.
2. Milli-Q water 500 mL.
3. Glacial acidic acid 50 mL.

2.2.5 Buffer for Incubation with Serum (CRIE)

1. Phosphate-buffered saline (PBS), 1 L:
2. NaCl Mw 58.44 8.0 g.
3. KCl Mw 74.55 0.2 g.
4. Na_2HPO_4, $2H_2O$ Mw 175.98 1.44 g.
5. KH_2PO_4 Mw 136.06 0.2 g.
6. Buffer for CRIE incubations (serum, biotin-aIgE, ^{125}I-streptavidin).
7. PBS, 0.1% HSA, 0.05% Tween (5 days' shelf life at +5 °C).
8. Washing buffer for CRIE:
9. PBS, 1% Tween.

2.2.6 Biotin-aIgE (ALK, Hørsholm, Denmark)

1. 20 μL/Plate of a dilution 10 ng/μL

2.2.7 Isotope for CRIE

1. Isotope: ^{125}I-streptavidin Code IRC-140 (Institute of Isotopes Co., Ltd., Budapest, Hungary).
2. Bottle with 500 μL containing 50 μCi or 0.1 μCi/μL on activity date. Use 0.4 μCi/plate.

2.2.8 Standard Developing and Fixing Solutions for Medical X-Ray Film

1. Processing (e.g., AGFA G150 Developer and AGFA G354 Fixing Bath).

2.2.9 X-Ray

1. X-ray cassettes, e.g., Lanex, Kodak X-Omat with regular screens.
2. Kodak X-ray film, MXG ref. 1666007.

3 Methods (*See* Notes 1 and 2)

3.1 CIE (Crossed Immuno-electrophoresis) (See Note 3)

3.1.1 First-Dimension Electrophoresis (Fixed 1. Dimension)

1. Mark a 5 × 7 cm glass plate with identification numbers (e.g., year, month, and no.).

   Turn the plate upside down and clean with ethanol. Place it on a leveled surface and apply 5.3 mL of hot agarose.
2. After thorough setting, punch a well as indicated on the template (Fig. 4a) and apply antigen.
3. Place the glass plate on the cooled surface (approx. 15 °C) of the electrophoresis apparatus, oriented as indicated in Fig. 4a. Connecting bridges of eight layers of paper wicks moistened with electrode buffer are established. The wicks should overlap the gel plate by approx. 0.5 cm.
4. Switch on the current and adjust the voltage across the gel to 10 V/cm. Continue electrophoresis for 25–30 min.

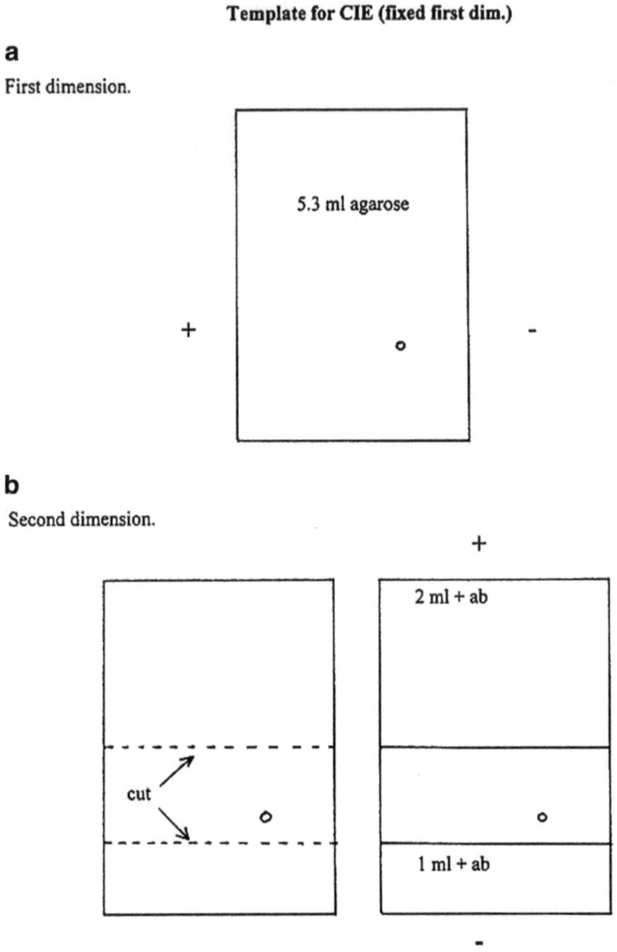

Fig. 4 Template for standard CIE indicating position of well, anode (+), and cathode (−) for the first dimension (**a**) and dimensions of antibody-containing gels for the second dimension (**b**)

3.1.2 Second-Dimension Electrophoresis

1. Cut away gel according to the template (Fig. 4b). Place the plate on the leveled surface.
2. Pour 1 mL agarose mixed thoroughly with the antibodies on the cathodic side of the first-dimensional gel.
3. Pour 2 mL agarose mixed with antibodies on the anodic side of the first-dimensional gel.
4. After thorough setting place the plate on the cooled surface of the electrophoresis apparatus and connect it to buffer reservoirs with five layers of paper wicks. The wicks should overlap the gel by approx. 0.5 cm.
5. Adjust the voltage to 2 V/cm. Place a glass plate on top of the wicks to avoid water to condense on the gel and perform electrophoresis overnight.

*3.1.3 Pressing and Washing of the Plates (See **Note 4**)*

1. Place the glass plates on a filter paper and fill all wells with distilled water (avoid air bubbles, which may cause rupture of the gel). Cover the gel with a wet filter paper (paper wick) and press the plates under several layers of filter paper (use large sheets, which can be air-dried and reused), a thick glass plate, and a load of 3–4 kg.
2. Renew the upper layers of filter paper after 10 min and press again.
3. Transfer the plates to a container with excess 0.1 M NaCl for 15–30 min (washing) and press again as above.
4. Dry the plates in a stream of hot air.

*3.1.4 Staining and Destaining (See **Note 5**)*

1. Stain the plates for approx. 5 min in Commassie Brilliant Blue staining solution.
2. Immerse the plates for a few seconds in distilled water to remove a great deal of the surplus stain.
3. Destain the plates twice in successive baths until the optimal destaining is reached (approx. 15 min).
4. Dry the plate in hot air.
5. Turn gel side down and write sample numbers and other information on the plate. Only write on the glass side.

3.2 Variations of CIE (See Note 6)

3.2.1 CLIE (Crossed-Line Immunoelectrophoresis)

1. Run the one-dimensional electrophoresis as described in Subheading 3.1.1.
2. Cut and remove the intermediate gel (Fig. 5).
3. Pipet a sample of the protein to be investigated into a test tube and heat it in the water bath. Apply agarose to a total volume of 0.9 mL. Mix the gel and sample and pour it in the slit between the first-dimension strip and the upper gel.
4. Allow the newly cast gel to settle before cutting and removing the anodic part of the gel. Apply the antibody-containing gels and run the electrophoresis as described in Subheading 3.1.2.

3.2.2 CIIE (Crossed Intermediate Gel Electrophoresis)

1. Run the one-dimensional electrophoresis as described in Subheading 3.1.1.
2. Cut and remove the intermediate gel (Fig. 5).
3. Pipet an antibody (polyclonal) into a test tube and heat it in the water bath. Apply agarose to a total volume of 0.9 mL. Mix the gel and antibody and pour it in the slit between the first-dimension strip and the upper gel.
4. Allow the newly cast gel to settle before cutting and removing the anodic part of the gel. Apply the antibody-containing gels and run the electrophoresis as described in Subheading 3.1.2.

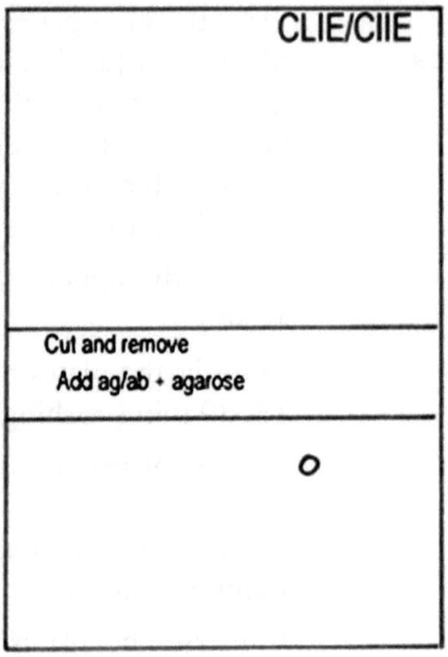

Fig. 5 Template for CLIE and CIIE indicating the position of the intermediate gel during second-dimension electrophoresis

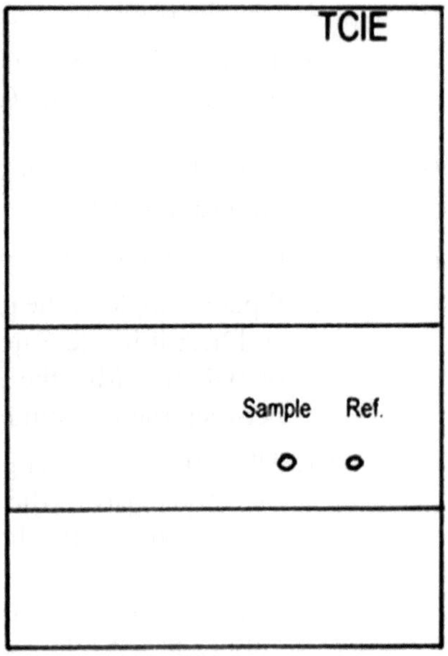

Fig. 6 Template for TCIE indication position of the two parallel wells for the first-dimension electrophoresis

3.2.3 TCIE (Tandem Crossed Immunoelectrophoresis)

1. Cast a plate for the first-dimension electrophoresis as described in Subheading 3.1.1.
2. Punch two wells alongside each other in the first-dimension gel according to the template in Fig. 6.
3. Follow the instructions for CIE as described in Subheading 3.1.

3.3 Crossed Radio-Immuno-electrophoresis and Allergogram

3.3.1 CRIE (See Note 7)

1. Choose the optimized CIE standard conditions for the extract in question and perform one CIE for each serum sample to be tested.
2. After pressing and washing (*see* Subheading 3.1.3) the plates are dried in a stream of cold air. This is important, as heat can denature the proteins, which may lead to loss of their biological activity.
3. To make reproducible results run all plates before serum incubation.

3.3.2 Incubations and Autoradiography

1. The plates are placed in small plastic boxes, which fit the size of the plate (5.3 × 7.3 cm) gel side up, and incubated with a mixture of serum (200–500 μL) and PBS, 0.1% HSA, and 0.05% Tween. Each plate should be totally submerged in a total volume of 8 mL. Before incubation each box is labeled with serum or plate number. Incubate overnight at room temperature (RT) without stirring.
2. Wash each plate directly in the incubation box for 4 × 10 min with approx. 4 × 10 mL PBS and 1% Tween.
3. Incubate with biotin-labeled aIgE (ALK, Hørsholm, Denmark); 200 ng/plate, overnight at RT, in a total volume of 8 mL PBS, 0.1% HSA, and 0.05% Tween.
4. Repeat the washing procedure (4 × 10 min with PBS, 1% Tween). Incubate with ^{125}I-streptavidin (Budapest, Hungary) 0.4 μCi/plate ~4 μL; 2 h at RT in a total volume of 8 mL PBS, 0.1% HSA, and 0.05% Tween. Repeat the washing procedure (3 × 10 min with PBS, 1% Tween, 1 × 2 min with distilled water).
5. Remove the plates from the individual boxes and dry them. Clean the glass side with ethanol and place in an X-ray cassette gel side up. In a darkroom place an X-ray film (Kodak MXG) on top of the plates and expose at −80 °C for 1 day, 3 days, and 10 days, for a total of 14 days.

Following autoradiography all CIE plates are washed for approx. 10 min in distilled water dried and stained (Subheading 3.1.4). Mark the position of the CRIE plates on the X-ray film with a pencil and label each autoradiography (well to the left) with plate no., serum ID, and exposure time and cut the individual X-rays apart with a pair of scissors.

3.3.3 Standard Picture, Scoring, and Allergogram

1. Choose one of the stained CIE plates and use it as the reference plate. Draw a standard picture. The precipitates are then numbered from right to left according to the peak of each precipitate (Fig. 2c).
2. A table with patient numbers and precipitate numbers is used to record the scorings. The stained CIE plate and the three

corresponding autoradiograms from each patient are then, in sequence, compared to the standard picture, and the IgE-binding precipitates visible on the X-ray film are identified.

3. When a precipitate is visible after 1 d score 3 (strong) is given, after 3 d score 2 (moderate), and after 10 d score 1 (weak).
4. Finally the allergogram is constructed as a histogram using the precipitate numbers from the standard picture and the number of patients reacting to each precipitate. On each column the number of patients reacting with the three different scores (1, 2, or 3) is indicated (Fig. 2d).
5. An allergen is classified as a major allergen if at least 50% of the patients show strong or moderate IgE binding. Other clearly specific IgE-binding allergens are classified as minor allergens.

3.4 Quantification of Antigens (See Note 8)

3.4.1 QIE (Quantitative Immunoelectrophoresis)

1. Label four 5 × 5 cm glass plates in the upper right-hand corner with identification numbers. Turn the plates upside down and place them on a leveled surface. Clean with ethanol.
2. Pipet 3.5 mL agarose in each plate.
3. After thorough setting, punch wells according to the template (Fig. 7).
4. Apply, e.g., three concentrations of the standard and one concentration of the sample.
5. Perform the electrophoresis as described in Subheadings 3.1.1, 3.1.2, 3.1.3, and 3.1.4.

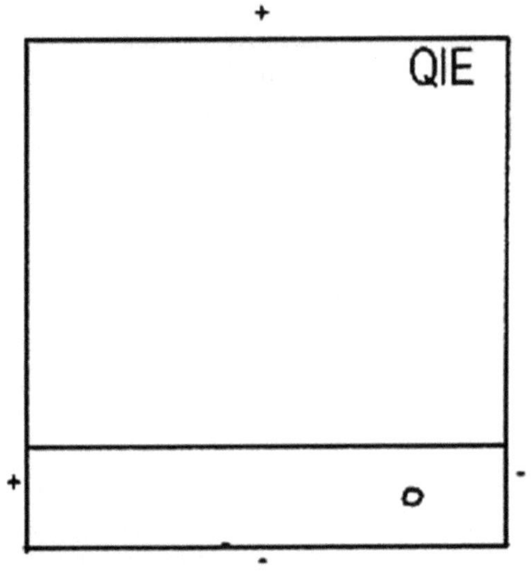

Fig. 7 Template for QIE indicating anode (+) and cathode (–) for both first- and second-dimension electrophoresis

3.4.2 RIE (Rocked Immunoelectrophoresis)

1. Label the glass plate (e.g., 10 × 7 cm) in the upper right-hand corner with identification number. Turn the plate upside down and place it on a leveled surface. Clean the plate with ethanol.
2. Pipet antibody into a test tube and heat it in the water bath (56 °C). Pipet 11 mL of agarose into the tube and mix the gel and the antibody (seal the tube with Parafilm and invert four times). Pour the antibody-containing agarose onto the glass plate (avoid air bubbles).
3. After thorough setting, punch wells 1.5 cm from the lower edge of the plate, Fig. 8a. Well size adjusted to the volume is to be applied.
4. Place the plate on the cooled surface on the electrophoresis apparatus as indicated in the template. Connecting bridges of five layers of filter paper are established. Switch on the current and adjust the voltage across the gel to 2 V/cm.
5. Apply the same volume of all samples. Place a glass plate on top of the wicks to avoid water to condense on the gel. Continue electrophoresis overnight.
6. Press and stain the plate as described in Subheadings 3.1.3 and 3.1.4.

3.4.3 SRID (Single Radial Immunodiffusion)

Prepare the gel as described in Subheading 3.4.2. Punch the wells equally spread on the plate (Fig. 8b), and apply the samples. Place the plate in a humid chamber for approx. 40 h. Press and stain the gel as described in Subheadings 3.1.3 and 3.1.4.

3.4.4 Calculation of Results

RIE and SRID: Measure the area of each precipitate. Draw a standard curve and read each sample.

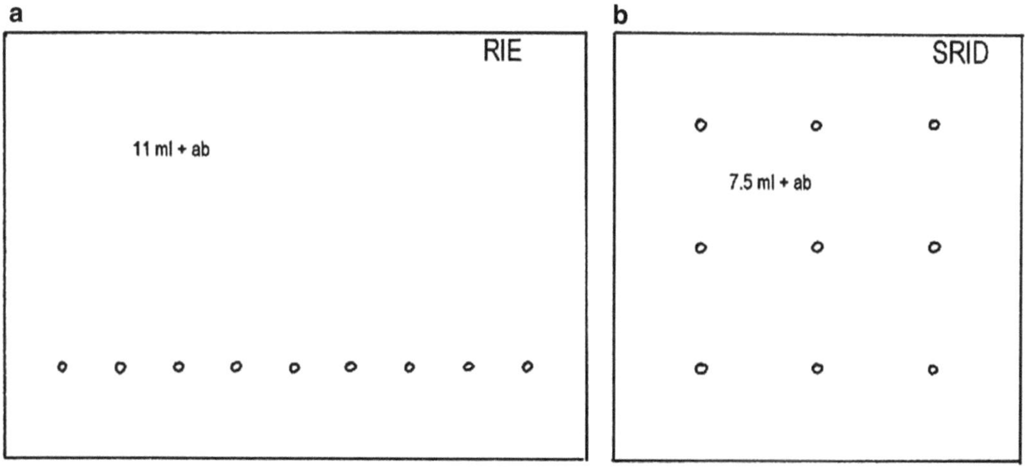

Fig. 8 Template for RIE (**a**) and SRID (**b**)

QIE: Measure the area limited by the precipitate to be quantified on the four plates. Use the line between the first-dimension gel and the antibody-containing gel as a baseline for the precipitate. Draw a standard curve and read the sample.

3.5 Fused Rocket Immuno-electrophoresis (FRIE)

1. Mark and clean a glass plate (e.g., 7 × 10 cm). Pour 11 mL agarose onto the plate.
2. After thorough setting cut away the upper and lower parts of the gel according to the template (Fig. 9).
3. Pipet antibody into two test tubes and heat them in the water bath. Pipet 5.5 mL agarose into the tube for the anodic gel and 1.5 mL agarose for the cathodic gel. Mix the gel and the antibody and pour the mixture on the glass plate.
4. Punch wells in the middle section (not containing antibody) according to the template (Fig. 9) and apply samples from each fraction (from a fractionation experiment) starting as indicated on the template.
5. Place the plate on the cooled surface of the electrophoresis apparatus and connect it to buffer reservoirs with five layers of paper wicks. The wicks should overlap the gel by approx. 0.5 cm.
6. Adjust the voltage to 2 V/cm. Place a glass plate on top of the wicks and continue electrophoresis overnight.
7. Press and stain the gel as described in Subheadings 3.1.3 and 3.1.4.

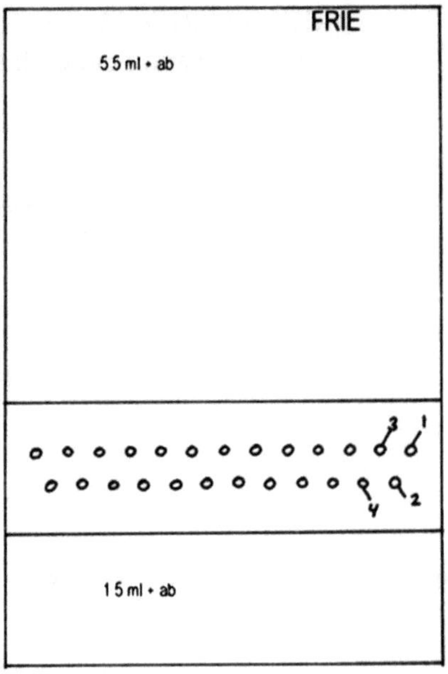

Fig. 9 Template for FRIE indicating position of wells and succession of the fractions applied

4 Notes

1. When starting to work with an unknown antigen/antibody (ag/ab) system, several parameters have to be established before the final conditions for the standard CIE picture are selected. Plates sized 5 × 7 cm have been found convenient to work with. Ag migration in the first dimension: Make sure that no ags run further than 3.5 cm toward the anode or 1.5 cm toward the cathode. As a control run the first dimension for, e.g., 10 and 30 min.

   Ag and ab concentrations: Adjust empirically the ratio between antigen and antibody so that a majority of the precipitates have a suitable size.

   Adjustments of the pattern: Initial examination of the CIE system may lead to adjustment of the gel dimensions. Positioning of the well is dependent on the mobility of the antigens in question. The size of the intermediate gel may be adjusted or a second ab may be included in this. If no antigens run toward the cathode, the antibody-containing cathodic gel can be spared and the first-dimension gel moved to the edge of the glass plate.

   Agarose: The type of agarose can be changed. Usually agarose-type HSA with electroendosmosis (Mr = −0.13) is used. In rare occasions, agarose-type HSB (Mr = −0.07) or HSC (Mr = −0.02) may be more suitable.

2. Instead of glass plates, coated plastic sheets cut in suitable sizes can be used.

   Disposable plastic tubes can replace glass test tubes, but they are difficult to incubate in a rack in the water bath.

   Use a (rotating) diamond pen to scratch the labels into the glass plate for identification.

   After use the agarose gel may be stored at 5 °C and used again after boiling.

   Heat the pipet to 56 °C before pipetting the agarose. When not used, store the pipet in a tall cylinder glass placed in the water bath to keep the pipet hot. Work fast! The agarose will set quite quickly.

   The size of the well must correspond to the sample volume. Use a gel puncher (e.g., 5, 10, or 15 μL size) connected to a vacuum pump (water jet stream or mechanical pump).

   Always keep the anode to the same side in the apparatus. Cut the paper wicks to fit the size of the glass plates to cover. The current is measured in V/cm. Use a probe with a fixed distance between the electrodes connected to a voltmeter for the calculation of V/cm. Place a glass plate on top of the wicks during the overnight electrophoresis. Moisture from the air will condense on top of the upper glass plate instead of on the gel, which may cause fluffy precipitates.

The buffer in the electrophoresis vessels can be used for approximately six runs before renewal is necessary (first and second dimensions included in one run).

All volumes of agarose gel are calculated from the area in cm2 and the thickness of the gel. The thickness is adjusted so that the first cast gel on a plate is a little higher than the next. First-dimension gel: 1.5 mm. Intermediate gel: 1.4 mm. Ab gel (anode): 1.3 mm.

Pipet the antibody into a test tube and heat the tube for approx. 10 s in the water bath before applying the agarose. Let the agarose run along the side of the test tube. Avoid air bobbles when agarose and antibody are mixed. Pay attention to the temperature in the water bath; temperatures above 60 °C will denature the antibodies. If air bubbles are present in the newly cast gel they may be removed (punctured) immediately with a clean pipet tip.

In order to reduce background staining, nonprecipitated proteins are removed by repeated pressing and washing. The use of purified immunoglobulins instead of crude antisera also reduces background staining.

3. The method described above uses a fixed first dimension directly on the glass plate, on which the antibody subsequently is applied. If several plates have to be performed in parallel a transferred one dimension may be preferred. In that case, several one-dimension strips can be performed side by side on a larger plate, separated (with a long razor blade), and transferred to the final plates where intermediate gel and antibody-containing gels are cast. Care should be taken comparing plates run under the two different conditions (transferred and fixed first dimension).

   Check and adjust the voltage once during electrophoresis, e.g., after 15 min. Beware of the shock hazard.

4. The paper wick directly on the plates may stick to the gel. In that case, moisten the paper with distilled water and remove it carefully starting in one corner. Check with a touch of a fingertip that the gels are still on the glass plates. Pour on more water if the gel sticks to the paper.

   Put saline in a suitable box, place a paper wick in the bottom (easier to get the plates up again!), and carefully place the plates in the box. Do not move the box. The gels might slide off the plates.

   Dry in cold air if the proteins should retain their biological activity for subsequent incubation with, e.g., serum (CRIE).

5. Stain with gel side up. Use a special rack accommodating several plates. Keep the staining and destaining solutions in tight plastic boxes for reuse.

The destaining solution can be regenerated passing through a filter with activated charcoal and can be reused several times.

If the gels by accident are destained too excessively, they can be restained. The best result is obtained if the plates are not dried before restaining.

6. Make a 2% agarose gel if more than 400 μL must be applied in the intermediate gel.
7. The dried plates can be stored at +5 °C for several months in a sealed plastic box or wrapped in tinfoil. Place a piece of filter paper or a soft tissue between the plates to avoid scratching of the dried agarose gels.

   The amount of ^{125}I-streptavidin/plate is calculated from the activity date given on the product specification sheet. 4 μL/Plate is used on activity reference date = 0.

Day from activity date	μL/8 per CRIE plate
−10	28
−8	29
−6	30
−4	31
−2	31
0	32 (=4 μL/plate)
2	33
4	34
6	34
8	35
10	36
12	37
14	38

The washed and dried plates are placed edge by edge in the cassette not leaving any space between them. This will ease the cutting of the film later. Start in the upper right-hand corner. Make sure that the plates do not slide in the cassette; keep it horizontal at all times.

Label the film in one edge with a pencil with date and cassette number. Expose the film in the freezer; the low-exposure temperature (−80 °C, alternatively −20 °C) will lead to stronger X-ray staining.

Before each film is developed remove the cassette from the freezer in ample time to allow complete equilibration at RT; otherwise condensed water will damage the X-ray film.

Standard developing and fixing solutions for medical X-ray film processing and procedures from the manufacturer are used.

The standard CIE picture is either drawn during projecting a stained CRIE plate in a photo magnifier or printed from a digitally scanned plate. Check the picture carefully with the stained CRIE plates to ensure that all precipitates are visible on the standard picture.

If it is difficult to recognize a CRIE precipitate on the X-ray film when individual patients are scored, it may help also to look at the stained CIE plate from which the standard picture was drawn.

Very often particular precipitates are visible only on the autoradiogram and not on the Coomassie-stained plates. This is because of lower sensitivity in the Coomassie staining. These precipitates are drawn on the standard picture with dotted lines and numbered.

All autoradiograms should be scored by two individuals. In case of discrepancies, the scoring is re-evaluated.

The CRIE technique can also be performed with biotin-labeled αIgE followed by avidin-AP (alkaline phosphatase-conjugated avidin) and substrate. This method is much faster because autoradiography is avoided; however, the relative intensity in staining is lost. Furthermore, unspecific binding is more pronounced by using this method. The method is, however, useful if a fast analysis of an individual serum or a serum pool is wanted or when monitoring, e.g., an allergen purification.

8. The humid chamber for diffusion of the SRID plate is made by placing paper napkins or filter paper moistened with distilled water in a tight box. Leave at room temperature and beware of one-sided heat from, e.g., laboratory equipment, which will disturb the shape of the precipitates.

   The height of the rockets (RIE) and d × d (diameters perpendicular to each other) of the SRID correlate with the area limited by the precipitates.

   A more precise method to work out the area is to determine it electronically or place the plate in a photo magnifier, draw the precipitates on paper, cut them out, and weigh.

References

1. Løwenstein H (1978) Quantitative immunoelectrophoretic methods as a tool for the analysis and isolation of allergens. Prog Allergy 25:1
2. Axelsen NH, Krøll J, Weeke B (1973) A manual of quantitative immunoelectrophoresis. Methods and applications. Scand J Immunol 2(Suppl 1):1

Chapter 5

Standardization of Allergen Extracts

Jørgen Nedergaard Larsen and Sten Dreborg

Abstract

Allergens are molecules with the capacity to elicit IgE responses in humans. When stimulated with allergens, most allergic patients respond with production of IgE specific for several proteins/allergens in the source material. The standardization of allergen extracts is essential in order to control variability and to achieve consistency and reproducibility in a clinical setting.

Because the IgE binding capacity of an allergen extract is related to the content of one or a few major allergens, it is important that the standardization procedure ensures consistency, not only in the overall IgE binding potency, but also in the content and ratio of individual major allergens. Owing to the complexity of allergen extracts, a key element in standardization of allergen extracts is the use of standards.

This chapter describes the principles for standardization of allergen extracts to be used by research laboratories. Other chapters in this volume describe in vitro methods in detail.

Key words Allergen extracts, Allergen standardization, Major allergen, In vitro, In vivo

1 Introduction

Allergen extracts, such as grass pollen extract or house dust mite extract, are used for allergen-specific diagnosis and treatment of allergic disease. In the production of allergen extracts, it is essential to apply standardization in order to control the variability in naturally occurring source materials, and achieve consistency and reproducibility for optimal safety and efficacy in clinical use. In the widest sense, standardization includes controlling the entire production chain of processes including qualifications of collectors of raw materials, quality of collected raw materials, establishment of robust and reproducible production procedures in compliance with "good manufacturing practice" (GMP) or "Good Laboratory practice" (GLP) regulations, and formulation of allergen extracts intended for clinical use in allergy diagnosis, in vivo as well as in vitro, and in allergen immunotherapy/vaccination. Standardization,

Penny Lympany and Meinir G. Jones (eds.), *Allergy: Methods and Protocols*, Methods in Molecular Biology, vol. 2020, https://doi.org/10.1007/978-1-4939-9591-2_5,

however, is not a precisely defined term, as different qualities of standardization are in current use by various laboratories and manufacturers of allergen extracts. It is therefore essential that even scientific laboratories describing new allergens, new aspects, or new processes establish internal standards that can be used and referenced in future work in a transparent manner.

Allergen molecules are present in inhaled particles, foods, insect venoms, etc. They are defined by the capacity to elicit IgE responses in humans. By far most allergen molecules are proteins, readily soluble in water, and presented to the immune system after extraction on the moist surfaces of the airways, in the gastrointestinal tract or in the bloodstream. Allergic patients respond to allergen exposure with immediate symptoms initiated by allergen-IgE interaction and in most cases accompanied by prolonged allergic inflammation in the airways, the gastrointestinal tract, and/or the skin.

The allergic reaction is allergen specific and reinforced by cells and molecules of the adaptive immune system. Thus, the active fraction of an allergen extract is the protein fraction, and batch-to-batch standardization is particularly focused on control of the protein fraction including control of the total allergenic potency, antigen and allergen profile, as well as stability, assuring relevant composition and potency in clinical use during an appropriate period of time.

Any protein in a source material has the potential to elicit an IgE response; however, in practice the IgE binding capacity of an allergen extract is related to the content of one or a few major allergens, i.e., allergens to which a majority of patients react with IgE [1]. It is therefore important that the standardization procedure ensures consistency, not only in the overall IgE binding potency, but also in the content and ratio of individual major allergens.

Owing to the complexity of allergen extracts, a key element in standardization of allergen extracts is the use of standards [2]. In Europe, each laboratory and manufacturer establishes an in-house reference (IHR) preparation for each source material. The IHR must be thoroughly characterized by in vitro methods as a basis for equilibration of subsequent batches, and the biological activity of the IHR should be determined by in vivo methods in humans. The IHR eliminates the need for in vivo methods in batch-to-batch standardization, which can be performed by comparing new batches to the IHR using in vitro methods exclusively.

This chapter describes the principles for standardization of allergen extracts suitable for allergen-specific management of allergy, i.e., diagnosis and immunotherapy, whereas other chapters in this volume describe methods in detail. Chemical modification of allergen extracts sometimes used for immunotherapy is not included, as well as single allergen molecules, purified native or recombinant.

2 Materials

2.1 Selection of Human Sera

A critical reagent in the study of new or established allergen extracts is constituted by human serum samples. The availability of adequate amounts of serum with broad specificity to all relevant allergens present in the source material should be secured. The selection of raw material and the selection of suitable sera is an interdependent process. Sera from a number of patients clinically sensitive to the allergen source in question should be collected and tested against selected raw materials by, e.g., immunoblotting. Subsequently, sera suitable for detection of specific allergens should be characterized, and a pool of sera containing IgE specificities detecting all relevant allergens should be established. When mixing sera, care should be taken to ensure that sufficient amounts of sera containing IgE against minor allergens are included.

The individual serum samples and the serum pool should be stored for future documentation and batch control in small aliquots at −20 °C.

2.2 Selection of Source Materials

Inhalant allergens are present in airborne particles derived from natural allergen sources. These particles constitute the material to which humans are exposed, and the aim of raw material selection is to provide materials containing the same active allergens in a manageable form. In most cases, the optimal source material is rather obvious, but in some cases the allergen source is still debated (e.g., cat saliva/pelt/dander or mouse urine/dander).

The source materials should be selected with attention to the need for specificity and for inclusion of all relevant allergens in sufficient amounts [2].

The collection of the source materials should be performed by qualified persons, and reasonable measures must be employed to assure that collector qualifications and collection procedures are appropriate to verify the identity and quality of the source materials. This means that only specifically identified allergenic source materials that do not contain avoidable foreign substances should be used in the manufacture of allergenic extracts. Means of identification and limits of foreign materials should meet established acceptance criteria for each source material. Where identity and purity cannot be determined by direct examination of the source materials, other appropriate methods should be applied to trace the materials from their origin. This includes complete identity labeling and certification from competent collectors. The processing and storage of source materials should be performed to ensure that no unintended substances, including microbial organisms, are introduced into the materials.

When possible, source materials should be fresh and stored in a manner that minimizes or prevents decomposition. Records should describe source materials in as much detail as possible, including the particulars of collection, pretreatment, and storage.

2.3 Specific Aspects of Source Materials

Specific aspects of the most important raw material categories are briefly discussed below.

2.3.1 Pollens

The natural sources of inhalant allergens from plants are the pollens. Pollen may be obtained either by collection in nature or from cultivated fields or greenhouses. The collection may be performed by several methods, such as vacuuming or drying flower heads followed by grinding. The pollen may be cleaned either by passing through sieves of different mesh sizes or by flotation. Finally, pollens are dried under controlled conditions and stored in sealed containers at −20 °C. The maximum level of accepted contamination with pollen from other species is 1% by number, and a maximum of 0.5% of any individual foreign pollen [3]. Pollen should be devoid of flower and plant debris, with a limit of 5% by weight. Pollens may show large variation in quantitative composition depending on season and location of growth, and in order to achieve a relatively constant composition, harvests from different years should, after thorough characterization in vitro, be pooled for the production of allergen extracts.

2.3.2 Acarids

House dust mites are grown in pure cultures. Source materials are either pure mite bodies (PMB) or whole-mite cultures (WMC). Extracts based on WMC include material from mite bodies, eggs, larvae, and fecal particles as well as mite decomposition material and contain all the material to which a mite-allergic patient is exposed under natural conditions. The source material may be enriched in particles particularly common in inhaled air, such as fecal particles. The culture medium should ideally be antigen free, or contaminants from the culture medium should be shown not to be allergenic. The PMB extract avoids extensive contamination with debris from the culture medium. Clinical trials comparing vaccines based on WMC and PMB extracts have shown similar clinical efficacy in specific allergy vaccination [4], although they were underpowered to demonstrate clinically relevant differences.

2.3.3 Animals

Allergens of animal origin may be present in various sources (e.g., dander, serum, saliva, or urine). The allergens to which humans are exposed depend on the normal behavior of the animal and, therefore, cannot be generalized. In each case, the optimal source or mix of sources of allergens from animals should be thoroughly investigated using a large panel of sera from allergic patients. Whether derived from dander or deposited from body fluids, most allergens are present in the pelt. Source materials should be collected only from animals that are declared healthy by a veterinarian at the time of collection. When sacrificed animals are used, the conditions for storing should minimize postmortem decomposition until the source materials can be collected. The optimal source materials are often dander. Hair proteins are insoluble and therefore irrelevant. Urine, saliva, milk, or meat may be adequate sources in particular cases. Use of whole pelt would increase the proportion of serum proteins, which are unwanted as they are generally of low allergenic activity and may displace more important allergens from dander and saliva. Because of the quantitative differences in the yield of the various allergens from different dog breeds [5], a mixture of material from different breeds should be selected representing a balanced content of the major allergens [6].

2.3.4 Insects

The optimal source for insect allergens is dependent on the natural route of exposure (i.e., inhalation, bite, or sting). Where whole insects or insect debris is inhaled, the whole insect body is selected as allergen source. In the case of biting or stinging insects, saliva or venom, respectively, is the proper allergen source.

2.3.5 Fungi

Molds should be grown under controlled conditions. The harvested raw materials should consist of mycelia and spores. Owing to difficulties in maintaining a constant composition of fungal cultures, it is recommended that extracts should be derived from several independent cultures of the same species. The primary inoculum should be obtained from established fungal culture banks, i.e., American Type Culture Collection (ATCC, http://www.atcc.org/) or Central Bureau Schimmelcultures (CBS, http://www.cbs.knaw.nl/). As the composition of mold extracts may vary even under seemingly similar growth conditions, mixing of several strains from the same species can be considered [7, 8].

The cultivation medium should be synthetic or at least devoid of allergenic constituents (i.e., intact proteins). Culturing should be conducted under aseptic conditions to reduce the risk of contamination by microorganisms or other fungi, and controls must include tests for suspected toxins.

2.3.6 Foods

Foods constitute a diversified area, and the supply of standardized allergen extracts is scarce. Foods are often derived from various subspecies, grown under a broad variety of conditions reflecting geographical variation. In addition, foods are often cooked prior to ingestion, and the cooking procedures may differ geographically. Consequently, the source of allergen exposure, qualitative as well as quantitative, is highly variable [9].

Ideally, source materials for food allergen extracts should reflect local subspecies, conditions, and habits for the cultivation, harvesting, storing, and cooking of the foods. However, ingested foods are increasingly derived from distant parts of the world. A solution to these problems may be to combine materials from as many sources as possible, reflecting variation in as many parameters as possible.

The difficulties in producing consistent and reproducible food allergen extracts have resulted in many clinicians using untreated foods from retail trade for diagnosis by the prick–prick method [10]. Examples are fresh fruit, cow's milk, and hen's egg. Undiluted cow's milk and hen's egg have the best documented diagnostic properties [11].

A further problem in food allergen extract production is the presence in many foods of natural or microbial toxins, pesticides, antibiotics, preservatives, and other additives that may be concentrated in the manufacturing process. The use of organic source material should therefore be preferred.

3 Methods

3.1 Preparation of Allergen Extracts

Allergen–IgE binding involves the interaction of molecular surfaces of allergens and IgE antibodies having contours exactly fitting each other [12]. Because the structure of the molecular surface of the allergen and thus the IgE-binding epitopes are vulnerable to protein denaturation, procedures used for the preparation and storage of allergen extracts/vaccines should avoid organic solvents, elevated temperatures, and extreme pH and ionic conditions. The extraction should be performed under conditions resembling the physiological conditions in the human airways (i.e., pH and ionic strength) and suppressing possible proteolytic degradation and microbial growth [13]. The optimal extraction time is always a compromise between yield and degradation/denaturation of the allergens, and special attention should be drawn to the fact that different allergens are released with different kinetics [14]. In general, processing time should be minimized and extraction performed at low temperature.

Low-molecular-weight, i.e., below 5000 Da, nonantigenic material should be removed from the extract by dialysis, ultrafiltration, or size-exclusion chromatography. Any substance excluded from the final product should be shown to be nonallergenic. The production procedure should include procedures to measure and exclude below-defined thresholds for known toxins, viral particles, and free histamine or other physiologically active substances.

The final extract should be stored under conditions that impede deterioration of the allergenic activity either by lyophilizing the extract or by storage at low temperatures (i.e., −20 °C to −80 °C), possibly in the presence of stabilizing agents, such as 50% glycerol, nonallergenic proteins (e.g., certified human serum albumin), or other stabilizers.

3.2 IHR Preparations and Standards

3.2.1 IHR Preparations

A particularly important aspect of the standardization procedure is the IHR. In Europe, the IHR is prepared by the individual laboratory or manufacturer, whereas in the United States, the US Food and Drug Administration (FDA) authorizes general standards of some common allergens for the purpose. The IHR is used by manufacturers/laboratories for equilibration of the potency and composition of each batch of manufactured extract [15–17]. By this procedure the batch-to-batch standardization can be performed by comparison to the IHR using in vitro techniques exclusively avoiding use of in vivo methods. The establishment of an IHR and subsequent production of new batches related to the IHR are illustrated in Fig. 1.

When a robust extraction procedure has been defined, three batches of the extract should be produced in order to verify consistency and reproducibility of the production processes. The three batches are compared, and if consistency is achieved one is selected to represent the new IHR, which is subsequently dispended into freeze-dried aliquots of suitable size. The IHR should be carefully defined including assessment of dry weight, protein content, and composition as well as major allergen content preferentially by internationally recognized methods, and total allergenic activity by in vitro methods (Fig. 1). Furthermore, the biological activity of the IHR should be established by in vivo methods [18–20]. The dispensing into aliquots can be based on dry weight, as other methods are less precise, e.g., protein by Lowry, or too expensive for routine use, e.g., automated amino acid analysis.

The determination of total allergenic activity by in vivo methods, most often by skin prick testing (SPT) [18], is laborious and should be used exclusively for the establishment of IHR preparations. For standardization of subsequent batches major allergen determination with a validated assay is sufficient, as the biological

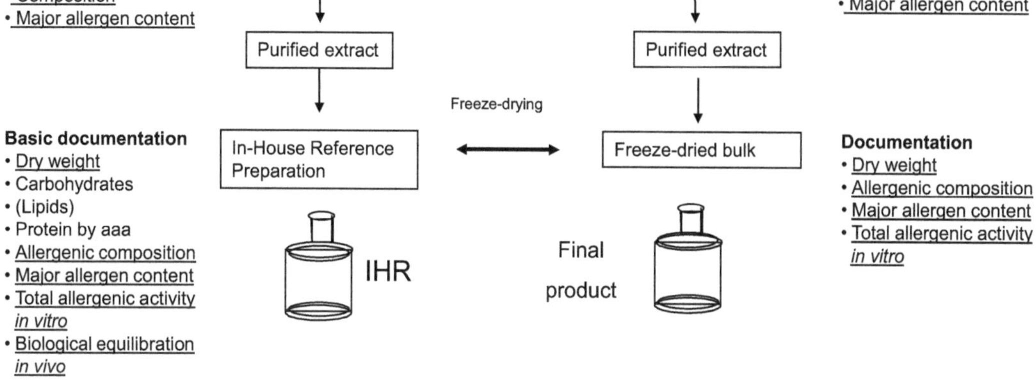

Fig. 1 Standardization of allergen extracts. The principle for establishment of an in-house reference (IHR) preparation to the left and standardization of subsequent batches, calibrated against the IHR. Different methods can be applied to determine the total allergenic composition. Figure modified from [18]

activity has been shown to correlate with the major allergen content [21]. A determination of the total allergenic potency by IgE-based in vitro methods should also be included. If in vitro methods alone are used for the establishment of the potency of the IHR, comparison is best made with the International Standard. Research laboratories investigating new allergen source materials may omit the in vivo potency estimation, but should follow the rest of the standard procedures and store IHR as well as serum pools and individual sera used for characterization.

3.2.2 International Standards (IS)

Allergen extract standardization ideally requires use of two types of standards for each source material, an IHR preparation as described above and an IS. IS of allergen extracts is obtainable from the National Institute of Biological Science and Control, NIBSC, London, the United Kingdom, and was produced under the auspices of the WHO according to guidelines established by the Allergen Standardization Sub-Committee under the International Union of Immunological Societies (IUIS). IS enables comparison of specific activities of products from different manufacturers and can be used as calibrators by new producers and laboratories.

IS is, however, only available for the following allergen extracts: *Ambrosia artemisiifolia* (short ragweed) [22], *Phleum pratense* (timothy grass) [23], the house dust mite *Dermatophagoides pteronyssinus* [24], *Betula verrucosa* (birch) [25], and *Canis familiaris* (dog) [26]. Additional standards were planned for the mold *Alternaria alternata* [27], for the grasses *Cynodon dactylon* (Bermuda grass) [28], and *Lolium perenne* (ryegrass) [29], *Felis domesticus* (cat), and the house dust mite *Dermatophagoides farinae*, but unfortunately this initiative was stopped prematurely due to lack of general acceptance.

3.3 Units and Measure

The strength or potency of an allergen extract relies on the magnitude of the response it will elicit in human allergic subjects. Allergic patients respond individually to allergen extracts because they are sensitized to different allergens in the source material and the degree of sensitivity differs from patient to patient as well as for each allergen in the extract. Because allergen extracts from different producers differ in composition there is no straightforward relationship between potency and response when considering allergen extracts from different manufacturers. This paradox poses an inherent problem in the labeling of allergen extracts, as the potency of different extracts cannot be compared in a meaningful manner.

Direct skin testing of human allergic subjects is the predominant in vivo method for the assessment of allergen extract potency [18] and also constitutes the principle underlying the establishment of biological units of allergen extract potency [19]. Patient selection criteria are important, as all potency measures will be dependent on the patient panel, and skin sensitivity may vary up to a factor of 10,000 among patients.

In Europe, SPT has been used for estimating the biological activity of allergen extracts. The aim is to equilibrate the potency between extracts of different inhalant allergen extracts [30]. When performing a potency test at least 20 consecutive patients attending a specialist clinic should be included. The concentration inducing a weal of the same size as that of histamine dihydrochloride, 10 mg/mL, is estimated by parallel-line bioassay. The median concentration constitutes 10,000 biological units (BU/mL) [20]. This method was adopted by the Nordic Council on Medicines as the Nordic Biological Unit, BU/ml or HEP [19]. With proper patient selection the unit has been shown to be reproducible between different regions of Europe [20]. European manufacturers use their own company-specific units, most of which are based on the same method [18].

In the United States, the FDA/CBER uses a unit based on intradermal testing with the allergen extract and subsequent measurement of the flare rather than the weal size. The "intradermal end point" is expressed as the number of threefold dilutions producing a summed erythema diameter of 50 mm. Furthermore, the CBER in the United States proposed the "bioequivalent allergy unit" (BAU). The method for assigning BAU is named the $ID_{50}EAL$ method, i.e., "intradermal threefold dilution for 50 mm sum of erythema diameters determines bioequivalent allergy unit." The mean value of 20 highly sensitive individuals defines the potency of the allergen extract [31].

Labeling of the potency of allergen extracts based on the microgram amount or, more correctly, the millimolar concentration of major allergen has been proposed, as the major allergen content correlates with the biological activity [21]; that is, 10 μg of major allergen corresponds to 10 HEP or 10,000 BU/mL within a range of ±2, i.e., 5–20 μg [20, 21]. Using the same well-characterized antibodies, IHR, and validated methodology, and with similar extract composition, determination of major allergen content can replace other methods for potency declaration [32]. However, in most cases the composition of test materials varies between laboratories and the content of a single major allergen does not reflect the overall potency between marketed allergen extracts from different companies.

Research laboratories investigating new allergen sources should primarily set up methods to determine the composition and major allergen content using well-defined and published methods enabling comparison between studies in a transparent manner.

3.4 Stability Testing

Criteria, methods, and limits for stability should be established. In Europe, a total allergenic activity in the interval between 50% and 150% of the IHR is accepted, whereas the US authorities use limits of 50–200% of the labeled activity. Methods used to assess the potency should have a demonstrated higher precision, which is not always trivial. The reference should be the IHR stored, preferably freeze-dried, at −70 °C or lower. For stability assessment, the extract should be stored at several different temperatures to assure safe storage at room temperature, in a refrigerator, and at −20 °C. Accelerated degradation studies designed to measure the kinetics of breakdown of the allergen extract can be performed by incubation at multiple high temperatures.

Researchers should ensure small aliquots of the material be stored at −70 °C for future comparisons.

3.5 Batch-to-Batch Control

Having established an IHR preparation, batch-to-batch standardization is performed by calibrating new freeze-dried batches in bulk with the IHR before dispensing into vials for distribution. Batch-to-batch standardization includes, apart from determination of dry weight, three steps:

1. Assessment of allergenic composition to ensure the presence in the final product of all allergens present in the source material: Techniques used include crossed (radio)-immunoelectrophoresis (CIE/CRIE) [33], sodium dodecyl sulfate-polyacrylamide gel electrophoresis (SDS-PAGE) [34], and immunoblotting [35], as well as isoelectric focusing (IEF) [36]. CIE has the advantage of being a semiquantitative technique, and a reproducible precipitation pattern will ensure constant ratios between all major antigenic components. Immunoblotting allows semi-quantification by scanning.
2. Quantification of specific major allergens to ensure that essential allergens are present in constant ratios: Techniques used include quantitative immunoelectrophoresis (QIE) [33] and enzyme-linked immunosorbent assay (ELISA) [37].
3. Quantification of the total allergenic activity to ensure that the overall potency of the extract is constant: Techniques used include several variations of in vitro allergen specific IgE inhibition assays, such as the radioallergosorbent test (RAST) [38] and RAST inhibition assays.

In batch-to-batch standardization, in vitro laboratory techniques are used to compare individual batches to the IHR, which should be matched in every aspect; *see* Fig. 2.

3.6 Conclusion

Allergen extracts are complex mixtures derived from natural source materials and as such prone to natural variation. Standardization is necessary to control variation and ensure consistency and reproducibility for the safety and efficacy of specific allergy disease management. Batch-to-batch standardization is performed by comparison of new batches to established standards assessing complexity, major allergen content, and IgE binding.

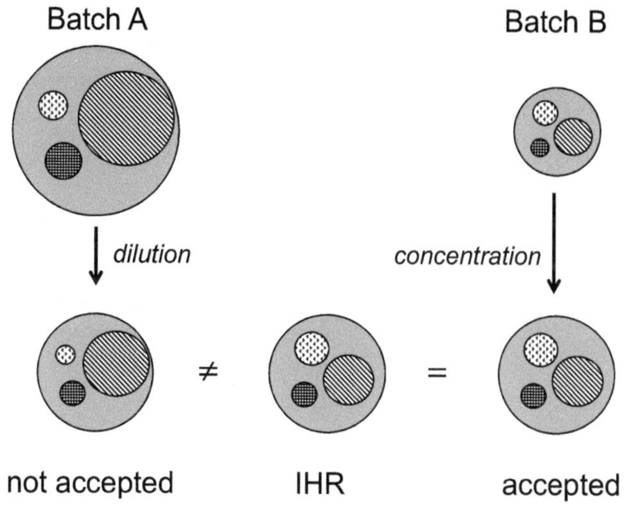

Fig. 2 Complexity of allergen extracts represented by a model with three major allergens. The area of shaded circles represents the relative potency of individual components. The area of outer circles represents the total allergenic potency of the extracts. The total allergenic potency of batches A and B may be adjusted by dilution or concentration, but still the composition of the extracts may vary stressing the importance of the measurement of individual components. Figure modified from [39]

3.7 Checklist for Standardization of Allergen Extracts

1. **Establish criteria for raw material quality.**
   Criteria should define standard procedures for collection and storage of raw materials and thresholds for contamination with bacteria, viruses, and suspected toxins.
2. **Collect serum samples.**
   Serum from a group of patients with clinical sensitivity to the allergen source under study should be collected and characterized.
3. **Select supplier of raw materials.**
   Suppliers of raw materials should document qualifications of experts, e.g., mycologists, acarocologists, and palynologists, and collection procedures to ensure optimal quality and absence of infectious particles.
4. **Select relevant raw materials.**
   Source materials from different suppliers and different growth conditions should ideally be included in initial screenings.
5. **Perform test extractions.**
   Allergenic raw materials are complex. Empirical testing of the following parameters is essential: extraction buffer composition, time, and temperature.

6. **Select individual sera and establish serum pool.**

   Select individual sera with relevant IgE in suitable concentration for characterization of the allergen extract, and establish a serum pool.

7. **Remove low-molecular-weight components by dialysis or filtration.**

   Excluded material should be verified to be nonallergenic in IgE binding assays.

8. **Establish criteria for batch-to-batch variability.**

   Assess the robustness of the extraction procedure by performing three batches, and verify that the variability is below predefined limits.

9. **Define the IHR.**

   The IHR should be characterized with respect to dry weight, allergen complexity, major allergen content, and total IgE binding potency. Biological activity should ideally be determined by skin testing. When major allergens are well characterized, in vivo biological standardization can be replaced by major allergen determination as a basis for adjusting the potency to a suitable level.

10. **Assess stability of the IHR.**

    Methods to be used and criteria for the precision of assays used for stability assessment should be the same as those used for documenting the IHR.

11. **Batch control.**

    Production batches should be produced according to the established production processes, and the freeze-dried product should be calibrated to the IHR assessing complexity, major allergen content, and total IgE binding capacity.

References

1. King TP, Hoffman D, Løwenstein H et al (1994) Allergen nomenclature. WHO/IUIS Allergen Nomenclature Subcommittee. Int Arch Allergy Immunol 105:224–233
2. Løwenstein H (1987) Selection of reference preparation. IUIS reference preparation criteria. Arb Paul Ehrlich Inst 80:75–78
3. European Directorate for the Quality of Medicines and HealthCare. Monograph on Allergen Products, European Pharmacopoeia 01/2010:1063
4. Wahn U, Schweter C, Lind P, Løwenstein H (1988) Prospective study on immunologic changes induced by two different Dermatophagoides pteronyssinus extracts prepared from whole mite culture and mite bodies. J Allergy Clin Immunol 82:360–370
5. Lindgren S, Belin L, Dreborg S, Einarsson R, Pahlman I (1988) Breed-specific dog-dandruff allergens. J Allergy Clin Immunol 82:196–204
6. Uhlin T, Reuterby J, Einarsson R (1984) Antigenic/allergenic composition of poodle/Alsatian dandruff extract. Allergy 39:125–133
7. Steringer I, Aukrust L, Einarsson R (1987) Variability of antigenicity/allergenicity in different strains of *Alternaria alternata*. Int Arch Allergy Appl Immunol 84:190–197
8. Wallenbeck I, Aukrust L, Einarsson R (1984) Antigenic variability of different strains of *Aspergillus fumigatus*. Int Arch Allergy Appl Immunol 73:166–172

9. Lemanske RF, Taylor SL (1987) Standardized extracts, foods. Clin Rev Allergy 5:23–36
10. Dreborg S, Foucard T (1983) Allergy to apple, carrot and potato in children with birch pollen allergy. Allergy 38:167–172
11. Verstege A, Mehl A, Rolinck-Werninghaus C et al (2005) The predictive value of the skin prick test weal size for the outcome of oral food challenges. Clin Exp Allergy 35:1220–1226
12. Davies DR, Padlan EA, Sheriff S (1990) Antibody–antigen complexes. Annu Rev Biochem 59:439–473
13. Løwenstein H, Marsh DG (1981) Antigens of *Ambrosia elatior* (short ragweed) pollen. I. Crossed immunoelectrophoretic analyses. J Immunol 126:943–948
14. Marsh DG (1987) Differential rates of allergen release: an important consideration in the preparation of allergenic extracts. Arb Paul Ehrlich Inst 80:47–57
15. Løwenstein H (1980) Physico-chemical and immunochemical methods for the control of potency and quality of allergenic extracts. Arb Paul Ehrlich Inst 75:122–132
16. Einarsson R, Dreborg S (1987) Manufacturers' criteria for in-house references. Arb Paul Ehrlich Inst Georg Speyer Haus Ferdinand Blum Inst Frankf A M 80:131–138
17. Løwenstein H (1994) Methods used to develop standards. Arb Paul Ehrlich Inst 87:49–57
18. Dreborg S (1993) Standardization of allergenic preparations by in vitro and in vivo methods. Allergy 48(Suppl 14):63–70
19. Nordic Council on Medicines (1989) Guidelines for registration and standardization of allergenic extracts. NLN Publication No 23, 1–48
20. Dreborg S, Basomba A, Belin L et al (1987) Biological equilibration of allergen preparations: methodological aspects and reproducibility. Clin Allergy 17:537–550
21. Dreborg S, Einarsson R (1992) The major allergen content of allergenic preparations reflect their biological activity. Allergy 47:418–423
22. Helm RM, Gauerke MB, Baer H et al (1984) Production and testing of an international reference standard of short ragweed pollen extract. J Allergy Clin Immunol 73:790–800
23. Gjesing B, Jäger L, Marsh DG, Løwenstein H (1985) The international collaborative study establishing the first international standard for timothy (*Phleum pratense*) grass pollen allergenic extract. J Allergy Clin Immunol 75:258–267
24. Ford A, Seagroatt V, Platts-Mills TAE, Løwenstein H (1985) A collaborative study on the first international standard of *Dermatophagoides pteronyssinus* (house dust mite) extract. J Allergy Clin Immunol 75:676–686
25. Arntzen FC, Wilhelmsen TW, Løwenstein H et al (1989) The international collaborative study on the first international standard of birch (*Betula verrucosa*) pollen extract. J Allergy Clin Immunol 83:66–82
26. Larsen JN, Ford A, Gjesing B et al (1988) The collaborative study of the international standard of dog, *Canis domesticus*, hair/dander extract. J Allergy Clin Immunol 82:318–330
27. Helm RM, Squillace DL, Yunginger JW, Members of the International Collaborative Trial (1988) Production of a proposed international reference standard *Alternaria* extract II. Results of a collaborative trial. J Allergy Clin Immunol 81:651–663
28. Baer H, Anderson MC, Helm RM et al (1986) The preparation and testing of the proposed international reference (IRP) Bermuda grass (*Cynodon dactylon*)-pollen extract. J Allergy Clin Immunol 78:624–631
29. Stewart GA, Turner KJ, Baldo BA et al (1988) Standardization of rye-grass pollen (*Lolium perenne*) extract. An immunochemical and physicochemical assessment of six candidate international reference preparations. Int Arch Allergy Appl Immunol 86:9–18
30. Aas K, Backman A, Belin L, Weeke B (1978) Standardization of allergen extracts with appropriate methods. The combined use of skin prick testing and radio-allergosorbent tests. Allergy 33:130–137
31. Turkeltaub PC (1987) Biological standardization based on quantitative skin testing - the ID_{50} EAL method (intradermal dilution for 50 mm sum of erythema diameters determines the allergy unit). Arb Paul Ehrlich Inst Georg Speyer Haus Ferdinand Blum Inst Frankf A M 80:169–173
32. van Ree R, Chapman MD, Ferreira F et al (2008) The CREATE project: development of certified reference materials for allergenic products and validation of methods for their quantification. Allergy 63:310–326
33. Løwenstein H (1978) Quantitative immunoelectrophoretic methods as a tool for the analysis and isolation of allergens. Prog Allergy 25:1
34. Laemmli UK (1970) Cleavage of structural proteins during the assembly of the head of bacteriophage T4. Nature 227:680–685
35. Kyhse-Andersen J (1984) Electroblotting of multiple gels: a simple apparatus without buffer tank for rapid transfer of proteins from polyacrylamide to nitrocellulose. J Biochem Biophys Methods 10:203–209

36. Brighton WD (1975) Profiles of allergen extract components by isoelectric focussing and radioimmunoassay. Dev Biol Stand 29: 362–369
37. Engvall E, Perlmann P (1972) Enzyme-linked immunosorbent assay, ELISA. III. Quantitation of specific antibodies by enzyme-labelled anti-immunoglobulin in antigen-coated tubes. J Immunol 109:129–135
38. Ceska M, Eriksson R, Varga JM (1972) Radioimmunosorbent assay of allergens. J Allergy Clin Immunol 49:1–9
39. Larsen JN, Houghton CG, Vega ML, Løwenstein H (2014) Manufacturing and standardizing allergen extracts in Europe. In: Lockey RF, Ledford DK (eds) Allergens and allergen immunotherapy, 5th edn. CRC Press, New York, pp 289–305

Chapter 6

Quantifying Human Innate Cytokine and Chemokine Responses Ex Vivo via Pattern Recognition Receptor Stimulation

Natascha Fitch, Stephanie J. Marshall, William P. Stefura, Rishma Chooniedass, Allan B. Becker, and Kent T. HayGlass

Abstract

Linkages between human innate immune capacity, the environment in which we live, and the development of clinical tolerance versus a spectrum of disease phenotypes are a major focus of inflammatory disease research. While extensive epidemiologic evidence indicates key roles for the microbiome and other environmental factors, the underlying mechanisms that explain how these stimuli lead to a given clinical phenotype remain speculative. Here we review strategies for characterizing human cytokine production ex vivo in response to innate immune receptor stimulation with defined ligands. Human cytokine and chemokine biomarker data provides a tool to test hypotheses on the relationship between innate immune capacity in vivo and expression of current or future clinical phenotypes. The most important limitations of experimental strategies that have been used to date are reviewed. Detailed experimental protocols are provided for characterization of pattern recognition receptor (PRR)-driven stimulation with a panel of bacterial (TLR4, TLR5) and viral (TLR3, TLR7/8, RIG-I/MDA5) ligands to assess the role played by human pro-inflammatory, anti-inflammatory, Th1-like, and Th2-like responses. The importance of characterizing human innate immune phenotypes extends beyond discovery-based research to development of improved strategies for prevention or inhibition of chronic inflammatory diseases, improved design of immunization programs, and more effective cancer immunotherapy.

Key words Pattern recognition receptors, Innate immunity, TLR, RLR, Human, Cytokine, Chemokine, Allergy, Autoimmunity, Cardiovascular disease, Immunization

1 Introduction

Research since the mid-1990s has transformed our view of the innate immune response from being a relic of our evolutionary history [1, 2]. Recognition of its role as a pivotal determinant of adaptive immunity and clinical outcomes is now widespread. Much effort is directed toward understanding how we interact with our microbially rich environment, including our microbiome, to yield good health versus disease. Extensive opportunities exist for

Penny Lympany and Meinir G. Jones (eds.), *Allergy: Methods and Protocols*, Methods in Molecular Biology, vol. 2020,
https://doi.org/10.1007/978-1-4939-9591-2_6,

translational research on the role that innate immunity plays in shaping clinical outcomes, with particular attention devoted to innate immunity's role in shaping predisposition toward, or current expression of, chronic inflammatory diseases.

In a diverse population of healthy individuals, why do some develop transient or persistent inflammatory disorders while others remain healthy? While the human genome has a large influence on innate immune phenotype [3], the individual's history of environmental exposure to various innate immune stimuli is pivotal in determining innate immune status. One hypothesis is that there is a causal relationship between an individual's innate immune potential in early life, the particular environmental triggers they encounter (both positive and negative), subsequent development of innate phenotypes (i.e., pro- or anti-inflammatory bias), and clinical outcomes in both the short term and much later in life. While strong epidemiologic evidence supports the importance of interactions between environment, innate immune capacity, time of exposure, and other key variables [4–6], our actual understanding of the mechanisms involved, hence opportunities at which one might intervene, still remains basic, with much to be done [7–9].

The importance of characterizing human innate immune phenotypes extends beyond discovery-based research for prevention of chronic inflammatory diseases, to improved design of immunization programs [10–12] as well as monitoring and improving of cancer immunotherapy [13].

Pattern recognition receptors (PRR) serve as the eyes of the innate immune response. One of the most ancient, conserved, and evolutionarily common elements of the immune system, they sense conserved molecular motifs in pathogenic and nonpathogenic microbes. As well as recognizing conserved microbial signatures, they respond to cellular stress with autophagy, a major area of immune regulation [14]. Major families of PRR include Toll-like receptors (TLR), Nod-like receptors (NLR), RIG-like receptors (RLR), C-type lectin receptors, and cytosolic DNA-sensing receptors, such as RNA polymerase III, DAI, and AIM2. Ubiquitous in innate immune cells, they can also be expressed by adaptive immune cells and structural cells such as epithelial and smooth muscle cells [15, 16]. Pattern and intensity of PRR expression are highly regulated by the environment and activation state of the cell, so broad generalities regarding lineage-specific expression are of limited use.

PRR-selective agonists have been isolated or created for most PRR and are readily available commercially. This provides the opportunity to determine innate immune status in individuals of different clinical phenotypes, or of populations of healthy neonates who will subsequently go on to exhibit health or disease as they age. Despite the recognition that there exist some 40–50 different pattern recognition receptors, and the broad availability of experimental ligands for most, the majority of studies which have sought linkages between differential human innate immune capacity, immune outcomes, and clinical outcomes have focused (exclusively) on TLR4. Studies examining putative differences in other bacterial (TLR5, NOD) or viral (TLR3, TLR7/8, RLR) receptors and their function make up much less than 10% of total PubMed citations in this area. Thus, ~17,000 research publications exist for TLR4, with only ~900 for TLR8 and ~500 for RLR in 2018. There is no a priori reason why TLR4 should be "the" determining, or even one of the more important, PRRs in determining human health outcomes. We speculate that this narrow focus on a single PRR has been a major hindrance to progress to date.

Here we provide specific recommendations on (a) identification and clinical phenotyping of study participants, (b) optimal blood sample handling, (c) isolation of PBMC and monocyte subpopulations, (d) optimization of primary culture conditions to assess innate immunity, (e) strategies for utilization of PRR ligands, and (f) a summary of useful cytokine/chemokine/biomarker readouts for different PRRs along with typical ranges of responses seen in sample healthy populations. The methods presented are equally applicable to analyses of the healthy phenotype or healthy aging [17–19] and a broad variety of human chronic immune inflammatory disorders (allergic, autoimmune, cardiovascular diseases, IBD, etc.) where differential innate immune capacity is hypothesized to underlie the ultimate development of clinical status.

2 Materials

2.1 Who to Recruit?

Full protocols on clinical characterization are beyond the scope of this chapter, but we strongly emphasize the need for careful planning (carefully developed inclusion/exclusion criteria, feasibility, logistics) and clinical characterization of the human population to be examined before beginning recruitment and laboratory work. This is for several reasons. Well-characterized, apparently homogeneous, healthy human populations exhibit much greater variability in immune responses than do inbred animal models (Fig. 1). Thus in a typical experiment with inbred mice, individuals in the same experimental group usually differ by less than twofold. A human population, being much more genetically, immunologically, and environmentally diverse, usually exhibits a five- to tenfold range of cytokine responses. This underlines the need for sufficient power through recruitment of appropriate population sizes to have the power to draw useful, reproducible conclusions. Many human immunology studies are underpowered.

Secondly, it is well established that individuals with a given clinical phenotype (i.e., "allergic asthma" or "healthy/asymptomatic controls") arrived at that status via different mechanistic pathways [20, 21]. Many studies have been marred by inclusion of

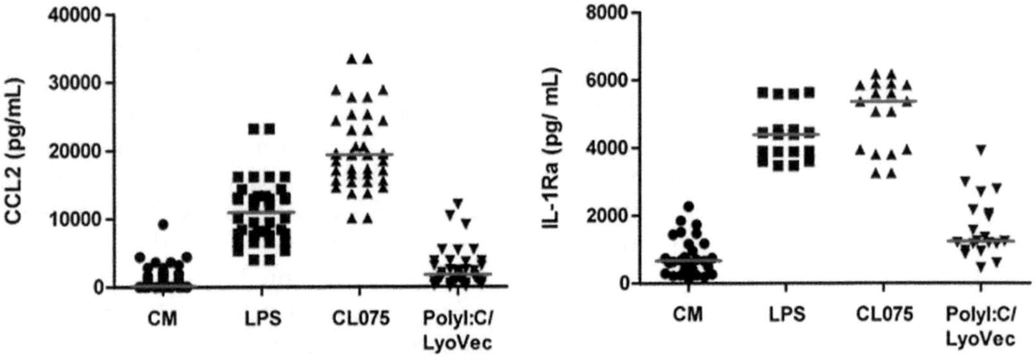

Fig. 1 Breadth of cytokine responses characteristic of a clinically homogeneous, asymptomatic human population upon PRR stimulation. Primary PBMC were stimulated for 24 h in culture medium (black circles), LPS for TLR4 (black squares), CL075 for TLR7/8 (black triangles), or polyI:C/lyovec for RLR activation (black inverted triangles). Cytokine levels for a representative pro-inflammatory and anti-inflammatory cytokine were determined by ELISA (CCL2) or Meso Scale (IL-1Ra). Each symbol represents an independent experiment performed with a unique donor (n = 20–40)

dissimilar individuals within a nominally homogeneous population, which is then subjected to detailed molecular analysis. For all of these reasons, careful discussion between senior investigators to define and integrate clinical and basic science needs is absolutely essential as a first step.

Thirdly, most immune responses within individuals are stable over weeks (data not shown and [22]). Variations due to circadian rhythm are dwarfed by inter-individual differences. In practice, this means that it is not necessary to recruit dozens or hundreds of individuals at the same time of day over the duration of a study, an almost impossible logistical challenge.

Finally, an important limitation to any human study is the very limited amount of material obtained ex vivo, hence the number of culture conditions that can be examined. Here we focus on examination of representative bacterial (TLR4, TLR5) and viral (TLR3, TLR7/8, RIG-I/MDA5) PRR ligands where we developed and validated protocols for assessing pro-inflammatory, anti-inflammatory, Th1, Th2, Th9, and Th17-like biomarkers of activation.

2.2 Isolation of Peripheral Blood Mononuclear Cells

1. 10 mL Sodium Heparin BD Vacutainer tubes REF#367874.
2. 2.0 mL Microcentrifuge tubes (i.e., Nunc), conical upright with O-ring screw caps.
3. Salines, 0.85%.
4. Polystyrene tubes (15 mL and 50 mL, Falcon BD).
5. 10 mL Serological sterile plastic pipette (Falcon BD).
6. Ficoll-Paque™PLUS (GE-Healthcare Bio Sciences, Uppsala, Sweden).

7. Pasteur Pipet Borosilicate Glass Cotton Plugged Disposable 9″ (VWR, Rador PA).
8. Culture media (RPMI-1640 medium, 10% fetal bovine serum (*see* **Note 1**), 1% 200 mM L-glutamine, Lonza, 1% antibiotic-antimycotic, 55 μM 2-mercaptoethanol, Invitrogen).
9. 50 mL Reagent Reservoir Polystyrene Sterile (Corning Incorporated, Corning NY).
10. RNA*later* (Ambion, Life Technologies).
11. Tissue Culture Microwell 96-U-bottom plates with lid (Nunclon D SI).
12. Thermowell aluminum plate sealing tape (plate sealers) for 96-well plates (Corning).
13. Sterile culture tubes, polystyrene 12 × 75 mm (Simport).
14. Human CD14 Selection Kit (Stemcell Technologies, Vancouver, Canada).
15. CD14+ Media (PBS, 2% fetal bovine serum, 1 nM EDTA) (Stemcell Technologies).
16. Flow cytometry buffer (1× PBS, 1% fetal bovine serum).
17. Fluorochrome-conjugated anti-CD14 Ab (Biolegend, San Diego, CA).
18. TC10 System Sample Slide Dual Chamber (BioRad, Hercules, CA).
19. TC10 hardware (*see* **Note 2**) (BioRad).

3 Methods

3.1 Clinical Characterization/Information Tracking

Procedures for data tracking and sharing vary widely between individual research groups. It is important to ensure that a single, consistent nomenclature and SOP are used throughout, thereby preventing confusion regarding individual subjects, assigned experimental grouping (i.e., asymptomatic/healthy, allergic vs. nonallergic asthma), sampling time, in vitro stimuli, etc. These need to be expressly developed, made public within the group, and adhered to.

3.2 Isolation of Fresh Human PBMC

Following study approval by the local REB and having obtained written informed consent from each individual, fresh peripheral blood is taken into EDTA-, citrate-, or heparin-containing tubes (typically 2 mL of 2.5% EDTA for 40–50 mL blood in Falcon 50 mL tubes or using vacutainers) by venipuncture (*see* **Note 3**). While blood processing should take place within 24 h, we have found minimal differences in the innate cytokine/chemokine protein responses examined below when PBMC were isolated and stimulated after 2, 6, or 24 h. By 48 h, sample and data integrity are often severely compromised (data not shown).

1. Whole blood is centrifuged at 500 × *g* for 10 min to separate plasma from blood cells.
2. Whole-blood plasma is stored in 1.5 mL aliquots in Nunc tubes at −20 °C indefinitely.
3. Blood samples are diluted 1:1 with 0.85% saline solution, mixed (to obtain higher cell yields), and layered onto 3.5 mL of Ficoll-Paque™PLUS. This can be sterilely pre-prepared in 15 mL polystyrene tubes stored at 4 °C in the dark for many months (foil wrapped or within a box). Ficoll must be brought to room temperature before use in isolating PBMC (*see* **Note 4**).
4. Samples are centrifuged for 30 min at 600 × *g* for separation of PBMC from red blood cells and granulocytes. Ensure that the "no brake" setting is used or PBMC "buffy coat" layer will be disrupted and difficult to harvest.
5. PBMC are removed using a pasture pipette and resuspended in ~10 mL 0.85% saline.
6. Cells are centrifuged at 250 × *g* for 10 min and all but ~0.3–0.5 mL supernatant is removed and discarded.
7. Repeat wash step using ~10 mL saline.
8. Isolated PBMC are resuspended in 2 mL culture media (if processing a starting volume of ~20–30 mL blood).
9. Cells are counted via hemocytometer or, for high-volume laboratories, using BioRad TC10 automated cell counter to determine cell concentration. Ensure that cell counts are within the most linear part of the reproducible range of the instrument used for counting, optimally 1–30 million PBMC/mL for reproducibility.

Typically, ~1–2 million PBMC/mL of original blood volume are obtained following Ficoll fractionation when working with adult donors. Pediatric samples (aged 1–5) typically yield 2–3 times this number of cells per mL of blood.

3.3 Monocyte Isolation

If primary monocytes are sought, the Stemcell CD14 Selection Kit provides a simple and efficient method for separation (positive selection described below) of CD14+ monocytes from PBMC.

1. Complete previous PBMC isolation **steps 1–7**. However, at **step 8** resuspend PBMC in 200–500 μL of CD14+ media.
2. Transfer cells to 5 mL polystyrene tube.
3. Add EasySep-positive selection cocktail at 100 μL/mL of PBMC cells. Mix well and allow cells to sit undisturbed at room temperature for 15 min.

4. Mix EasySep magnetic nanoparticles in reagent vial to ensure that suspension is homogenous. Add 50 μL/mL to PBMC, mix, and allow cells to sit at room temperature for 10 min.
5. Bring cell volume to 2.5 mL using the room-temperature CD14+ media. Mix by swirling gently.
6. Place the 5 mL tube containing 2.5 mL total volume (no cap) into the magnet and allow it to sit for 5 min at room temperature.
7. Invert tube (still in magnet) in one motion, pouring off the supernatant in one continuous motion. This step removes CD14− cells. Keep tube inverted for 2 or 3 s, but ensure that you do not remove or blot off any drops.
8. Remove the 5 mL tube from magnet and resuspend enriched CD14+ cells in 2.5 mL of CD14+ media. Mix the cell suspension and return to magnet. Set aside for 5 min.
9. Repeat **steps** 7 and **8** and then **step** 7 once more so that cells have had three cycles of enrichment.
10. Resuspend enriched CD14+ monocytes in 0.5 mL of culture media.

Determine cell concentration using hemocytometer or TC10 automated cell counter. Yield should be ~5–10% of total PBMC initially used, or 3–4 million CD14+ cells from 40 million starting PBMC. Cell death from this process is 0–10% maximum. Process (*see* Method below) yields >90% CD14+ in the enriched population, with CD14-depleted populations containing <1% CD14+ cells.

3.4 Flow Cytometry Assessment of Enrichment Efficacy

1. Prior to use of EasySep cocktail, set aside two aliquots of PBMC cells in 5 mL polystyrene tubes (~10^4 and ~3×10^4) to be used for unstained and CD14+-stained PBMC controls.
2. Complete monocyte isolation protocol **steps 2–9**.
3. Resuspend enriched monocyte population in 0.5 mL flow cytometry buffer (PBS/1% FBS).
4. Count monocyte cells using hemocytometer or TC10 counter and determine yield.
5. Aliquot ~3×10^4 cells CD14+ cells in 5 mL polystyrene tube.
6. Bring all cell aliquots up to ~300 μL for staining using flow cytometry buffer.
7. Add 5 μL of fluorochrome-conjugated anti-CD14 Ab to (a) PBMC control (to assess the percentage of CD14+ cells in the starting PBMC population of that individual) and (b) enriched monocyte population (purity should be >90% by flow cytometry) and, if using CD14-depleted population for culture, (c) the frequency of contaminating CD14+ cells should be determined in this group also.
8. Place the cell aliquots on ice for 30 min and analyze by flow cytometry, without washing.

3.5 Preparation of Innate Stimuli Prior to Primary Cell Culture

For logistical efficacy and to minimize variation between experiments, most stimuli are added to culture plates prior to PBMC isolation and stored frozen, sealed with aluminum plate sealers. These are thawed and used when needed. This allows maximal efficiency and consistency when large numbers of patient samples are to be used, and decreases effects due to repeated freezing and thawing of PRR ligand stocks. Storing ligand stocks at 4x the desired final concentration ensures that all plates contain the same lot of ligand, and allows for easy calculation of cell concentrations when using a final well volume of 200 μL.

Importantly, while we find the ligands above are stable to freeze/thawing at least four times, the stimulatory activity of polyI:C/LyoVec is dramatically affected by each freeze-thaw cycle, losing 30–50% activity with each cycle. 5′ppp-dsRNA is also not stable upon freeze-thaw. Thus, for RLR assessment, these lyophilized reagents need to be reconstituted and stored at 4 °C beginning on the first day of usage. Minimal loss of activity is evident in reconstituted material until ~14 days. After this point the stimulus loses bioactivity rapidly, so is unreliable. Note that freeze-thawing reconstituted polyI:C lyovec also results in a substantial loss of bioactivity.

3.6 Primary Cell Culture

1. Isolated PBMC or monocytes are plated at 350,000 and 150,000 cells per well, respectively, in 96-well U-bottom plates in triplicate (*see* **Note 5**). This cell number provides readily quantified, reproducible responses to all of the PRR ligands examined here while maximizing the number of experimental conditions that can be examined from a given volume of blood.
2. Incubate cultures at 37 °C in a 5% CO_2 environment for 24 h. While 20–30 h are all appropriate for strong protein and mRNA responses, the time selected for harvest should be kept within 1 h for all subjects in a study.
3. 180 μL/well cell-free supernatants from cultured cells are then collected and stored at −20 °C in sealed plates used for later cytokine and chemokine analyses (*see* **Note 6**).
4. Cell pellets are stored in 100 μL RNA*later* (in preference to Trizol) for subsequent total RNA extraction and QPCR analysis of mRNA expression.

3.7 General Comments to Enhance Effectiveness

The need for optimization of culture conditions prior to embarking on extensive studies must be reiterated. The major variables that need to be experimentally determined are the optimal number of fresh cells required per well, optimal antigen/PRR ligand concentrations for stimulation, the period of culture, and the anticipated intensity of the response for the readouts to be examined. In practice, we find that 350,000 PBMC/well, using a 96-well plate, is sufficient for most PRR ligands (Table 1).

Table 1
PRR ligand concentrations and cytokine biomarker expression by human PBMC

Pattern recognition receptor	Stimulus	Concentration	Effective Th1 or Th2-immunity readouts	Validated pro-inflammatory readouts	Validated anti-inflammatory readouts
TLR4	LPS (*E. coli* 0111:B4)	0.4–4 ng/mL	CXCL10; CCL22, CCL17	CCL2, CXCL8, TNFα, IL-1β, IL-6	IL-10, sTNF-RI, sTNF-RII IL-1Ra
TLR5	Flagellin	5 μg/mL	ND	CCL2, CXCL8, TNFα, IL-1β	IL-10
TLR3	PolyI:C	25 μg/mL	IFNγ	Type I IFNs, CCL2 CXCL8	IL-1Ra
TLR7/8	CL075 (3 M002)	2 μg/mL	CXCL10; CCL22	Type I IFN, CCL2, CXCL8, CCL8, CXCL10	IL-10 sTNF-RI, sTNF-RII IL-1Ra
RLR (MDA5 and RIG-I)	PolyI:C/ lyovec 5′ppp-dsRNA	100–250 ng/ mL	ND	Type I IFN, CCL8, CXCL10	IL-1Ra, EBI3 (IL-27/35) IL-1Ra

PRR ligand concentrations that consistently result in substantive protein responses following short-term primary culture of PBMC or enriched monocytes, directly ex vivo ($n > 500$ humans of different ages). Suggested readouts are provided for pro/anti-inflammatory or Th1/Th2-like biomarkers. Most are readily quantified at both mRNA (QPCR) and protein (ELISA or Meso Scale) levels in both healthy and allergic populations. Which biomarkers are optimal for any given research study is determined by the question addressed
ND not determined

The optimal antigen/ligand concentration needs to be determined empirically for each PRR ligand. Concentrations recommended by commercial vendors are typically 10–1000-fold higher than is needed (and are most commonly based on stimulation of one type of cell line) in order to obtain a "strong" response. Thus, while LPS is often used in culture at 100 ng–1 ug/mL, strong responses are consistently at 0.1–0.4 ng/mL for human PBMC. These much lower concentrations may reflect human physiology more accurately, whereas the extent to which stimulation with massively supraoptimal concentrations reflect typical human biology is questionable.

Spontaneous production of cytokine in antigen-unstimulated cultures needs to be considered. For most cytokines, culture in medium alone yields very low, essentially irrelevant levels of background. Some cytokines (i.e., CCL2, CXCL8, CCL5, and IL-1Ra) are routinely detectable at low but significant levels in negative controls at 24 h, so should be quantified for some or all samples.

3.8 Analysis of Cytokine and Chemokine Production

Selecting which biomarkers of activation to utilize for different PRR is a key step in experimental design. While there is some overlap, different PRR elicit different patterns of cytokine and chemokine production. This is further complicated by the fact that the same PRR ligand can elicit different responses in different cell types (i.e., TLR5 eliciting TSLP in keratinocytes and not PBMC, polyI:C eliciting TSLP in epithelial cells and not PBMC). Detailed reviews of the nature and function of different immunomodulatory molecules are useful in experimental design [23]. Detailed methods for quantifying the levels of cytokine and chemokine production elicited by PRR activation are beyond the scope of this chapter. Readers are referred to other chapters in this volume.

3.9 Statistical Analysis

Many researchers are not experts in statistics and, as such, may apply a single tool (Student's t-test) to analyze all of their data. This practice is often mathematically inappropriate and results in loss of sensitivity (Fig. 2). Particularly for humans, where normal (Poisson) distributions are uncommon, using Student's t-tests (and the implicit assumptions about the data that accompany this decision) provides incorrect p-values if applied to non-normally distributed data. A detailed discussion of statistics is beyond the scope of this publication, but the following flowchart provides essential assistance to obtain correct analysis of data sets. If in any doubt, a biostatistician should be consulted before analyzing and presenting your data.

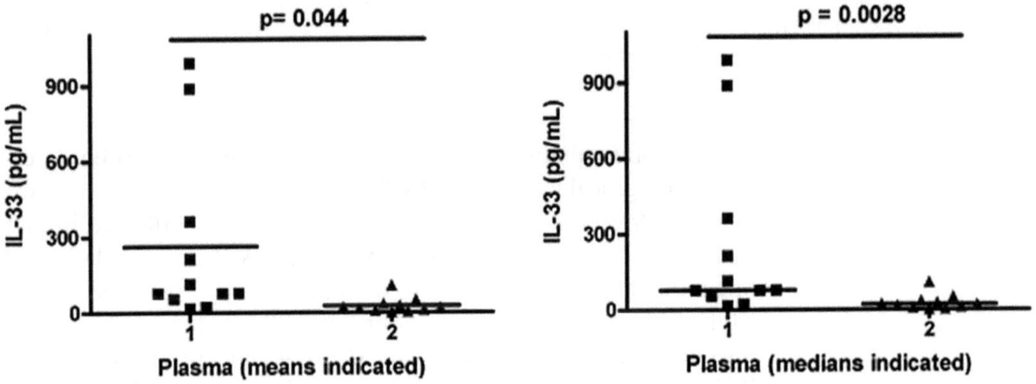

Fig. 2 Why it is essential to determine if a normal (Gaussian or Poisson) distribution exists before conducting statistical analyses. One data set was analyzed using different statistical tests to determine the statistical significance of differences between groups 1 and 2. In panel A, mean values are 263 vs. 28 pg/mL, yielding borderline significance with Student's t-test. In panel B, median values *of the same data set* are 78 vs. 21 pg/mL, yielding a Mann–Whitney of $p = 0.0028$. Conclusion: It is essential to determine if data sets under analysis exhibit a normal distribution before undertaking statistical analysis. The effects of improper analysis can be even more pronounced with incorrect paired analyses (i.e., examining cytokine production in individuals pre/posttreatment). In cases where both data sets are normally distributed, p-values obtained with parametric (i.e., Student's t-test) and nonparametric tests (i.e., Mann–Whitney) are usually very similar

1. *Are the data sets normally distributed?* Many programs (i.e., Graph Pad Prism) incorporate an automated test to provide a yes/no answer to the normality of data sets. The D'Agostino and Pearson normality test should be applied to determine whether each set examined is normally distributed.
2. *If yes, and ALL data sets being compared exhibit a normal distribution:* When comparing different populations (i.e., men to women, asthmatics to non-asthmatics) Student's t-test, or ANOVA if multiple comparisons are made, is appropriate. If comparing different treatments *within* a population (i.e., cells from the same individuals stimulated with two different stimuli) then paired samples should be compared using paired t-tests.
3. *If no, some or all data sets being compared are not normally distributed:* It is extremely common that some or all sets of immunological data from outbred, highly diverse human populations (unlike inbred models) are not normally distributed. For such nonparametric data sets, one must utilize nonparametric tests or, alternatively, log transform the data and utilize parametric tests. Both approaches are equally acceptable. Among nonparametric tests, Mann-Whitney is appropriate for different populations (i.e., cross-sectional analyses) of unpaired data. For paired data (i.e., medium vs. stimulated cells from the same individuals, or longitudinal analyses of the same individuals' responses at different times), the test of choice is a two-tailed Wilcoxon matched pairs test.
4. *Does the **frequency** of responsive individuals provide additional information relative to that obtained from the intensity of responses?* For strong stimuli, or readily detected readouts where the great majority of the population provides a response, frequency assessments add no value. However, where only a subset of individuals generate a detectable response, Fisher's exact test provides useful quantitative comparison on the frequency of individuals capable of responding in different populations (i.e., [24]).

4 Notes

1. Some investigators prefer to use commercial human AB serum in preference to fetal bovine serum (FBS). This is a matter of personal preference. We recommend the latter for several reasons: (a) FBS elicits extremely low-background cytokine or proliferative responses which can confound; (b) vitamin D, a well-established modulator of innate immunity, is found at highly variable levels in human serum, adding an additional confounder; and (c) many of the cytokines/chemokines being

examined in culture are also routinely present in human AB serum. The diverse impacts that these have on human responses under resting or PRR-stimulated conditions are difficult to control for. Bovine cytokines are not active on human cells. Whichever source of serum is used, careful prescreening should be performed first and sufficient material bought for an entire study. In our hands, serum-free or other defined media provide inferior nutrition and poorer responses in culture.

2. We make use of either the TC10 automated cell counter or the hemocytometers to determine cell concentration of PBMC samples. Both work effectively.
3. Much discussion concerns the optimal anticoagulant to use, with concerns about the potential impact of using a biological agent (heparin) versus calcium chelators (i.e., EDTA). In practice all can provide a useful strategy, but we recommend that a lab or consortium commits to a single anticoagulant for the duration of a study.
4. Fresh blood must be layered carefully so as not to disturb the Ficoll-blood interface. It should be centrifuged within 5–10 min after layering. An important tip for layering Ficoll is to wet the sides of the 15 mL tube by gently rolling the tube; this will help the blood trickle down the sides of the tube to the interface.
5. Various cell concentrations can be used. Our practice is to use 350,000 PBMC/well (of which 3–10% are CD14+ monocytes, depending on the donor) to balance cell availability with the desire to examine multiple PRR ligands. 150,000 isolated CD14+ cells are sufficient to provide robust, reproducible responses.
6. Use of aluminum plate sealers is essential as they eliminate sublimation. Sublimation increases the apparent concentration of proteins per volume of supernatant and therefore dramatically alters conclusions from experiments.

Acknowledgments

We thank the many researchers and volunteers who have participated as well as Caroline Graham for editorial assistance. This work was funded by CIHR (Canadian Institute for Health Research) operating grants, the Canada Research Chairs program, and AllerGen NCE.

References

1. Lemaitre B, Nicolas E, Michaut L et al (1996) The dorsoventral regulatory gene cassette spatzle/toll/cactus controls the potent antifungal response in Drosophila adults. Cell 86(6):973–983
2. Medzhitov R, Preston-Hurlburt P, Janeway CA Jr (1997) A human homologue of the Drosophila Toll protein signals activation of adaptive immunity. Nature 388(6640):394–397
3. Patin E, Hasan M, Bergstedt J et al (2018) Natural variation in the parameters of innate immune cells is preferentially driven by genetic factors. Nat Immunol 19(3):302–314. https://doi.org/10.1038/s41590-018-0049-7
4. Blander JM, Longman RS, Iliev ID et al (2017) Regulation of inflammation by microbiota interactions with the host. Nat Immunol 18(8):851–860
5. Martinez FD (2014) The human microbiome. Early life determinant of health outcomes. Ann Am Thorac Soc 11(Suppl 1):S7–S12
6. Azad MB, Konya T, Maughan H et al (2013) Infant gut microbiota and the hygiene hypothesis of allergic disease: impact of household pets and siblings on microbiota composition and diversity. Allergy Asthma Clin Immunol 9(1):15
7. Prince BT, Mandel MJ, Nadeau K et al (2015) Gut microbiome and the development of food allergy and allergic disease. Pediatr Clin N Am 62(6):1479–1492
8. Proal AD, Albert PJ, Marshall TG (2013) The human microbiome and autoimmunity. Curr Opin Rheumatol 25(2):234–240
9. Proal AD, Albert PJ, Marshall TG (2014) Inflammatory disease and the human microbiome. Discov Med 17(95):257–265
10. Kuroda E, Coban C, Ishii KJ (2013) Particulate adjuvant and innate immunity: past achievements, present findings, and future prospects. Int Rev Immunol 32(2):209–220
11. Boraschi D, Castellano LRC, Italiani P (2017) Editorial: interaction of nanomaterials with the immune system: role in nanosafety and nanomedicine. Front Immunol 8:1688
12. Schultze JL, Aschenbrenner AC (2019) Systems immunology allows a new view on human dendritic cells. Semin Cell Dev Biol 86:15–23. https://doi.org/10.1016/j.semcdb.2018.02.017
13. Goldberg JL, Sondel PM (2015) Enhancing cancer immunotherapy via activation of innate immunity. Semin Oncol 42(4):562–572
14. Dolasia K, Bisht MK, Pradhan G et al (2018) TLRs/NLRs: shaping the landscape of host immunity. Int Rev Immunol 37(1): 3–19
15. Lei-Leston AC, Murphy AG, Maloy KJ (2017) Epithelial cell inflammasomes in intestinal immunity and inflammation. Front Immunol 8:1168
16. Hirota JA, Knight DA (2012) Human airway epithelial cell innate immunity: relevance to asthma. Curr Opin Immunol 24(6):740–746
17. Castelo-Branco C, Soveral I (2014) The immune system and aging: a review. Gynecol Endocrinol 30(1):16–22
18. Gubbels Bupp MR (2015) Sex, the aging immune system, and chronic disease. Cell Immunol 294(2):102–110
19. Kollmann TR, Levy O, Montgomery RR et al (2012) Innate immune function by toll-like receptors: distinct responses in newborns and the elderly. Immunity 37(5):771–783
20. Wenzel SE (2012) Asthma phenotypes: the evolution from clinical to molecular approaches. Nat Med 18(5):716–725
21. Holgate ST (2013) Immune circuits in asthma. Curr Opin Pharmacol 13(3):345–350
22. Campbell JD, Stinson MJ, Simons FE et al (2001) In vivo stability of human chemokine and chemokine receptor expression. Hum Immunol 62(7):668–678
23. Akdis M, Burgler S, Crameri R et al (2011) Interleukins, from 1 to 37, and interferon-gamma: receptors, functions, and roles in diseases. J Allergy Clin Immunol 127(3):701–721 e1-70
24. Thottingal TB, Stefura BP, Simons FE et al (2006) Human subjects without peanut allergy demonstrate T cell-dependent, TH2-biased, peanut-specific cytokine and chemokine responses independent of TH1 expression. J Allergy Clin Immunol 118(4):905–914

Chapter 7

Improved Methods for Quantifying Human Chemokine and Cytokine Biomarker Responses: Ultrasensitive ELISA and Meso Scale Electrochemiluminescence Assays

William P. Stefura, Caroline Graham, Larisa Lotoski, and Kent T. HayGlass

Abstract

ELISAs and similar immunoassays are a backbone of biomedical research and clinical practice. Here we review the major factors to consider in the development and application of ultrasensitive ELISAs for analysis of human immune responses in plasma, serum, urine, or tissue culture supernatants. We focus on cytokine and chemokine biomarkers of health and chronic inflammatory diseases including allergy, asthma, autoimmunity, and cardiovascular disease. Detailed protocols for ELISA and Meso Scale Discovery assays (an improved variant of ELISA) are provided for 15 cytokines and 11 chemokines that play immune-regulatory roles in human innate and adaptive immunity. Protocols have been individually optimized to yield ultrasensitive limits of detection and quantification. Major factors enhancing immunoassay sensitivity, precision, and reproducibility, as well as key pitfalls in assay design and execution, are critically reviewed.

Key words Cytokine, ELISA, Meso Scale discovery (MSD), Primary culture, Antigen-specific, Pattern recognition receptor, Innate, Adaptive, Human, Asthma, Allergy

1 Introduction

As of 2019, some 750,000 peer-reviewed publications for "cytokine or chemokine" are identified on PubMed. 100,000 are cited in a search of "cytokine or chemokine AND biomarker." Clearly, this is a major strategy throughout biomedical research and clinical practice to provide insight into the balance between health and disease at the level of the individual. Biomarkers have characteristics that can be objectively quantified as a validated indicator of normal biological processes, pathogenic processes, or pharmacological responses to therapeutic intervention. Neither diagnostic nor predictive biomarkers need to be causally related to underlying disease mechanisms as long as they provide trustworthy linkage to outcomes (current or future clinical status), or, for instance, allow the prediction of subgroups of individuals likely to be responsive to particular therapies. Biomarkers should have utility across most, or

Penny Lympany and Meinir G. Jones (eds.), *Allergy: Methods and Protocols*, Methods in Molecular Biology, vol. 2020, https://doi.org/10.1007/978-1-4939-9591-2_7,

all, of the population—not only in individuals at the extremes of clinical phenotype [1–3]. With greatly improved tools available for quantifying immunomodulatory molecules such as cytokines and chemokines, this strategy is widely used in many disciplines [4–11]. Similarly, among researchers focused on elucidating underlying disease mechanisms rather than biomarker discovery and validation, quantifying immunoregulatory cytokine and chemokine protein responses can explain differences in immune activation that may lead to pathogenesis (or maintenance or resolution) of chronic inflammatory diseases in humans.

While many tools are available for assessing cytokine and chemokine production, the most commonly used is ELISA. Some 60 years ago the radioimmunoassay (RIA) was invented. Its creation led to a Nobel Prize in 1977. Yalow and Roslyn [12] refused to patent the assay, which evolved to a modern ELISA, in order to better facilitate widespread uptake by researchers. It remains one of the most reliable and widely used techniques in biomedical research and practice.

In this chapter, we provide practical steps to integrate ELISA strategies into research programs focused on human biology. We review the main factors in development and application of ultrasensitive ELISAs used for analysis of human cytokine and chemokine responses. We specify conditions and provide detailed protocols that have been optimized to quantify some 26 cytokines and chemokines that are of demonstrated relevance to human immune regulation, and that exhibit potential as biomarkers of health and disease.

1.1 Meso Scale Discovery Assays Versus ELISA

For laboratories seeking high throughput for larger studies (i.e., birth cohorts), a variety of industrial scale, yet affordable, options exist. We have substantial experience with Meso Scale Discovery (MSD) assays (www.mesoscale.com). This technology is similar to ELISA, but is based on electrochemiluminescence detection, rather than light absorption. MSD offers several advantages over conventional ELISA. These include (a) a very large range of linearity (typically 4–6 orders of magnitude vs. two for most ELISA titrations), thereby circumventing a need to conduct series of dilutions for each sample analyzed; (b) smaller sample volumes, conserving difficult-to-obtain clinically derived material; (c) improved multiplexing capacity, circumventing challenges that occur with many bead-based flow cytometry analyses; (d) decreased intra-assay variation within data sets compared to even high-proficiency ELISA operators; (e) decreased inter-assay variation within data sets; and (f) increased speed and higher sample handling capacity.

To balance this, the main challenges we have observed to date are as follows: (a) initial start-up costs for equipment are not trivial, as they are for ELISA, and (b) costs per sample are high if carrying out assays of only a few samples at a time (i.e., <10 samples).

Collectively, for university-scale research laboratories or groups seeking analyses of medium to large numbers of tissue culture, urine, or plasma/serum samples (>50 samples at a time), this offers a marked improvement over conducting batches of 20+ ELISA plates at a time.

1.2 Key Factors Affecting Assay Sensitivity and Reproducibility

Standards: The same standard (supplier and lot) needs to be used throughout a study, as lot-to-lot, or supplier-to-supplier, variation is often substantial. 100 pg/mL from supplier A is rarely the same as 100 pg/mL from supplier B. Comparison between, for instance, two IL-4 preparations from different sources can easily be 100-fold different in terms of specific activity.

Stimuli: The availability of ultrasensitive assays is a double-edged sword. Ultrasensitivity allows use of physiologically relevant ligands (i.e., antigens, peptides) for analysis of Ag-specific responses rather than pharmacologic reagents (PMA/calcium ionophore, anti-CD3/28) that yield intense cytokine production by virtually all cells. Since the frequency of T cells specific for any single Ag represents only a tiny fraction (usually <1%) of total T cells, specific stimulation is clearly better to characterize such responses. Different cell signaling pathways (and very different conclusions [13]) are also elicited by antigen compared to pattern recognition receptor selective ligands or pharmacologic stimulation. Similarly, in the analyses of urine or plasma/serum, ultrasensitive assays offer the sensitivity needed to identify and reliably quantify such low-concentration analytes. Detection limits of <1 pg/mL versus the 10–30 pg/mL characteristic of many fast, but relatively insensitive commercial ELISAs can make the difference between original discoveries and a failed project where many samples yield "undetectable" or unreliable values.

Pipetting accuracy: Pipetting is so simple and universal that it becomes a major source of error. Any ultrasensitive technique is highly sensitive to systematic error. Because measuring small volumes by micropipetor is so routine, it is not always carried out with precision. To reinforce the need for accuracy and to provide a quantifiable indicator of an individual's level of precision, we routinely have all new trainees/staff quantify pipetting skill when first entering the laboratory. CVs need to be well under 10%. While conventional ELISAs deliver high-quality results with conventional pipetting techniques, for MSD assays, a higher level of precision is required due to the higher sensitivity and low sample volumes used. The manufacturer recommends utilization of reverse pipetting. We have found that it does substantially reduce inter-assay variance (*see* **Note 1**).

Reagent usage: The assays described below are configured using the minimum amount to minimize cost. Use of higher concentrations of capture and development reagents can increase sensitivity by one- or twofold. Similarly, there is a linear relationship between how long an ELISA develops and the sensitivity of that assay. Cytokines, such as IL-5, IL-9, or IL-13, are produced at relatively high levels (typically 10–1000 pg/mL) after in vitro stimulation of PBMC with recall Ags. These ELISAs can be read at 1 h. For cytokines produced at low levels (i.e., IL-4), assays are allowed to develop up to 9 h. In all cases, the greater the difference between the absorbance of the maximum concentration of the standard and the background (all reagents except the analyte), the better the precision of the assay.

Sample storage: We do not find differences in samples kept at −20 °C or −80 °C for 2 years. A more important concern is sublimation, which dramatically alters cytokine concentrations in the remaining supernatant. This is prevented by ensuring that plates used to store supernatants do not have large numbers of empty wells (using sterile distilled water), using plate sealers, and prompt analysis.

2 Materials

2.1 ELISA Buffers (See Note 2)

1. Coating buffer: 1.59 g Na_2CO_3, 2.93 g $NaHCO_3$ made up to 1 L with double-distilled water. Add NaN_3 to 0.02% and adjust pH to 9.6.
2. Blocking buffer: PBS containing 0.17% BSA, 0.02% NaN_3. Adjust pH to 7.4.
3. Wash buffer: PBS containing 0.05% Tween-20. Adjust pH to 7.4.
4. Dilution buffer: PBS containing 0.085% BSA, 0.05% Tween-20, 0.02% NaN_3. Adjust pH to 7.4.
5. Substrate buffer: 122 mg $MgCl_2{\cdot}6H_2O$, 117 mL diethanolamine. No NaN_3. $MgCl_2$ is dissolved in 800 mL double-distilled water prior to addition of diethanolamine. Diethanolamine may require warming at 37 °C to liquefy. Adjust final pH to 9.8 and volume to 1 L. Keep this buffer in a dark bottle at 4 °C, as it is light sensitive. We utilize one *p*-nitrophenyl phosphate (PNPP) tablet (Sigma #S0942-200TAB) per 5 mL buffer.

2.2 ELISA Immunological Reagents

ELISA antibodies and reagents listed below are available from multiple sources including BD Biosciences (http://www.bdbiosciences.com), Biolegend (http://www.biolegend.com), eBioscience (http://www.ebioscience.com), R&D Systems (http://www.rndsystems.com), PeproTech (http://www.peprotech.com), and Serotec (http://www.serotec.co.uk). Prices vary considerably for very similar products. In several instances, the clones producing the Abs are available from the ATCC (http://www.atcc.org), providing a more cost-effective approach for labs which will make frequent use of particular assays. We have listed combinations of clones and conditions which we find provide highly sensitive assays. While many excellent ELISA plates are available, we have consistent success (high protein binding, low backgrounds, amenable to 50 μL sample and reagent volumes, and excellent reproducibility) with Costar 96-well EIA/RIA polystyrene plates (Corning Inc. #3369).

2.2.1 Measurement of Human IFNγ Levels

1. Capture: Mouse anti-human IFNγ (Biolegend clone MD-1).
2. Standard: Human rIFNγ, catalog number Gxg01–902-535. Available from NCI at 80,000 IU/ampoule. Commercial standards are also readily available.
3. Detection: Biotinylated mouse anti-human IFNγ (Biolegend clone 4S.B3).

2.2.2 Measurement of Human IL-1β Levels

1. Capture: Mouse anti-human IL-1β (Antibody Solutions).
2. Standard: Human rIL-1β (PeproTech #200-01B). Detection: Biotinylated mouse anti-human IL-1β (Antibody Solutions).

2.2.3 Measurement of Human IL-1 Receptor Accessory Protein (IL-1RAcP)

1. Capture: Goat anti-human affinity-purified polyclonal IL-1RAcP/IL-1R3 (R&D Systems).
2. Standard: Human rIL-1RAcP/IL-1R3/FcChimera (R&D Systems).
3. Detection: Biotinylated goat anti-human affinity-purified polyclonal IL-RAcP/IL-1R3 (R&D Systems).

2.2.4 Measurement of Human IL-2 Levels

1. Capture: Rat anti-human IL-2 (BD Biosciences clone MQ1-17H12).
2. Standard: IL-2, human, Jurkat-derived 86/504 at 100 IU/ampoule available from NCI or NIBSC or human rIL-2, ISRO 851 at 1000 IU/ampoule.
3. Detection: Biotinylated mouse anti-human IL-2 (BD Biosciences clone B33–2).

2.2.5 Measurement of Human IL-4 Levels

1. Capture: Mouse anti-human IL-4 (BD Biosciences clone 8D4–8).
2. Standard: Human rIL-4 WHO standard 88/656 available from NCI or NIBSC at 1000 U/ampoule. Commercial standards are also readily available.
3. Detection: Biotinylated rat anti-human IL-4 (BD Biosciences clone MP4-25D2).

2.2.6 Measurement of Human IL-5 Levels

1. Capture antibody: Rat anti-mouse/human IL-5 (Biolegend clones JES1-39D10 or TRFK5).

2. Standard: Human rIL-5 or rIL-5 WHO standard 90/586 from NCI or NIBSC at 5000 U/ampoule. Commercial standards are also readily available.
3. Detection: Biotinylated rat anti-human IL-5 (Biolegend clone JES1-5A10).

2.2.7 Measurement of Human IL-6 Levels

1. Capture: Mouse anti-human IL-6 (Biolegend clone MQ2-13A5).
2. Standard: Human rIL-6 (i.e., PeproTech #200–06 or similar from other suppliers).
3. Detection: Biotinylated mouse anti-human IL-6 (Biolegend clone MQ2-39C3).

2.2.8 Measurement of Human IL-9 Level

sp.lympany@hotmail.couk

1. Capture: Mouse anti-human affinity-purified IL-9 (Biolegend clone MH9A4).
2. Standard: Human rIL-9 (PeproTech).
3. Detection: Biotinylated mouse anti-human affinity-purified IL-9 (Biolegend clone MH9A3).

2.2.9 Measurement of Human IL-10 Levels

1. Capture: Rat anti-human IL-10 (Biolegend clones JES-9D7 or JES3-19F1).
2. Standard: IL-10 WHO Reference Reagent 93/722 available from NIBSC at 5000 U/ampoule or human rIL-10 from commercial source. Commercial standards are also readily available.
3. Detection: Biotinylated rat anti-human IL-10 (Biolegend clone JES3-12G8).

2.2.10 Measurement of Human IL-11 Levels

1. Capture: Mouse anti-human IL-11 (R&D Systems clone 22616.1).
2. Standard: Human rIL-11.
3. Detection: Biotinylated goat anti-human IL-11 polyclonal (R&D Systems).

2.2.11 Measurement of Human IL-13 Levels

1. Capture: Rat anti-human IL-13 (Biolegend or BD Biosciences clone JES10-5A2).
2. Standard: Human rIL-13 (PeproTech#200–13) or human rIL-13 WHO Reference Reagent 94/622 available from NIBSC at 1000 U/ampoule.
3. Detection: Biotinylated mouse anti-human IL-13 (BD Biosciences clone B69–2).

2.2.12 Measurement of Human IL-17A Levels

1. Capture: Goat anti-human IL-17A polyclonal (PeproTech).
2. Standard: Human rIL-17A (PeproTech #200–17).
3. Detection: Biotinylated goat anti-human IL-17A polyclonal (PeproTech).

2.2.13 Measurement of Human IL-33 Levels

1. Capture: Rabbit anti-human IL-33 polyclonal (PeproTech).
2. Standard: Human rIL-33 (PeproTech #200–33).
3. Detection antibody: Biotinylated rabbit anti-human IL-33 polyclonal (PeproTech).

2.2.14 Measurement of Human TGF-β1 (See Note 3)

1. Capture antibody: Rat anti-mouse/human/pig TGF-β1 (BD Biosciences clone A75–2).
2. Standard: Human rTGF-β1 (PeproTech #100-21R) or human rTGF-β1 standard 89/514 at 3000 U/ampoule from NCI or NIBSC.
3. Detection: Biotinylated rat anti-mouse/human TGF-β1 (BD Biosciences clone A75–3).

2.2.15 Measurement of Human TNFα Levels

1. Capture antibody: Mouse anti-human TNFα (Biolegend clone MAb-1 or PeproTech).
2. Standard: Human rTNFα (PeproTech #300-01A).
3. Detection: Biotinylated mouse anti-human TNFα (Biolegend clone MAb11 or PeproTech).

2.2.16 Measurement of Human CCL2 (MCP-1) Levels

1. Capture: Mouse anti-human MCP-1 (BD Biosciences #23231D, clone 10F7.2, or PeproTech polyclonal).
2. Standard: Human rMCP-1 (BD Biosciences or PeproTech).
3. Detection: Biotinylated mouse anti-human MCP-1 polyclonal (BD Biosciences or PeproTech).

2.2.17 Measurement of Human CCL3 (MIP-1α) Levels

1. Capture: Mouse anti-human MIP-1α (R&D Systems #MAB670, clone 14215.41, or PeproTech polyclonal).
2. Standard: Human rMIP-1α (PeproTech #300–08).
3. Detection: Biotinylated goat anti-human MIP-1α (R&D Systems #BAF270 or PeproTech polyclonal).

2.2.18 Measurement of Human CCL5 (RANTES) Levels

1. Capture: Mouse anti-human RANTES (R&D Systems #DY278).
2. Standard: Human rRANTES (R&D Systems #DY278).
3. Detection: Biotinylated goat anti-human RANTES (R&D Systems #DY278).

2.2.19 Measurement of Human CCL8 (MCP-2) Levels

1. Capture: Rabbit anti-human MCP-2 polyclonal (PeproTech #500-P35).
2. Standard: Human rMCP-2 (PeproTech #300–15).
3. Detection: Biotinylated rabbit anti-human MCP-2 polyclonal (PeproTech #500-P35Bt).

2.2.20 Measurement of Human CCL11 (Eotaxin) Levels

1. Capture: Mouse anti-human Eotaxin (R&D Systems #MAB320, clone 43911.11).
2. Standard: Human rEotaxin (PeproTech #300–21).
3. Detection: Biotinylated goat anti-human Eotaxin polyclonal (R&D Systems #BAF320).

2.2.21 Measurement of Human CCL17 (TARC) Levels

1. Capture: Mouse anti-human TARC (R&D Systems #MAB364, clone 54026.11, or PeproTech polyclonal).
2. Standard: Human rTARC (PeproTech #300–30).
3. Detection: Biotinylated goat anti-human TARC polyclonal (R&D Systems #BAF364 or PeproTech).

2.2.22 Measurement of Human CCL22 (MDC) Levels

1. Capture: Mouse anti-human MDC (R&D Systems #MAB336, clone 57226.11, or PeproTech).
2. Standard: Human rMDC (R&D Systems #336-MD).
3. Detection: Biotinylated chicken anti-human MDC polyclonal (R&D Systems #BAF336 or PeproTech).

2.2.23 Measurement of Human CXCL8 (IL-8) Levels

1. Capture: Mouse anti-human IL-8 (Biolegend #514601, clone BH0814, or PeproTech polyclonal).
2. Standard: Human rIL-8 (Biolegend #561001).
3. Detection: Biotinylated mouse anti-human IL-8 (Biolegend #508502, clones JK8–2 or BH0840, or PeproTech polyclonal).

2.2.24 Measurement of Human CXCL9 (MIG) Levels

1. Capture: Mouse anti-human MIG (R&D Systems #MAB392, clone 49106.11, or PeproTech polyclonal).
2. Standard: Human rMIG (PeproTech #300–26).
3. Detection: Biotinylated goat anti-human MIG polyclonal (R&D Systems #BAF392 or PeproTech).

2.2.25 Measurement of Human CXCL10 (IP-10) Levels

1. Capture: Mouse anti-human IP-10 (R&D Systems #MAB266, clone 33036.211, or PeproTech polyclonal).
2. Standard: Human rIP-10 (PeproTech #300–12).
3. Detection: Biotinylated goat anti-human IP-10 polyclonal (R&D Systems #BAF266 or PeproTech).

2.2.26 Measurement of Human CXCL11 (I-TAC) Levels

1. Capture antibody: Rabbit anti-human I-TAC polyclonal (PeproTech #500-P132).
2. Standard: Human rI-TAC (PeproTech #300–46).
3. Detection: Biotinylated rabbit anti-human I-TAC polyclonal (PeproTech #500-P132Bt).

2.3 Meso Scale Discovery (MSD) Reagents

Every MSD kit includes reagents specific to that assay. Always dilute buffers to proper concentrations before beginning an assay and store as instructed (http://www.mesoscale.com). The following is a list of reagents one should expect to receive with a MSD kit.

1. Blocker buffer: included in certain assays; prepare as instructed in specific assay protocols.
2. Read buffer: received from MSD at 4× concentrations; dilute with deionized water before use.
3. Assorted diluent buffers: received ready-to-use from MSD (*see* **Note 4**).
4. Calibrators: received from MSD lyophilized or at a stock concentration; prepare using suggested diluents.
5. Detection antibody mix: mixes are generally received at a 50× concentration and should be diluted with provided diluents to a working concentration; mixes are light sensitive and should be wrapped in foil when received.

3 Methods

3.1 Quantifying Intra-assay Variability Due to Pipetting Error

Pipetting errors are dismissed as "problems that beginners have—not me." However, this is the single most common reason for assay failure or high variability. Pipetting errors are cumulative, compounding problems by increasing variability throughout the assay. Therefore, the coefficient of variation (CV) needs to be <3% at each step for each investigator.

Before beginning ELISA (or almost any other biomedical research technique!), variability in operator pipetting or pipet malfunction must be assessed. To do so, ELISA solution from previous assays is used as a source of chromogen. For PNPP, a substrate for alkaline phosphatase, this yields a bright yellow solution that can be used to generate readings in the microplate plate reader, allowing one to determine how precisely and reproducibly one measures volumes. The same can be done with any chromogen (i.e., leftover solutions from HRP ELISAs). For, a diagram of suggested plate design and sample data, *see* Table 1.

1. Using P200 or similar equipment, pipet eight 50 μL and eight 100 μL volumes of expired ELISA solution into 96-well ELISA plates, using columns 1 and 3, respectively (running up and down plate).
2. In column 2, pipet two 50 μL volumes of expired ELISA solution in the top two wells.
3. In column 4, pipet two 100 μL volumes of expired ELISA solution in the top two wells.

Table 1
Determination of coefficient of variation: sample data

Row	1	2	3	4	5	6	7
A	0.899	0.919	1.779	1.764	3.887	3.866	3.869
B	0.934	0.887	1.766	1.779	3.280	3.251	3.276
C	0.912		1.757		1.660	1.682	1.697
D	0.927		1.762		0.869	0.871	0.861
E	0.907		1.771		0.437	0.429	0.43
F	0.893		1.770		0.229	0.225	0.223
G	0.905		1.747		0.121	0.122	0.115
H	0.919		1.802		0.067	0.067	0.061
Mean absorbance (405–690 nm)	0.912	0.903	1.769	1.772			
CV (%)	1.5	2.5	0.9	0.6			

4. In columns 5–7, add 50 μL dilution buffer to all 24 wells (three columns of eight wells each), and then pipet 50 μL expired ELISA solution into the top three wells. Carry out twofold dilutions of this solution down the plate. Discard the 50 μL extra from the last well.
5. Using microplate reader, determine the absorbance values at 405 nm (or more commonly 405–690 nm background) for each data set.
6. Using plate reader software (or by transferring data to SPSS, Prism, Excel, or similar software), determine the CV—the variability in dispensing and titrating samples—as a check on pipetting technique. Because errors are cumulative and ELISA is a multistep process, errors in dispensing samples and reagents need to be below 3% for maximal sensitivity and reproducibility. If worse than 3%, practice is required. A similar check should be performed with multichannel pipettors, as individual channels can become defective. Pipettor accuracy should be checked at least every 3 months and a record kept.

3.2 Ultrasensitive ELISA Protocol (See Note 5)

Once it has been established that operator technique (or old unserviced pipettors) adds minimal variability to the assay, the optimized assay conditions below will provide excellent sensitivity (*see* **Note 6**). Specific capture and development reagents, standards, and their suggested concentrations are described (*see* **Note 7**).

1. Coat ELISA plate with 50 μL capture antibody in high pH coating buffer at a predetermined optimal concentration, generally between 50 ng/mL and 2 μg/mL (*see* **Note 8**). All four

plate sides are tapped four to five times each to ensure uniform coating of every well. For maximum sensitivity, the plate is incubated overnight at 4 °C.

2. Plates with a sealing lid should be kept in a plastic box lined with wet paper towels to minimize evaporation, hence variability in edge wells (*see* **Note 9**).
3. Blocking, using 75 μL/well blocking buffer, is carried out at 37 °C for 1–3 h in a moist box (*see* **Note 10**). We find no difference in background between these times. The time is used to prepare samples for the next step. Wash four times manually or using a plate washer. Afterwards, bang plate dry three times on paper towels to avoid dilution of the next series of reagents added to the plate.
4. A standard curve in dilution buffer is generated on each assay plate (*see* **Notes 11** and **12**). The titration range is determined by the anticipated intensity of sample values.
5. Each experimental sample is titrated in dilution buffer from an empirically determined optimal starting dilution (typically between 1:2 and 1:10) for a series of four twofold 50 μL dilutions running down the plate (i.e., 1:2, 1:4, 1:8, 1:16) (*see* **Notes 13** and **14**). This allows ~20 sample titrations per plate. Initial dilutions should not sit in the starting well for more than 2–3 min before carrying out this titration, usually with a multichannel pipettor, or resulting curves will not be linear. A sample of dilution buffer alone is generally included in wells A2, A3, and A4.
6. Sample incubation is 3 h at 37 °C or overnight at 4 °C in a covered moist box. Maximal sensitivity is obtained following overnight incubation. Wash 4× as previously described. Bang dry on paper towels.
7. Biotinylated development Ab in dilution buffer is added at a predetermined optimal concentration, usually between 50 ng/mL and 2 μg/mL, using 50 μL/well (*see* **Note 15**). Incubation can be 3 h at 37 °C or overnight at 4 °C in a covered moist box. Maximal sensitivity is obtained with overnight incubation. Wash 4×, and bang dry 3× on paper towels afterwards.
8. Streptavidin–enzyme conjugate is added at a predetermined optimal concentration to maximize signal while minimizing background. In our experience, streptavidin-alkaline phosphatase used at 1:1000–1:5000 with 50 μL/well is useful. Incubation (45 min at 37 °C) is followed by washing (4×), banging dry (3×), and addition of 50 μL/well PNPP in substrate buffer at RT.
9. Assay progress is monitored visually with readings (405–690 nm) taken between 45 min and 6 h of assay development, depending on the sensitivity required.

10. A standard curve is calculated using the data obtained by serial dilution of the standard, with the cytokine concentration on the *x*-axis (log) and the absorbance on the *y*-axis (linear) to generate a sigmoidal curve. When carrying out sample data analysis, the mean of at least two unknown points (generally 3–4 points) falling on the linear component of the standard curve of that plate is required. The calculated values should not differ from one another by more than ~15–20%, typically much less (*see* **Note 16**). Mean values ± standard error for that sample should be reported. Inter-assay variability (the same samples titrated in an independent assay on another day) should be explicitly determined for a proportion of the samples to confirm reliability of the data/operator/assay. Sensitivity is defined in each assay as the beginning of the linear portion of the standard's titration curve (*see* **Notes 11** and **12**).

3.3 Optimized Conditions for Analysis of Human Cytokine Levels in Culture Supernatants or Plasma

3.3.1 IFNγ

1. Using Subheading 3.2 protocol, add capture Ab, mouse anti-human IFNγ, at 2 μg/mL.
2. Use standard human rIFNγ and titrate from 20 U/mL to 0.15 U/mL.
3. Typically, dilute antigen-driven culture samples from 1:2. Titrate polyclonally stimulated cultures from 1:10. Plasma levels are usually below detection.
4. Use detection Ab, biotinylated mouse anti-human IFNγ, at 0.5 μg/mL.
5. Read plate after 4 h with substrate for useful sensitivity of 0.15–0.3 U/mL.

3.3.2 Il-1β

1. Using Subheading 3.2 protocol, add capture Ab, mouse anti-human IL-1β, at 0.5 μg/mL.
2. Use standard human rIL-1β and titrate from 500 pg/mL to 3.9 pg/mL.
3. Typically, dilute antigen-driven culture samples from 1:4. Plasma levels are usually below detection.
4. Use detection Ab, biotinylated mouse anti-human IL-1β, at 0.15 μg/mL.
5. Read plate after 1 h with substrate for useful sensitivity of 3.9 pg/mL.

3.3.3 IL-1R Accessory Protein (AcP)

1. Using Subheading 3.2 protocol, add capture Ab, goat anti-human IL-1RAcP/IL-1R3, at 0.25 μg/mL.
2. Use standard human rIL-1RAcP/IL-1R3/Fc chimera and titrate from 1000 pg/mL to 7.8 pg/mL.
3. Dilute plasma samples from 1:300.

4. Use detection Ab, biotinylated goat anti-human IL-1RAcP/IL-1R3, at 0.05 μg/mL.
5. Read plate after 4 h with substrate for useful sensitivity of 7.8 pg/mL.

3.3.4 Il-2

1. Using Subheading 3.2 protocol, add capture Ab, rat anti-human IL-2, at 2 μg/mL.
2. Use standard IL-2 and titrate from 10 U/mL to 0.078 U/mL.
3. Antigen-driven samples are diluted 1:2, whereas polyclonally stimulated cultures are diluted 1:10. Plasma levels are usually below detection.
4. Use detection antibody, biotinylated mouse anti-human IL-2, at 1 μg/mL.
5. Read plate after 5–6 h with substrate for sensitivity of 0.078–0.15 U/mL.

3.3.5 Il-4

1. Using Subheading 3.2 protocol, add capture Ab, mouse anti-human IL-4, at 0.7 μg/mL.
2. Use standard human rIL-4 and titrate from 125 pg/mL to 0.98 pg/mL.
3. Use antigen-driven samples either neat or at 1:2 dilution, and polyclonally stimulated samples at 1:3 dilution. Plasma levels are usually below detection.
4. Use detection antibody, biotinylated rat anti-human IL-4, at 0.5 μg/mL.
5. Read plate after 4–6 h with substrate to obtain sensitivity of 0.98 pg/mL or ~0.006 U/mL of WHO standard 88/656.

3.3.6 Il-5

1. Using Subheading 3.2 protocol, add capture Ab, rat anti-mouse/human IL-5, at 0.5 μg/mL.
2. Use standard human rIL-5 and titrate from 200 pg/mL to 1.56 pg/mL.
3. Use antigen and polyclonally driven samples from 1:3 dilution.
4. Use detection antibody, biotinylated rat anti-human IL-5, at 0.25 μg/mL.
5. Read plate after 3 h with substrate for sensitivity of 1.56 pg/mL.

3.3.7 Il-6

1. Using Subheading 3.2 protocol, add capture Ab, mouse anti-human IL-6, at 0.4 μg/mL.
2. Use standard human rIL-6 and titrate from 2000 pg/mL to 15.6 pg/mL.

3. Antigen-driven samples are diluted from 1:4, whereas polyclonally stimulated cultures are diluted from 1:10. Plasma samples are diluted from 1:2.
4. Use detection antibody, biotinylated mouse anti-human IL-6, at 0.125 μg/mL.
5. Read plate after 2–3 h with substrate for sensitivity of 15.6 pg/mL.

3.3.8 IL-9

1. Using Subheading 3.2 protocol, add capture Ab, mouse anti-human IL-9, at 1 μg/mL.
2. Use standard human rIL-9 and titrate from 300 pg/mL to 2.3 pg/mL.
3. Antigen-driven samples are diluted from 1:4.
4. Use detection antibody, biotinylated mouse anti-human IL-9, at 0.25 μg/mL.
5. Read plate after 2–3 h with substrate for sensitivity of 2.3 pg/mL.

3.3.9 IL-10

1. Using Subheading 3.2 protocol, add capture Ab, rat anti-human IL-10, at 0.35 μg/mL.
2. Use standard human rIL-10 from 1000 to 7.8 pg/mL.
3. Use antigen-driven samples from 1:4 dilution and polyclonally stimulated cultures at 1:10 dilution. Plasma samples are diluted from 1:2.
4. Use detection antibody, biotinylated rat anti-human IL-10, at 0.05 μg/mL.
5. Read plate after 2 h for sensitivity of 7.8 pg/mL or ~0.01 WHO 93/722 U.

3.3.10 IL-11

1. Using Subheading 3.2 protocol, add capture Ab, mouse anti-human IL-11, at 1.5 μg/mL.
2. Use standard human rIL-11 and titrate from 500 pg/mL to 3.9 pg/mL.
3. Antigen-driven samples are diluted from 1:2.
4. Use detection antibody, biotinylated mouse anti-human IL-11, at 0.08 μg/mL.
5. Read plate after 3–4 h with substrate for sensitivity of 7.8 pg/mL.

3.3.11 IL-13

1. Using Subheading 3.2 protocol, add capture Ab, rat anti-human IL-13, at 0.4 μg/mL.
2. Use standard human rIL-13 from 1000 pg/mL to 15.6 pg/mL.

3. Use antigen-driven cultures at 1:4, polyclonally stimulated at 1:10.
4. Use detection Ab, biotinylated mouse anti-human IL-13, at 0.25 μg/mL.
5. Read plate after 4–6 h with substrate for sensitivity of 15.6 pg/mL.

3.3.12 IL-13 Ultrahigh-Sensitivity Assay

Typical food antigen-driven responses (i.e., peanut specific) fall between 10 and 200 pg/mL, so altered ELISA conditions may be used to yield an assay with higher sensitivity.

1. Using Subheading 3.2 protocol, add capture antibody, rat anti-human IL-13, at 1 μg/mL.
2. Use standard human rIL-13 from 200 pg/mL to 1.56 pg/mL.
3. Use detection Ab, biotinylated mouse anti-human IL-13, at 0.2 μg/mL.
4. Read plate after 6 h with substrate for sensitivity of 1.56 pg/mL.

3.3.13 IL-17A

1. Using Subheading 3.2 protocol, add capture Ab, goat anti-human IL-17A, at 0.125 μg/mL.
2. Use standard human rIL-17A from 4000 pg/mL to 62.5 pg/mL.
3. Use antigen-driven samples at a dilution of 1:3.
4. Use detection Ab, biotinylated goat anti-human IL-17A, at 0.125 μg/mL.
5. Read plate after 4–6 h with substrate for sensitivity of 62.5 pg/mL.

3.3.14 IL-33

1. Using Subheading 3.2 protocol, add capture Ab, rabbit anti-human IL-33, at 0.5 μg/mL.
2. Use standard human rIL-33 from 500 pg/mL to 3.9 pg/mL.
3. Use antigen-driven samples at a dilution of 1:4.
4. Use detection Ab, biotinylated rabbit anti-human IL-33, at 0.0625 μg/mL.
5. Read plate after 4–6 h with substrate for sensitivity of 3.9 pg/mL.

3.3.15 TGF-β1

1. Using Subheading 3.2 protocol, add capture Ab, rat anti-mouse/human/pig TGF-β1, at 1 μg/mL.
2. Use standard human rTGF-β1 from 2000 pg/mL to 15.6 pg/mL.

3. Prior to assay, serum/culture samples are acidified to convert TGF-β1 from latent to active form for recognition in this assay. Incubate 50 μL of sample with 2 μL 1 N HCl for 15 min at room temperature; then add 2 μL 1 N NaOH. Carry out dilutions from 1:5 (which should be later calculated based on the actual dilution of 1:5.4, allowing for the addition of acid and base above).
4. Use detection Ab, biotinylated rat anti-mouse/human TGF-β1, at 0.25 μg/mL.
5. Read plate after 5 h with substrate for sensitivity of 15.6 pg/mL.

3.3.16 TNFα

1. Using Subheading 3.2 protocol, add capture Ab, mouse anti-human TNFα, at 0.25 μg/mL.
2. Use standard human rTNFα and titrate from 1000 pg/mL to 7.8 pg/mL.
3. Antigen-driven samples are diluted from 1:4, whereas polyclonally stimulated cultures are diluted from 1:10. Plasma levels are usually below detection.
4. Use detection Ab, biotinylated mouse anti-human TNFα, at 0.125 μg/mL.
5. Read plate after 3 h with substrate for sensitivity of 7.8 pg/mL.

3.3.17 CCL2 (MCP-1)

1. Using Subheading 3.2 protocol, add capture Ab, polyclonal anti-human CCL2, at 0.25 μg/mL (BD Biosciences or PeproTech).
2. Use standard human rMCP-1 and titrate from 500 pg/mL to 3.9 pg/mL.
3. Antigen-driven and polyclonally stimulated samples are diluted from 1:50. Plasma samples are diluted from 1:2.
4. Use detection Ab, biotinylated mouse polyclonal anti-human MCP-1, at 0.025 μg/mL (BD Biosciences or PeproTech).
5. Read plate after 3 h with substrate for sensitivity of 3.9 pg/mL.

3.3.18 CCL3 (MIP-1α)

1. Using Subheading 3.2 protocol, add capture Ab, polyclonal anti-human MIP-1α, at 0.35 μg/mL (R&D Systems) or 0.125 μg/mL (PeproTech).
2. Use standard human rMIP-1α and titrate from 1000 pg/mL to 7.8 pg/mL.
3. Antigen-driven and polyclonally stimulated samples are diluted from 1:10.

4. Use detection Ab, biotinylated goat anti-human MIP-1α, at 0.015 μg/mL (R&D Systems or PeproTech).
5. Read plate after 5–6 h with substrate for sensitivity of 7.8 pg/mL.

3.3.19 CCL5 (RANTES)

1. Using Subheading 3.2 protocol, add capture Ab, mouse anti-human CCL5, at 0.125 μg/mL.
2. Use standard human rRANTES and titrate from 1000 pg/mL to 7.8 pg/mL.
3. Antigen-driven samples are diluted from 1:4.
4. Use the detection antibody, biotinylated goat anti-human RANTES, at 0.005 μg/mL.
5. Read plate after 2–3 h with substrate for sensitivity of 7.8 pg/mL.

3.3.20 CCL8 (MCP-2)

1. Using Subheading 3.2 protocol, add capture Ab, rabbit anti-human MCP-2, at 0.06 μg/mL.
2. Use standard human rMCP-2 and titrate from 250 pg/mL to 1.95 pg/mL.
3. Antigen-driven samples are diluted from 1:5.
4. Use the detection Ab, biotinylated rabbit anti-human MCP-2, at 0.01 μg/mL.
5. Read plate after 2–3 h with substrate for sensitivity of 1.95 pg/mL.

3.3.21 CCL11 (Eotaxin-1)

1. Using Subheading 3.2 protocol, add capture Ab, mouse anti-human Eotaxin, at 0.35 μg/mL.
2. Use standard human rEotaxin and titrate from 500 pg/mL to 3.9 pg/mL.
3. Dilute plasma samples 1:4.
4. Use detection Ab, biotinylated goat anti-human Eotaxin, at 0.05 μg/mL.
5. Read plate after 3 h with substrate for sensitivity of 3.9 pg/mL.

3.3.22 CCL17 (TARC)

1. Using Subheading 3.2 protocol, add capture Ab, polyclonal anti-human TARC, at 0.25 μg/mL (R&D Systems) or 0.0625 μg/mL (PeproTech).
2. Use standard human rTARC and titrate from 500 pg/mL to 3.9 pg/mL.
3. Dilute antigen and polyclonally driven samples 1:10.
4. Use detection Ab, biotinylated goat anti-human TARC, at 0.05 μg/mL (R&D Systems) or 0.0313 μg/mL (PeproTech).
5. Read plate after 3 h with substrate for sensitivity of 3.9 pg/mL.

3.3.23 CCL22 (MDC)

1. Using Subheading 3.2 protocol, add capture Ab, polyclonal anti-human MDC, at 0.125 μg/mL (R&D Systems) or 0.1 μg/mL (PeproTech).
2. Use standard human rMDC and titrate from 1000 pg/mL to 7.8 pg/mL.
3. Dilute antigen and polyclonally driven samples 1:10. Dilute plasma samples from 1:5.
4. Use detection Ab, biotinylated chicken anti-human MDC, at 0.02 μg/mL (R&D Systems) or 0.125 μg/mL (PeproTech).
5. Read plate after 1 h with substrate for sensitivity of 7.8 pg/mL.

3.3.24 CXCL8 (IL-8)

1. Using Subheading 3.2 protocol, add capture Ab, mouse anti-human IL-8, at 1.5 μg/mL.
2. Use standard human rIL-8 and titrate from 1000 pg/mL to 7.8 pg/mL.
3. Dilute antigen-driven samples 1:25.
4. Use detection Ab, biotinylated mouse anti-human IL-8, at 0.03 μg/mL.
5. Read plate after 2–3 h with substrate for sensitivity of 7.8 pg/mL.

3.3.25 CXCL9 (MIG)

1. Using Subheading 3.2 protocol, add capture Ab, polyclonal anti-human MIG, at 0.25 μg/mL (PeproTech) or 0.350 μg/mL (R&D Systems).
2. Use standard human rMIG and titrate from 1000 pg/mL to 7.8 pg/mL.
3. Dilute antigen and polyclonally driven samples 1:10.
4. Use detection Ab, biotinylated goat anti-human MIG, at 0.1 μg/mL (PeproTech) or 0.015 μg/mL (R&D Systems).
5. Read plate after 3–5 h with substrate for sensitivity of 7.8 pg/mL.

3.3.26 CXCL10 (IP-10)

1. Using Subheading 3.2 protocol, add capture Ab, mouse anti-human IP-10, at 0.015 μg/mL (PeproTech) or 0.4 μg/mL (BD Biosciences).
2. Use standard human rIP-10 and titrate from 250 pg/mL to 1.95 pg/mL.
3. Dilute antigen and polyclonally driven samples 1:10. Dilute plasma samples from 1:2.
4. Use detection Ab, biotinylated goat anti-human IP-10, at 0.0625 μg/mL (PeproTech) or 0.05 μg/mL (BD Biosciences).
5. Read plate after 3–4 h with substrate for sensitivity of 1.95 pg/mL.

3.3.27 CXCL11 (I-TAC)

1. Using Subheading 3.2 protocol, add capture Ab, rabbit anti-human I-TAC, at 0.125 μg/mL.
2. Use standard human rI-TAC and titrate from 1000 pg/mL to 7.8 pg/mL.
3. Dilute urine samples 1:4.
4. Use detection Ab, biotinylated rabbit anti-human I-TAC, at 0.25 μg/mL.
5. Read plate after 3–4 h with substrate for sensitivity of 7.8 pg/mL.

3.4 Meso Scale Discovery Protocols

The following is a summary of the protocol for a typical 96-well MSD plate assay for one analyte (*see* **Notes 17** and **18**). For specific assay protocols, visit the MSD website.

1. Prepare a sample master plate 1 day in advance, seal with aluminum plate sealer, and store overnight at 4 °C. Alternatively, plates can be made in advance and frozen at −20 °C, and then thawed overnight at 4 °C before use. We have not assessed the stability of samples stored or frozen in MSD diluent. The plate should include all samples and controls at proper dilutions, as well as at least eight empty wells that will correspond to the locations of the serially diluted assay standards and negative ("zero") control (*see* **Notes 19** and **20**).
2. Prepare all assay reagents (blocking buffers, read buffers, etc.) at least 1 day in advance, and store at temperatures specified in the MSD protocols.
3. Validate that the MSD Imager is operating properly before beginning the MSD assay by using the demonstration test plate supplied with the imager.
4. Immediately before starting the MSD assay, serially dilute the MSD calibrator (or your laboratory standard) to create a standard curve (*see* **Notes 21** and **22**). Always include a well with only the buffer used to dilute the standards to serve as a negative control.
5. Add the standards and samples to the MSD plate, and incubate with shaking for 3 h (MSD assay plates arrive pre-coated with primary antibodies for analytes of interest). Alternatively, certain MSD assays can be incubated overnight without shaking.
6. Add the detection antibody to the MSD plate, and incubate with shaking for 3 h.
7. Wash the plate three times. Add the read buffer to the MSD plate using a reverse pipetting technique; read the plate using the MSD SECTOR Imager immediately following read buffer addition (*see* **Note 23**).

4 Notes

1. The process for reverse pipetting is as follows: Most brands of pipettors have two plunger positions for pipetting liquids. The first is calibrated to allow aspiration and dispensing of user-specified amounts of liquid (conventional pipetting). The second, or blowout position, enables one to expel residual liquid after the pipet has been pushed to the first position. A concern is that in the process of blowing out the residual drop, bubbles are commonly created in the dispensed liquid. Reverse pipetting circumvents this problem by avoiding creation of bubbles. The process is to push the pipet plunger past the first position to the second position before aspirating liquid into the tip, thereby aspirating slightly more liquid than the desired volume (overdraw). When then dispensing the desired volume from the tip, the pipet plunger is pushed to the first position only. This enables the researcher to precisely deliver the desired volume without creating bubbles. The precision of delivery is also enhanced, as the question of the residual drop in each tip is effectively dealt with.
2. All solutions are kept in a cold room (4 °C) and are stable for a minimum of 6 months.
3. Platelets, regular contaminants of Ficoll-isolated PBMC, release substantial amounts of TGF-β1 in culture, making analysis of Ag-driven TGF-β1 responses unreliable. TGF-β1 assessment is not recommended for primary culture cells, serum, or plasma.
4. Many diluents are of similar composition to basic culture media. We have found that in certain MSD assays (i.e., MCP-1, IL-10), laboratory culture media can be used interchangeably with Diluent 1.
5. Importance of maintaining and adhering to SOPs: Much time can be spent determining why an assay "did not work." We strongly encourage adherence to SOPs, with modifications/suggested improvements to protocols only added after group discussion and direct head-to-head comparison with the current technique. Without this, multiple variants of the same assay develop in the same laboratory. Sequential reagent checklists can also be useful in ensuring that individual steps are not omitted during a protocol.
6. In initially developing an ELISA, recall that arbitrarily pairing two cytokine-specific antibodies, or a polyclonal antibody, will not necessarily yield a useful assay. This is a largely empirical process that may require testing of several different antibody combinations to obtain an assay with high sensitivity. A sample

standard curve should be available on the vendor's website; if not, ask for one from the vendor's technical services.

7. Routinely, most ELISA reagents are reconstituted in PBS or PBS/BSA, as recommended by the manufacturer, then diluted with an equal volume of high-quality glycerol, and stored at −20 °C where they are stable for at least 1 year. Addition of glycerol allows the Ag, Ab, and enzyme conjugates to be stored at this temperature and used without undergoing the multiple freeze/thaw cycles that lead to degradation. Concentrations suggested by vendors (for ELISA, flow cytometry, etc.) are frequently two to five times higher than what is required. For assays to be used regularly, we strongly recommend an initial validation ELISA where the standard is titrated under recommended conditions (i.e., 1 μg/mL capture, 100 ng/mL development) and then also using twofold and fourfold less reagent. Sensitivity is rarely affected, and financial resources stretch much further.
8. A variety of high-binding immunoassay plates are commercially available. We have found substantial differences in their ability to bind capture antibody or Ag. Costar 3369 plates work effectively in our assays.
9. "Edge" effects, most commonly values that are too high, result from evaporation of edge wells. The solution is to ensure that plates are kept tightly wrapped in a humidified chamber (plastic box with wet paper towels) for all incubations. Also, if samples are allowed to sit in plate for an extended period prior to carrying out the dilutions, assay reproducibility is reduced.
10. Many blocking reagents (skimmed milk, bovine serum albumin (BSA), or gelatin) can be used. Recommended wash buffers sometimes utilize very high concentrations of BSA and Tween-20. In our experience, PBS with 0.05% Tween-20 is sufficient to minimize backgrounds with less cost and pollution of the environment than buffers containing up to 5% BSA and 2% Tween-20.
11. Biological standards are calibrated in units of biological activity which are established by consensus following exhaustive collaborative studies involving many laboratories. They have the advantage of allowing ready comparison of cytokine levels between different laboratories using a common standard. There is a hierarchy of standards, with the WHO International Standard being the primary standard. These standards are calibrated in arbitrary units, usually based on an initial functional bioassay, to provide a common standard that can be used to compare data internationally. It is important (but rare in practice) that secondary standards be calibrated against these primary standards. Secondary standards may be national or

regional standards, or working reference materials used in the laboratories of manufacturers, regulators, or others. WHO reference standards are available for most cytokines. There are only four "official" custodian laboratories for WHO International Standards, and these are NIBSC, CLB in the Netherlands, CDC, and NIH. NIBSC is a multidisciplinary scientific establishment located in the UK which has a national and international role in the standardization and control of biological substances used in medicine. As a WHO International Laboratory for biological standards, it prepares, evaluates, and distributes ampouled biological reference substances which serve the pharmaceutical, regulatory, and research communities as International Standards. Similarly, the BRB Preclinical Repository is a (US) NCI-sponsored facility which contains bulk cytokines, antibodies, and cytokine standards. Its purpose is to maintain a constant and uniform supply of high-quality reagents for scientists at nonprofit as well as commercial establishments. Information on low-cost distribution (nominal shipping charge) of these standards is available from the NIBSC at *www.nibsc.ac.uk/catalog/standards* or the US NCI at *www.ncifcrf.gov/brb/preclin*. Many laboratories choose to utilize recombinant standards from well-known manufacturers, and express their data in mass units based on that commercial preparation and lot. Because such standards vary widely in specific activity, some manufacturers have calibrated the specific activity of their standards against the WHO standard. Others utilize the bioassay of their choice to obtain specific activities. It should be recognized that 100 U/mL (or 100 pg/mL) in one assay is not necessarily equivalent to 100 U/mL (or 100 pg/mL) in a different assay or supplier lot. Comparison between, for instance, two IL-4 preparations from different sources can easily be 100-fold different in terms of specific activity.

12. When assay sensitivity is not sufficient for a given application, the first step is to compare the sensitivity of the standard curve generated with the literature or detailed above. Assuming that you obtain similar sensitivity to others, you need an estimate of the cytokine levels expected. Some cytokines are produced at substantial levels (i.e., IL-5, IL-9, IL-13) and chemokines (i.e., CCL17, CCL22) at even higher levels, while some, notably IL-4, are very tightly regulated and present at pg/mL levels in antigen-stimulated cultures.

13. If experimental values do not agree throughout the titration range, it is possible that the dilution range selected is not within the linear range of the assay. The titration of the samples needs to be adjusted so that more of the points lie on the linear component of the standard curve.

14. When a trainee is first gaining experience with ELISA, we provide coded samples of known concentration that fall within the range of values typically obtained in experimental work. These are titrated in duplicate until the accurate concentration (±10–15%) is reproducibly determined.
15. Development antibodies directly conjugated with enzyme are rarely used in ultrasensitive ELISA, as they do not provide adequate signal. Biotinylated reagents yield at least a tenfold increase in sensitivity. Avidin/streptavidin enzyme conjugates generally utilize alkaline phosphatase or horseradish peroxidase. The methods presented above use alkaline phosphatase with PNPP substrate, as it is inexpensive and stable, and generates a robust signal that increases linearly over many hours.
16. The most common reasons for duplicates which do not agree are poor titration precision/operator technique or defective pipets.
17. MSD also provides several multiplexing options (4-Spot, 7-Spot, 10-Spot, or V-Plex) that allow analysis of multiple proteins at once. However, it is important to determine if all potential analytes fall within the standardized MSD calibrator ranges or if dilutions need to be made.
18. Custom MSD kits are also available if one's protein of interest is not listed on the MSD website.
19. When planning a master plate, it is important to note that the MSD system reads the plate wells in blocks of four (wells A1, A2, B1, and B2 in typical 96-well plates, etc.).
20. In order to confirm acceptable intra-assay and inter-assay variation, it is important to include duplicates within each 96-well plate assay, as well as between different assays.
21. MSD calibrators may vary between batches; therefore, it is beneficial to use a laboratory standard (as discussed in **Note 11**) to use within the MSD assays if one will be conducting many assays over an extended period of time. If using a laboratory standard, it is important to include at least two high MSD calibrator dilutions (for example, 10,000 and 2500 pg/mL) within the plate for quality control. V-Plex assays are intended to circumvent this.
22. MSD assays have large detection ranges, so it is possible to serially dilute a standard curve up to eight times with up to fourfold dilutions to increase the detection limits of the assay.
23. It is important to read the MSD plate immediately following addition of read buffer, as the plate signal begins to decline after read buffer addition.

Acknowledgments

We thank the many colleagues and collaborators who have provided suggestions which aided in the development of these methodologies. We acknowledge funding from the CIHR (Canadian Institutes for Health Research) and the Canada Research Chairs program.

References

1. HayGlass KT (2012) Complex asthma endotypes, differential chemokine responses and birth cohort studies: solving equations with multiple variables. Clin Exp Allergy 42(11):1546–1548
2. HayGlass KT (2011) The quest for predictive immune biomarkers. Clin Exp Allergy 41(12):1656–1659
3. Maciejko L, Smalley M, Goldman A (2017) Cancer immunotherapy and personalized medicine: emerging technologies and biomarker-based approaches. J Mol Biomark Diagn 8(5):350
4. Alexis NE (2014) Biomarker sampling of the airways in asthma. Curr Opin Pulm Med 20(1):46–52
5. Tunceroglu H, Shah A, Porhomayon J et al (2013) Biomarkers of lung injury in critical care medicine: past, present, and future. Immunol Investig 42(3):247–261
6. Easton R, Balogh ZJ (2014) Peri-operative changes in serum immune markers after trauma: a systematic review. Injury 45(6):934–941
7. Massaro AN, Wu YW, Bammler TK et al (2018) Plasma biomarkers of brain injury in neonatal hypoxic-ischemic encephalopathy. J Pediatr 194:67–75 e1
8. Dhondalay GK, Rael E, Acharya S et al (2018) Food allergy and omics. J Allergy Clin Immunol 141(1):20–29
9. Prasad G, McCullough M (2013) Chemokines and cytokines as salivary biomarkers for the early diagnosis of oral cancer. Int J Dent 2013:813756
10. Rodney T, Osier N, Gill J (2018) Pro- and anti-inflammatory biomarkers and traumatic brain injury outcomes: a review. Cytokine 110:248–256. https://doi.org/10.1016/j.cyto.2018.01.012
11. Henriksen K, O'Bryant SE, Hampel H et al (2014) The future of blood-based biomarkers for Alzheimer's disease. Alzheimers Dement 10(1):115–131
12. Yalow RS, Berson SA (1960) Immunoassay of endogenous plasma insulin in man. J Clin Invest 39:1157–1175
13. Imada M, Simons FE, Jay FT et al (1995) Antigen mediated and polyclonal stimulation of human cytokine production elicit qualitatively different patterns of cytokine gene expression. Int Immunol 7(2):229–237

Chapter 8

Development of Mold Antigen-Specific Enzyme-Linked Immunosorbent Assays (ELISA) to Quantify Airborne Antigen Exposure

Eva Zahradnik and Monika Raulf

Abstract

Common methods to quantify molds in the environment are based on the detection of viable and nonviable fungal components using cultivation technique or assessment by microscopy. These methods are time consuming and laborious and require a high expertise and especially in airborne exposure studies they showed poor reproducibility. Therefore alternative techniques based on molecular or immunological tools attract wide interest. The development of specific ELISAs based on polyclonal antibodies to detect mold antigens in airborne samples starting with the extraction of the antigen material up to evaluation of the sandwich ELISA is summarized in this chapter.

Key words Antigen preparation, Polyclonal antibody production, Sandwich ELISA, Cross-reactivity check, Quantification of mold antigens, Air sampling

1 Introduction

Exposure to molds may induce various human disorders, such as infections, irritations, and allergic reactions. A large variety of sampling strategies and analytical methods are available for fungal exposure assessment [1]. The most widely used monitoring techniques are (1) the cultivation of fungi and the determination of colony-forming units, and (2) counting of fungal cells by microscopy. The main advantages of culture-based methods are the possibility to identify fungal species and higher sensitivity compared to microscopic counting. However, these methods do not identify several nonviable fungal fragments, which may also function as sources of allergens. Microscopic methods are independent of the viability of the organisms but have constricted potential for species classification. Furthermore, both techniques are of limited use in large epidemiological studies because they are time consuming and laborious, and require high expertise. Therefore, in recent years

Penny Lympany and Meinir G. Jones (eds.), *Allergy: Methods and Protocols*, Methods in Molecular Biology, vol. 2020, https://doi.org/10.1007/978-1-4939-9591-2_8, © Springer Science+Business Media, LLC, part of Springer Nature 2019 molecular methods based on polymerase chain reaction (PCR) or immunoassays (e.g., ELISA) based on antibodies specific for antigenic components play an increasing role.

The advantages of the ELISA technique are the speed, analytical sensitivity, and possibility to measure a large number of samples within a reasonable timeframe [2]. The most commonly used ELISA format for detecting substances in dust samples with high sensitivity is the sandwich assay. The antigen to be measured is bound between two specific non-interfering antibodies—the capture antibody and the biotin-labeled detection antibody. The detection of the biotinylated antibody is carried out via a streptavidin-enzyme conjugate that causes a color reaction after addition of a relevant substrate. The resulting color intensity is proportional to the amount of bound antigen and can be measured photometrically. The most commonly used enzymes are horseradish peroxidase (HRP) and alkaline phosphatase (AP). As a substrate, a variety of different chromogenic, chemifluorescent, or chemiluminescent substances are available. The choice of detection system including enzyme conjugate and substrate greatly influences the sensitivity level of the detection and depends on the instrumentation available for detection (e.g., spectrophotometer, fluorometer, or luminometer).

Either monoclonal or polyclonal antibodies may be used as the capture and detection antibodies in sandwich ELISA systems. Both work well for ELISA. Monoclonal antibodies are valued for their enormous specificity, purity, and consistency. However, the monospecificity of monoclonal antibodies may limit their usefulness. Small changes in the structure of an epitope can markedly affect the function. Polyclonal antibodies are heterogeneous and recognize a host of antigenic epitopes; the effect of change on single epitope is less significant. Their production is less expensive and less time consuming compared to monoclonals and polyclonals often have a high affinity for the antigen [3]. To obtain polyclonal antibodies with the greatest specificity, they can be affinity-purified using the immobilized antigen.

To assess the exposure to common allergens sources such as mites, cockroaches, cats, dogs, or rodents, generally monoclonal antibody-based ELISA against major allergens, e.g., Der p 1 or Fel d 1, are used as the gold standard technique [4, 5]. In the case of molds, the detection of single protein may be insufficient for exposure assessment. Because fungi are known to have varied expression of allergens/antigens (depending on environmental growth conditions) the absence of specific proteins does not necessarily prove the absence of those fungi. Monoclonal antibody-based ELISAs for major allergens of *Aspergillus fumigatus* (Asp f 1) and *Alternaria alternata* (Alt a 1) are commercially available; however, their application in the field seems to be limited. Surveys of Asp f 1 or Alt a 1 have often failed to detect these allergens in environmental dust samples [6, 7]. Therefore, a reliable assay for the measurement of fungal exposure levels should be able to detect the presence of fungi, even if they are not producing an allergen. This can be achieved by the use of polyclonal antibodies that recognize a variety of antigenic components from the same mold comparable to the antigen recognition in the human immune system. Additional advantages are sensitivity and robustness of the assays and the detection of several antigens which might be present simultaneously in airborne dust. A disadvantage of the polyclonal antibodies is their tendency to cross-react. Thus, extensive specificity testing of the developed assay has to be performed. Apart from the specificity, the assay to quantify antigens/allergens in air samples must be very sensitive because the concentrations of airborne allergens may be extremely low (pg/m^3 to ng/m^3 range).

The following method has been developed and applied for the measurement of airborne mold antigens from fungal species *Aspergillus fumigatus*, *Aspergillus versicolor*, *Penicillium chrysogenum*, and *Cladosporium herbarum* [8, 9]. These assays have been successfully used to assess the mold exposure in composting plants [10]. The assays in sandwich design are based on affinity-purified polyclonal antibodies against the whole soluble antigen spectrum extracted from the commercially available freeze-dried mold materials. This chapter reports the strategy for assay development including antigen preparation, production and purification of antibodies, assay setup, specificity check, quality control, and recommendations for sample analysis.

The main steps of sandwich ELISA development procedure are shown in Fig. 1.

2 Materials

2.1 Extraction of Fungal Antigens

1. Homogenizer (e.g., Schuett, Goettingen, Germany).
2. Ultrasonic bath.
3. Mold antigens: Lyophilized material containing spores and mycelia (inactivated by gamma radiation), e.g., from Allergon, Ångelholm, Sweden, or Greer, Lenoir, NY, USA (*see* **Note 1**).
4. Phosphate-buffered saline (PBS), tenfold concentrated: 1370 mM NaCl, 14.7 mM KH_2PO_4, 81 mM Na_2HPO_4, 27 mM KCl. Adjust pH to 7.4 if necessary. Store at room temperature. For use, dilute 1:10 with double-distilled water (ddH_2O).
5. Extraction buffer: PBS-0.05% Tween-20 (PBST).
6. Protease inhibitor cocktail tablet (e.g., Complete, Mini, EDTA free, Roche, Mannheim, Germany).
7. Cellulose filters, e.g., Whatman® 595 ½ Qualitative Filter Papers.

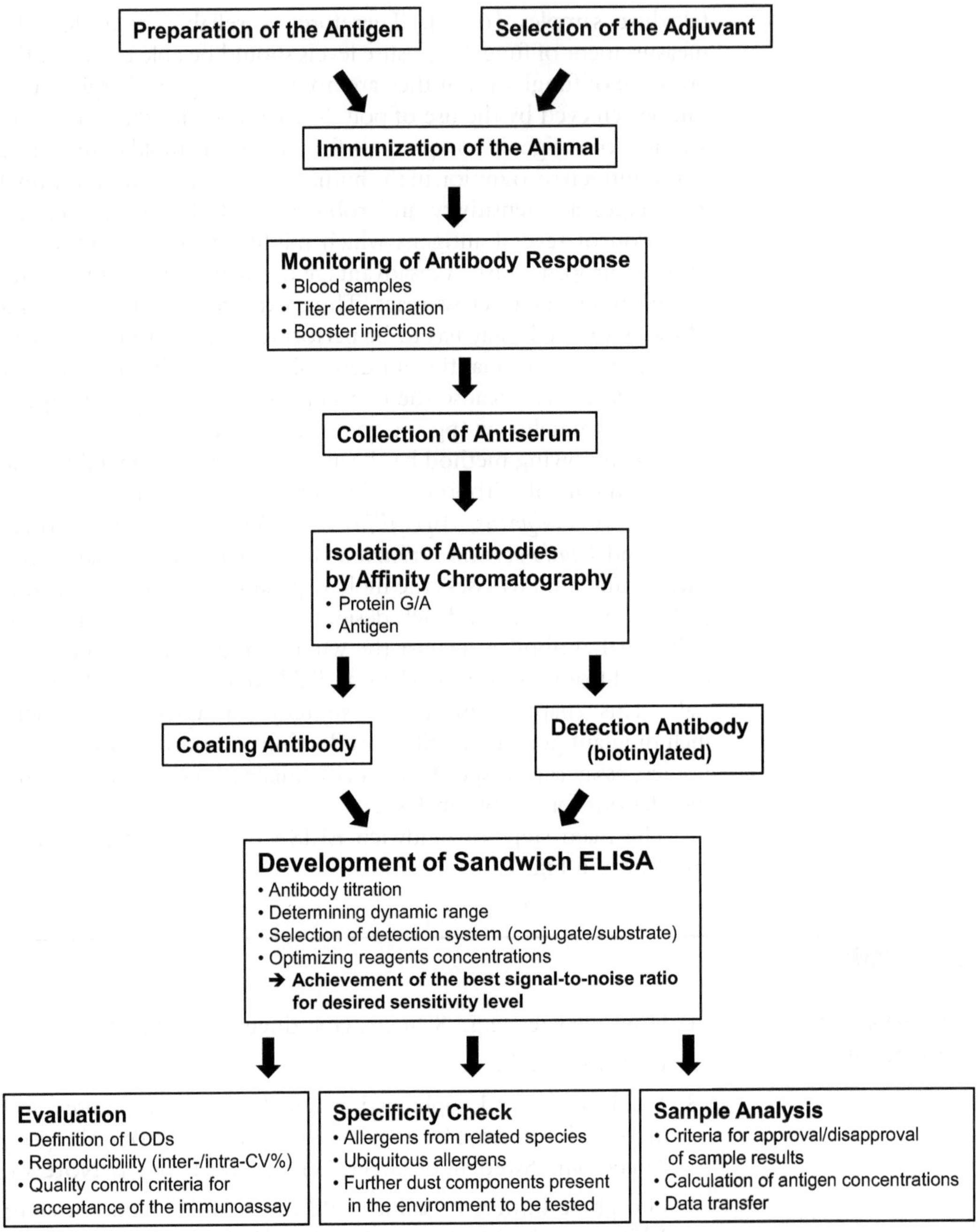

Fig. 1 Schematic steps of sandwich assay development procedure. *LOD* limit of detection, *CV* coefficient of variation

2.2 Production of Polyclonal Antibodies

1. Use 10–14-week-old female New Zealand White rabbit (*see* **Note 2**).
2. TiterMax® Classic or TiterMax® Gold adjuvant (TiterMax USA, Inc., Norcross, Georgia, USA) (*see* **Note 3**).

3. Mold antigen extract (0.5–1 mg/mL) (*see* **Note 4**).
4. Syringes (2 mL), 3-way stopcock and appropriate cannulas (18G–22G).
5. Winged infusion set Venofix® 21G (Braun, Melsungen, Germany).
6. Blood collection system, S-Monovettes 7.5 mL Z-Gel (Sarstedt, Nümbrecht, Germany).

2.3 Measurement of Antibody Titer (by ELISA)

1. Nunc™ MaxiSorp 96-well microtiter plates.
2. Microplate washer, e.g., HydroFlex™ (Tecan, Männedorf, Switzerland).
3. Microplate spectrophotometer, e.g., SPECTRAmax® (Molecular Devices, Sunnyvale, CA, USA).
4. Software program for analysis, e.g., Softmax®Pro (Molecular Devices).
5. Coating buffer: Carbonate-bicarbonate buffer, pH 9.6 (ten-fold concentrated). Prepare 1 M $NaHCO_3$ and 1 M Na_2CO_3 separately. Adjust the pH of the hydrogen carbonate solution by adding the bicarbonate solution until a pH of 9.6 is reached. For use in assay, dilute 1:10 with ddH_2O.
6. Blocking buffer: 1.5% Casein in PBST. Dissolve 1.5 g of casein in 1 L PBST by stirring overnight at 37 °C. The blocking solution can be frozen in 50 mL tubes and stored at −70 °C.
7. Wash buffer/dilution buffer: PBST.
8. Rabbit antiserum.
9. Alkaline phosphatase (AP)-conjugated goat-anti-rabbit IgG (whole molecule) (Sigma, Steinheim, Germany).
10. SIGMA FAST p-nitrophenyl phosphate (pNPP) tablets (Sigma): Dissolve the pNNP tablet and the enclosed buffer tablet in 5 mL ddH_2O.

2.4 Purification of Polyclonal Antibodies Using Affinity Chromatography

1. Protein G Sepharose columns (for whole IgG fraction; *see* **Note 5**) or antigen-coupled N-hydroxysuccinimide ester (NHS)-activated Sepharose columns (for antigen-specific IgGs, *see* **Note 6**) (HiTrap affinity columns, GE Healthcare, Munich, Germany).
2. Fast Protein Liquid Chromatography (FPLC) system, e.g., ÄTKA™ (GE Healthcare, Munich, Germany).
3. UV spectrophotometer.
4. Binding buffer: 20 mM Sodium phosphate, pH 7.0. Prepare 20 mM Na_2HPO_4 and 20 mM NaH_2PO_4 separately. Adjust the pH of the hydrogen phosphate solution by adding the dihydrogen phosphate solution until a pH of 7.0 is reached.

5. Elution buffer: 100 mM Glycine, pH 2.8.
6. Neutralization buffer: 1 M Tris, pH 9.0.
7. Rabbit antiserum.

2.5 Biotinylation of Antibodies

1. Slide-A-Lyse Dialysis Cassette 10,000–20,000 MWCO (Thermo Scientific, Rockford, IL, USA).
2. EZ-Link NHS-Biotin Reagents (Thermo Scientific).
3. Dimethyl sulfoxide (DMSO).
4. Affinity-purified antibodies (*see* **Note 7**).
5. Dialysis buffer: PBS, pH 7.4.

2.6 Sandwich ELISA

The ELISA equipment and buffers are similar as described in Subheading 2.3. Additional reagents needed are the following:

1. Coating antibody solution: Dilute the polyclonal antibodies (protein G-purified) in coating buffer pH 9.6 (approx. 0.5–2 μg/mL).
2. Standards and controls: A mold extract to which antibodies are specific should be used as a standard (ideally the same mold preparation as used for immunization). An extract of mold-free material may be used as negative control (e.g., soy or wheat flour). As a positive control, an extract containing a known amount of the antigen should be prepared, e.g., dust from mold-contaminated environment (*see* **Note 8**). The antigen concentration should be approx. at 50% of the standard curve range.
3. Detection antibody solution: Dilute the biotinylated polyclonal antibodies (antigen-affinity purified) in PBST, e.g., 1:1000.
4. Streptavidin-horseradish peroxidase conjugate, e.g., Streptavidin-Poly-HRP80 (Fitzgerald, Concord, MA, USA) diluted 1:10,000–20,000 in PBST (*see* **Note 9**).
5. Citrate buffer: Prepare 50 mM citric acid and 50 mM Na_2HPO_4 separately. Adjust the pH of the phosphate solution by adding the citric acid solution until a pH of 4.2 is reached.
6. ABTS substrate [2,2′-azino-bis(3-ethylbenzothiazoline-6-sulfonic acid)] tablets (Sigma, Steinheim, Germany): Dissolve the ABTS tablet in 12 mL citrate buffer and add 6 μL 30% H_2O_2.
7. Stop solution: 0.32% Sodium fluoride (NaF; Sigma, Steinheim, Germany).

3 Methods

3.1 Extraction of Fungal Antigens

1. Dissolve 500 mg raw mold material in 10 mL PBST plus protease inhibitor cocktail.
2. Disrupt the mold material with homogenizer at 2500 rpm for 10 min.
3. Sonicate for 3 min.
4. Incubate by rotation for 15 min.
5. Centrifuge for 20 min at 40,000 × *g* at 4 °C.
6. Filtrate the supernatant through cellulose filter paper.
7. Determine the protein concentration of the mold extract (*see* **Note 10**).
8. Store in aliquots at −80 °C.

3.2 Production of Polyclonal Antibodies

1. Prepare the antigen-adjuvant mixture using 3-way stopcock and two syringes. To prepare 1 mL immunizing emulsion, 500 μL antigen extract and 500 μL TiterMax are needed. It is important to add the antigen solution to the TiterMax in at least 2 volumes of 250 μL. It is recommended to push the aqueous antigen phase into the oil phase (TiterMax) first. Mix the two solutions by forcing the materials back and forth through the stopcock. After approximately 1 min a whipped-cream-like water-in-oil emulsion forms. Transfer the emulsion in one of the syringes and connect with sterile needle (22 gauge). Remove the air from the syringe before injecting (*see* **Note 11**).
2. Place the rabbit on a solid and *rough* surface. Avoid any smooth surfaces!
3. Clean the injection sites with 70% alcohol prior to injection.
4. Inject the antigen-adjuvant emulsion subcutaneously in 4 volumes of approx. 200 μL per injection near the dorsal shoulders.
5. After 4 weeks take a blood sample from the rabbit (usually 500 μL from ear artery using Venofix®) and check for antibody titer (*see* Subheading 3.3).
6. Boost with the same antigen dose emulsified in TiterMax 6 weeks after the first immunization.
7. After 4 weeks take a blood sample from the rabbit and check for antibody titer by ELISA.
8. If the antibody titer is not high enough, boost again with the second antigen dose in TiterMax.
9. Collect the blood by exsanguination 4 weeks after the last injection using S-Monovettes (*see* **Note 12**).
10. For serum separation, centrifuge the S-Monovettes for 10 min at 2500 × *g*.

3.3 Measurement of Antibody Titer

1. Coat the microtiter plate with mold extract diluted in coating buffer (10 μg/mL; 100 μL/well) overnight at 4 °C.
2. Incubate with blocking solution for 1 h at 22 °C (200 μL/well).
3. Wash the microtiter plate three times with 250 μL PBST per well.
4. Incubate with rabbit antiserum diluted in PBST for 2 h at 22 °C (100 μL/well). Use a long 1:2 dilution series, e.g., from 1:1000 to 1:1,000,000.
5. Wash three times with PBST.
6. Dilute AP-conjugated anti-rabbit IgG 1:20,000 in PBST and incubate for 2 h at 22 °C (100 μL/well).
7. Wash three times with PBST.
8. Add the pNPP substrate (100 μL/well).
9. Read the OD_{450nm} after 1 h.

3.4 Purification of Polyclonal Antibodies Using Affinity Chromatography

1. Connect the Protein G or antigen-NHS column (1 mL volume) to the FPLC system.
2. Wash the column with 10 column volumes of binding buffer at 1 mL/min.
3. Apply the serum by pumping it onto the column at a flow of 1 mL/min. For 1 mL columns, an application of 10 mL serum is suitable.
4. Collect the flow-through for a next run.
5. Wash with 10 column volumes of binding buffer or until no material appears in the effluent.
6. Elute with 10 column volumes of elution buffer (1 mL/min) and check $A_{280\ nm}$ for protein peak.
7. Collect the eluate in 1 mL fractions and add immediately 100 μL neutralization buffer to each fraction.
8. Wash the column with binding buffer and start the next run (*see* **Note 13**).
9. After last run, pool protein-containing fractions and determine protein concentration (*see* **Note 10**).

3.5 Biotinylation of Polyclonal Antibodies

1. Prior to biotinylation procedure the purified antibodies from Subheading 3.3. must be dialyzed to remove Tris buffer (*see* **Note 14**). Pipet antibody preparation into dialysis cassette and dialyze against PBS buffer with stirring at 4 °C overnight.
2. Dissolve the biotin reagent in DMSO at a concentration of 10 mg/mL (immediately before use).

3. Mix antibodies with a 30-fold molar excess of biotin reagent and incubate for 4 h at room temperature.
4. Dialyze the biotinylated antibodies against PBS to remove unbound biotin molecules!

3.6 Sandwich ELISA

3.6.1 General Procedure

1. Coat the microtiter plate with the coating antibody solution diluted in coating buffer (approx. 0.5–2 μg/mL; 100 μL/well) overnight at 4 °C.
2. Discard the antibodies and incubate with 1.5% casein (200 μL/well) for 1 h at 22 °C.
3. Wash the microtiter plate three times with 250 μL PBST per well.
4. Incubate for 1 h at 22 °C with standards, blanks, negative and positive controls, and samples diluted with PBST (100 μL/well). Use eight serial twofold dilutions of the mold extract in duplicate to obtain the standard curve. Use at least four blanks (PBST), controls in duplicate at predefined dilution, and samples in three serial twofold dilutions.
5. Wash three times with 250 μL PBST per well.
6. Dilute the biotinylated detection antibody, e.g., 1:1000 in PBST, and incubate for 1 h at 22 °C (100 μL/well).
7. Wash three times with 250 μL PBST per well.
8. Dilute HRP-conjugated streptavidin 1:10,000 in PBST and incubate for 1 h at 22 °C (100 μL/well).
9. Wash three times with 250 μL PBST per well.
10. Add 100 μL freshly prepared ABTS substrate and monitor the optical density (OD) at a wavelength of 414 nm.
11. Stop the color reaction with 100 μL/well NaF solution when the highest standard reaches OD_{414nm} of 2.8–3.0.
12. Read the OD_{414nm} and use a four-parameter fitted standard curve to calculate mold antigen concentrations of samples.

3.6.2 Assay Development: Optimizing Reagents and Reagent Dilutions

To develop an assay successfully (as described in Subheading 3.6.1), all reagents and their ideal concentrations must be established empirically (*see* **Note 15**).

1. For first experiments, use several dilutions of the coating and detection antibody (large serial dilution steps, e.g., 1:1000, 1:2000, 1:4000). Test each antibody combination with a long dilution series of the standard preparation (e.g., protein concentration from 100 ng/mL to 0.01 ng/mL) and at least four blank wells (zero standard). Some combinations will enhance sensitivity, and others will increase background. Choose the standard curve with the best signal-to-noise ratio that still gives an acceptable background. Determine the standard curve

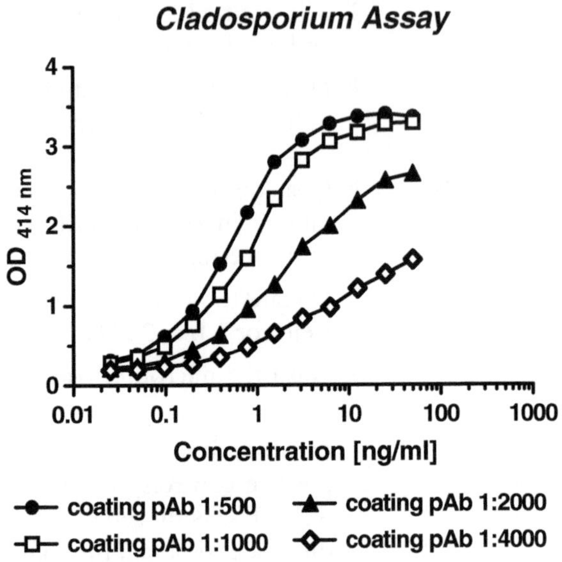

Fig. 2 Development of *Cladosporium* assay—Titration of the coating antibody (1:500–1:4000) at a constant dilution of detection antibody (1:5000) using a *Cladosporium herbarum* extract as a standard

range (generally eight serial twofold dilutions). The standard curve should utilize the majority of the OD range used with conjugate/substrate system. An example for antibody titration is given in Fig. 2.

2. For subsequent experiments, optimize the concentrations of both antibodies in minor dilution steps (e.g., 1:800, 1:1000, 1:1200). Choose the standard curve with the best signal-to-noise ratio again.
3. If the background of the standard curve with preferred sensitivity is too high, other blocking reagents may be used (*see* **Note 16**), number of washes can be increased (e.g., up to 5), or HRP-conjugate dilution should be optimized. The presence of a small amount of blocking agent in the antibody diluent (e.g., PBST-0.1% casein) helps to minimize background as well.
4. If the background of the standard curve is low and higher sensitivity is desired, instead of ABTS other substrates may be tested in combination with the streptavidin-poly-HRP conjugate (*see* **Note 17**).

3.6.3 Quality Control

After determining the final concentrations for all reagents, quality control criteria should be set up and used for acceptance of immunoassay (*see* **Note 18**).

1. *Calibration points*: Use all standard dilutions in duplicate and at least four blanks as zero standard.

2. *Curve fit: Use four-parameter logistic regression with the equation:*

$$y = D + \frac{A - D}{1 + \left(\frac{x}{C}\right)^B}$$

The four estimated parameters consist of the following:

A = the minimum value that can be obtained.

D = the maximum value that can be obtained.

C = the point of inflection (i.e., the point on the S-shaped curve halfway between A and D).

B = Hill coefficient (i.e., the slope of the curve at the inflection point C).

3. *Fit requirements*: All standard points should result in a four-parameter curve fit with $r^2 > 0.99$. Maximum one outlier of the standard points is allowed to be masked.
4. *Blanks*: Calculate the mean OD_{414nm} of the blank wells. The background OD should be smaller than 10% of the maximal OD. One clearly too high and deviating blank value is allowed to be masked.
5. *Lower limit*: Lower limit is defined by adding OD = 0.1 units to the parameter A (minimum of four-parameter fitted curve).
6. *Upper limit*: Use the smallest value of the following options:
   (a) OD = 3.
   (b) Maximal OD of standard values.
   (c) 90% of parameter D (maximum of four-parameter fitted curve).
7. *Limits of detection* (LODs): Lower and upper LODs are defined as the concentrations corresponding to lower and upper limit ODs, respectively.
8. *Negative control*: Negative control sample must be below lower LOD.
9. *Positive control*: Positive control sample should not deviate more than ±25% from the theoretical value (*see* **Note 19**).

If all criteria are fulfilled, the run is accepted.

3.6.4 Specificity Test

For polyclonal antibody-based assays, it is very important to assess the specificity and possible cross-reactions using a wide range of protein extracts from diverse antigen sources. An example for cross-reactivity check is given in Fig. 3. The extracts should be tested in several serial dilutions. A recommended starting concentration may be 1000–10,000-fold higher than the highest standard point.

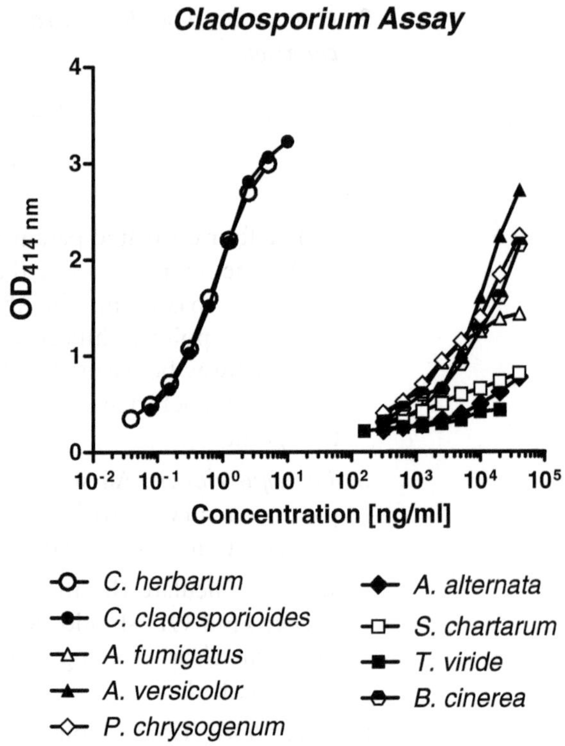

Fig. 3 Specificity of the *Cladosporium* sandwich ELISA based on tests using various extracts of diverse fungal species. *Cladosporium* assay was developed using affinity-purified polyclonal antibodies against antigens of the mold *Cladosporium herbarum*. However, antigens of closely related *Cladosporium cladosporioides* showed almost the same reactivity. Thus, the assay cannot discriminate between the two species. Other fungal extracts reacted only at high protein concentrations, demonstrating approximately 1000-fold less activity compared with *Cladosporium* extracts

1. Use extracts from phylogenetically related organisms, in this case diverse mold species from different genera (some proteins are highly conserved and may be widely shared among fungi).
2. Use extracts from ubiquitous allergens such as mites (in addition, mites are closely associated with mold growth).
3. Use extracts from antigen sources that are present in high concentration in dust samples from the environment to be tested, e.g., wheat flour in bakeries or animal epithelia in stables.

3.6.5 Analysis of Samples

Criteria for calculation of sample results and approval/disapproval of sample values should be defined. The following criteria are used routinely for our sandwich ELISA:

1. Test samples in three twofold serial dilutions (e.g., 1:10, 1:20, 1:40).
2. Sample concentrations are calculated by interpolation from the standard curve and corrected for sample dilution.

3. Final result is the average of concentrations at dilutions with OD values in working range.
4. CV% of OD values in range up to 25% is accepted. Samples with higher CV% are retested.
5. OD values in range must show a "logical order." That is, OD must be lower at higher dilutions and vice versa. If not, the result is discarded.
6. If all sample dilutions are <lower LOD or >upper LOD retest samples in lower or higher dilutions. Use freshly thawed new aliquot for each test (if possible).
7. Result is accepted when at least two dilutions are in range and CV% is <25%.
8. Result with only one dilution in range is accepted only for samples tested at a predefined lowest dilution or for undiluted samples.
9. Samples below the lower LOD are assigned a value of 2/3 of the detection limit.

4 Notes

1. If a mold material of a requested species is not commercially available, it can be purchased at the National Collection of Microorganisms and Cell Cultures of the respective country and cultivated on plates with protein-free CZAPEX-DOX medium. The exact cultivation conditions are dependent on fungal species. The mold material is harvested by scraping plates with a scalpel and extracted as described in Subheading 2.1. Please note that recultivation of the same mold strain could result in qualitatively and quantitatively variable expression of antigens. Therefore, the use of commercially available material (large amounts of the same batch) is preferred and advantageous because of better reproducibility of the results.
2. For the production of polyclonal antibodies, rabbits are most frequently used because of ease of handling and sufficient production of high-titer antiserum. If larger amounts of antibodies are required, other animals, e.g., goat or sheep, can be used. Meanwhile, immunizations are carried out by several companies using standardized protocols and procedures in different animal species (e.g., Antibody Development Services of Charles River Laboratories or Thermo Scientific). Critical steps in the production of antibodies including selection of the animal species, antigen-adjuvant preparation, and injection protocol are summarized in Ref. [11].

3. Other adjuvants like Freund's complete adjuvant (FCA), Freund's incomplete adjuvant (FIA), aluminum salts, or RIBI adjuvant system may be used. For detailed information *see* Ref. [12].
4. Usually the protein concentration of mold extracts from commercially available materials is low. To reach the required concentration of 0.5–1 mg/mL, the mold extract should be concentrated using, e.g., Centricon centrifugal filter devices, 3 MWCO (Millipore, Bedford, MA, USA). Another possibility to concentrate extracts is the freeze-drying process.
5. Instead of Protein G, Protein A columns may be used to purify rabbit antibodies with the same efficiency. Further details on the purification of the many different forms of antibodies, including examples and practical protocols, are described in the *Antibody Purification Handbook* (GE Healthcare, product Code 18-1037-46).
6. Antigen coupling should be done within pH range 6.5–9 and at protein concentration of 0.5–10 mg/mL. For detailed coupling procedure, please follow the manufacturer's instructions (GE Healthcare Instructions 71-7006-00 AX).
7. To prepare the biotinylated detection antibody for sandwich ELISA, we use generally the antigen-affinity-purified antibodies. Usually, this results in significantly improved specificity of the immunoassay.
8. Standard and control extracts should be prepared, calibrated, and diluted to suitable concentrations for easy use in the assay. Extracts with low protein concentrations should be stabilized with non-reacting protein such as casein or BSA. For instance, we dilute standard extracts generally in 1% casein to the concentration of 1 μg/mL. Stabilized extract may be stored in aliquots at −70 °C for several years. For each assay, freshly thawed new aliquot must be used.
9. The streptavidin-poly-HRP80 conjugate consists of five identical HRP homopolymer blocks (80 HRP molecules each) that are covalently coupled to multiple streptavidin molecules. It is designed to deliver the highest sensitivity and low background in immunoassays. It is compatible with chromogenic, fluorogenic, and chemiluminescent substrates. To our experience, it provides substantial signal amplification for most ELISA assays. Nevertheless, several poly-HRP-streptavidin conjugates (with diverse polymerization levels) are commercially available from other manufacturers (e.g., Thermo Scientific Pierce Streptavidin Poly-HRP Conjugate).

   Also other enzyme conjugates such as streptavidin-alkaline phosphatase may be used. The use of AP conjugates results often in lower sensitivity compared to HRP conjugates.

10. The protein content can be determined by the Bradford method (e.g., Bio-Rad protein assay kit) or the bicinchoninic acid method (e.g., Pierce™ BCA Protein Assay Kit).
11. For detailed emulsification procedure, please follow the step-by-step instructions of the manufacturer. A number of other emulsification methods are also described (www.titermax.com).
12. Exsanguination must be performed under general anesthesia and is best carried out by heart puncture. It should result in the death of the animal. When necessary, animals can be euthanized by an overdose of an anesthetic agent.
13. Using 1 mL HiTrap column and 10 mL serum, usually 3–4 runs are needed to isolate almost the whole IgG fraction from rabbit serum.
14. NHS-activated biotin reacts with primary amino groups (-NH_2). Therefore, buffers containing primary amines such as Tris must be avoided or exchanged into amine-free buffer such as PBS. An alternative to dialysis is the use of desalting columns (e.g., PD 10 columns, GE Healthcare, Munich, Germany).
15. In our experience, the combination of antibody pair concentrations and the detection system are major parameters which influence the assay sensitivity and background. Parameters such as incubation times, incubation temperature, use of a shaker during incubation, or washing technique can also be modified. These variations have mostly minor effects on ELISA results. Incubating plates in areas where environmental conditions vary should be avoided. Therefore, we recommend the use of an incubator with preferred temperature of 22–25 °C.
16. If the background of the assay (blank wells with dilution buffer) is too high other blocking reagents such as 2% bovine serum albumin (BSA) in PBST, 1% gelatin in PBST, or PBS-1% Tween 20 may be used.
17. A variety of colorimetric substrates are available for detecting peroxidase activity such as ABTS TMB (3,3′,5,5′-tetramethylbenzidine) and OPD (o-phenylenediamine dihydrochloride). These substrates vary in detection sensitivity, working range, and signal-to-noise ratios. The greatest sensitivity in ELISA applications is obtained mostly using chemiluminescent or chemifluorescent substrates (e.g., QuantaBlu Fluorogenic Substrate, Thermo Scientific). In our experience, the use of different substrates results usually in a minor signal amplification (e.g., two- to threefold). The highest amplification is achieved by the choice of the enzyme conjugate (10- to 20-fold) (*see* **Note 8**). However, note that the signal amplification correlates frequently with higher background.

18. The criteria described in Subheading 3.6.3 are used for most of our ELISAs based on polyclonal antibodies and poly-HRP-streptavidin plus ABTS as detection system. However, other criteria may be used. For example, the mean plus 3–5 times standard deviation of the blank values is commonly used as lower detection limit as well. Sometimes two positive controls (low and high) are applied in the assay. The criteria should be adapted depending on the detection system and type of antibodies used. For example, monoclonal antibody-based assays have generally lower background (<0.2 OD).
19. We use the positive control (in duplicate) to assess the reproducibility of the assay. Generally, at least 20 independent assays are needed to determine the intra-assay and inter-assay coefficient of variation (CV%).

References

1. Eduard W, Heederik D, Duchaine C et al (2012) Bioaerosol exposure assessment in the workplace: the past, present and recent advances. J Environ Monit 14:334–339
2. Crowther JR (2009) The ELISA guidebook. Humana Press, New York, NY
3. Lipman NS, Jackson LR, Trudel LJ et al (2005) Monoclonal versus polyclonal antibodies: distinguishing characteristics, applications, and information resources. ILAR J 46:258–268
4. Chapman MD, Vailes LD, Ichikawa K (2000) Immunoassays for indoor allergens. Clin Rev Allergy Immunol 18:285–300
5. Raulf M, Buters J, Chapman M et al (2014) Monitoring of occupational and environmental aeroallergens - EAACI position paper: concerted action of the EAACI IG occupational allergy and aerobiology & air pollution. Allergy 69:1280–1299
6. Ryan TJ, Whitehead LW, Connor TH et al (2001) Survey of the Asp f 1 allergen in office environments. Appl Occup Environ Hyg 16:679–684
7. Vailes L, Sridhara S, Cromwell O et al (2001) Quantitation of the major fungal allergens, Alt a 1 and Asp f 1, in commercial allergenic products. J Allergy Clin Immunol 107:641–646
8. Sander I, Zahradnik E, van Kampen V et al (2012) Development and application of mold antigen-specific enzyme-linked immunosorbent assays (ELISA) to quantify airborne antigen exposure. J Toxicol Environ Health Part A 75:1185–1193
9. Zahradnik E, Kespohl S, Sander I et al (2013) A new immunoassay to quantify fungal antigens from the indoor mould Aspergillus versicolor. Environ Sci Process Impacts 15:1162–1171
10. van Kampen V, Sander I, Liebers V et al (2014) Concentration of bioaerosols in composting plants using different quantification methods. Ann Occup Hyg 58:693–706
11. Leenaars M, Hendriksen CFM (2005) Critical steps in the production of polyclonal and monoclonal antibodies: evaluation and recommendations. ILAR J 46:269–279
12. Stills HF (2005) Adjuvants and antibody production: dispelling the myths associated with Freund's complete and other adjuvants. ILAR J 46:280–293

Chapter 9

Monocyte-Derived Dendritic Cells as Antigen-Presenting Cells in T-Cell Proliferation and Cytokine Production

Sun-Sang J. Sung

Abstract

Dendritic cells (DC) are the most potent antigen-presenting cells that link innate with adaptive immunity. They circulate the body and sample the microenvironments for maintaining homeostasis and for mounting T-cell responses against invading pathogens, foreign antigens, and aberrant self-proteins. In humans, DC derived from blood monocytes (MDC) by cytokine treatment provide the most abundant and versatile source for studying DC and T-cell biology, and for use as adjuvants in cancer therapy. In asthma patients, T-cell functions are studied by using autologous MDC as accessory cells for allergen presentation. The method for isolating T cells and monocytes from peripheral blood mononuclear cells (PBMC) and the stimulation of T cells to proliferate and produce cytokines by MDC are outlined in this chapter. The method can be applied to the functional studies of T cells and DC in other diseases.

Key words Monocytes, Dendritic cells, T lymphocytes, Antigen presentation, Allergen, Asthma, Human, Peripheral blood mononuclear cells, Der p 2, House dust mite

1 Introduction

Dendritic cells (DC) are mobile cells that shuttle between peripheral and lymphoid organs and are capable of sensing pathogens and internalizing foreign antigen or self neo-antigens for processing and presenting to naïve T cells (reviewed in [1–4]). The characteristic properties of DC are to prime naïve T cells, to migrate to target infection sites and lymphoid organs by expressing the appropriate chemokine receptors, to modulate their surface immune antigens and cellular functions by maturation to regulate immune functions, and to activate $CD8^+$ T cells by cross-presenting internalized pathogenic or cellular antigens [3, 4]. There are three main types of DC that differ in migration capabilities, and in efficiencies of $CD4^+$ and $CD8^+$ T-cell priming, regulatory T-cell induction, and cross-presentation. In humans, three main peripheral blood DC were found: the CD1c $(BDCA1)^+$ DC, the $BDCA2^+BDCA4^+$ plasmacytoid DC, and the CD141 $(BDCA3)^+XCR1^+$ DC which

Penny Lympany and Meinir G. Jones (eds.), *Allergy: Methods and Protocols*, Methods in Molecular Biology, vol. 2020, https://doi.org/10.1007/978-1-4939-9591-2_9,

are equivalent to the murine $CD11b^{hi}$ DC, the plasmacytoid $PDCA1^+B220^+GR1^+$ DC, and the $CD8^+/CD103^+$ DC, respectively [5–7]. The development of DC from bone marrow precursors involves intermediate cell types termed the monocyte and DC progenitors, the committed DC progenitors, and the pre-DC [8, 9]. The development from bone marrow progenitors to tissue DC is strongly Flt3 ligand and GM-CSF dependent. Monocytes have been shown to be a myeloid precursor that can develop into either a macrophage or a DC, depending on the environmental milieu [1, 10, 11]. In humans, the predominant cellular DC source for in vitro studies is the monocyte-derived DC (MDC) which is obtained by culturing isolated blood monocytes in GM-CSF plus IL-4 [1, 2, 12]. These cells are similar to freshly isolated DC in their abilities to prime T-cell efficiently, and they can be induced to undergo maturation by TNF, CD40 ligand, and toll-like receptor ligands such as LPS [12]. The ease of obtaining M-DC in large numbers has greatly facilitated the studies of DC functions in Ag presentation and T-cell subset stimulation, and in the therapeutic applications in human [13–15]. For studying antigenic responses by T cells in patients, the use of MDC is the most convenient and feasible because of the limited leukocyte numbers that can be obtained in a typical blood draw and the requirement for autologous DC for presentation due to MHC restriction [16]. This chapter outlines the preparation of DC and T cells from asthma patients and the measurements of allergen-specific T-cell responses including proliferation and cytokine production. This method can be readily adapted to studies of T-cell functions in other diseases.

2 Materials

2.1 PBMC Isolations

1. Anticoagulant acid citrate dextrose (ACD-A) solution: 22 g/L Trisodium citrate.$2H_2O$, 8 g/L citric acid.H_2O, 24.5 g/L dextrose. Sterilize by filtration (0.20 μm filter; Nalgene, Rochester, NY) and store at 4 °C (*see* **Notes 1** and **2**).
2. Ficoll-paque, density 1.077 g/L (Pharmacia, Piscataway, NJ): Store at 4 °C.
3. Ca^{2+}-Mg^{2+} solution: 0.25 M $CaCl_2$, 0.078 M $MgCl_2$, sterilize by filtration.
4. Phosphate-buffered saline (PBS): 1 part endotoxin-free 10 × PBS without Ca^{2+} and Mg^{2+} (Irvine Scientific, Santa Ana, CA), 9 parts endotoxin-free H_2O.

2.2 Isolation of $CD14^+$ Monocytes and MDC Derivation

1. Anti-CD14 monoclonal antibody (mAb) 63D3 (ATCC, Bethesda, MD).
2. Goat anti-mouse IgG magnetic microbeads (Miltenyi, Auburn, CA).

3. Miltenyi LS column and VarioMACS magnetic cell separation assembly.
4. Wash buffer for cell separation columns (PBS/BSA/EDTA): 0.5% Bovine serum albumin (BSA), 5 mM EDTA in PBS. Store at 4 °C. When ready to use, filter solution through a 0.2 μm 115 mL filter unit (Nalgene). Leave solution in vacuum in the filter unit for 15 min at room temperature to deaerate solution and store buffer on ice.
5. Human recombinant GM-CSF (PeproTech, Rocky Hill, NJ); 1×10^7 units/mg protein. Dissolve in RPMI 1640 with 10% fetal bovine serum at 10 μg/mL to 1 mg/mL. Aliquot in sterile freezing or Eppendorf tubes and store at −70 °C (*see* **Note 3**).
6. Human recombinant IL-4 (Dr. P. Isakson, Monsanto Co., St. Louis, MO); 2×10^7 units/mg protein. Dilute and aliquot as in GM-CSF.
7. Complete medium: RPMI 1640 (Life Technologies, Grand Island, NY), 2 mM L-glutamine, 100 U/mL penicillin, 100 μg/mL streptomycin, and 10% heat-inactivated (56 °C, 30 min), defibrinated autologous plasma (from stock 70% plasma; *see* Subheading 3.1, **step 4**).

2.3 T-Cell Purification for Ag-Specific Responses

1. Monoclonal antibodies against human CD19 (Pharmingen, San Diego, CA), CD56 (B159.5.2, Dr. G. Trinchieri, Wistar Institute, Philadelphia, PA), CD13 [16], and CD83 (Coulter Immunotech, Miami, FL).
2. Goat-anti-mouse IgG magnetic microbeads (Miltenyi, Auburn, CA), LS columns, VarioMACS magnetic sorting assembly, and PBS/BSA/EDTA column washing solution as described in Subheading 2.2, **item 4**.

2.4 MDC Antigen Presentation in T-Cell Proliferation

1. Antigens (Ag): Recombinant Der p 2 [16] at 2 mg/mL; tetanus toxoid at 1.4 mg/mL (Massachusetts Department of Health, Jamaica Plains, MA), dialyzed and sterile filtered; and phytohemagglutinin (PHA, Wellcome Diagnostics, Dartford, England) at 9 mg/mL.

2.5 T-Cell Ag-Specific Cytokine Production

1. Recombinant IL-2 (Hoffmann LaRoche, Nutley, NJ): Dissolve IL-2 in RPMI 1640 with 10% FCS at 10,000 U/mL. Aliquot in 2500 U/vial and store at −70 °C.
2. Ag as described in Subheading 2.4.
3. Der p 2 20mer overlapping set: A set of thirteen 20 mer Der p 2 peptides with 10 amino acid overlap between adjoining peptides is dissolved in H_2O at 1 mM and stored at −20 °C.

2.6 Assay of Th1 and Th2 Cytokines in Supernatants of Stimulated T Cells by ELISA

1. Nunc Maxisorp plates, 96-well (Thermo Scientific).
2. Paired anti-human (hu) IFN-γ, anti-huIL-4, and anti-huIL-5 capture and biotinylated detecting mAb (all from Biolegend, San Diego, Ca). Store in aliquots at −20 °C.
3. Standard recombinant huIFN-γ, huIL-4, and huIL-5 (all from Biolegend): Dissolve as 0.2 μg/mL in RPMI 1640 containing 10% FCS and store in 25 μL aliquots at −70 °C. Larger aliquots (e.g., 0.5 mL) can be used as stock aliquots and later re-aliquoted.
4. Streptavidin-horseradish peroxidase (HRP; Biolegend).
5. Coating buffer: 0.1 M Sodium bicarbonate solution, pH 8.2.
6. Plate-blocking solution: 5% BSA in PBS and 0.05% Tween 20 (Fisher Scientific, Pittsburgh, PA). Prepare fresh and allow BSA to dissolve for 1–2 h before use.
7. PBS/Tween plate-washing solution: 0.05% Tween 20 in PBS.
8. HRP substrate: *O*-phenylenediamine (0.4 mg/mL; Sigma Chemical Co, St. Louis, MO) in citrate-phosphate buffer, pH 5.0 (24.3 mL of 0.1 M citric acid and 25.7 mL of 0.2 M dibasic sodium phosphate per 100 mL buffer), and 80 μL H_2O_2 per 100 mL substrate solution. Prepare fresh for each measurement.
9. Stop solution: 3 N HCl.

3 Methods

The described procedure requires two donations of 200 mL of blood each with donations 7 days apart. Monocytes are purified from the PBMC of each donation for MDC generation. T responder cells are purified from the second donation. A complete experiment spans 13 and 17 days for T-cell proliferation and cytokine production, respectively.

3.1 PBMC Isolation (See Note 4)

1. Draw 7.5 mL ACD-A into each of the four 60 mL syringes with an 18 G needle.
2. Using a 19 G butterfly needle (Abbott Laboratories, N. Chicago, IL), draw 50 mL of blood in each syringe from the arm by venipuncture. Mix contents after each syringe is filled.
3. Put the blood into 50 mL conical centrifuge tubes. Spin blood at 450 × *g* for 15 min at 4 °C. Pipet out plasma and pool in 50 mL conical tubes. Avoid disturbing the white buffy coat cells on top of the packed red cells. Note the volumes of plasma and total blood.

4. To the plasma, add Ca^{2+}-Mg^{2+} solution (in mL) calculated by the empirical formula: 8.4 × plasma volume/total plasma plus red blood cell volume. Incubate plasma at 37 °C. If no clotting occurs after 1 h, add increments of 0.2 mL of Ca^{2+}-Mg^{2+} solution and continue the incubation. Centrifuge at 1400 × *g* for 30 min at 4 °C. Defibrinated plasma is aliquoted and stored at −20 °C. Use this plasma as 70% autologous plasma (*see* **Note 5**).
5. Pool the blood in a 500 mL sterile bottle. Add cold PBS to 420 mL.
6. Pipet 12 mL of Ficoll-Paque into each of the twelve 50 mL conical polypropylene tubes (Falcon 2070, B-D). Gently overlay the Ficoll-Paque with 35 mL of diluted blood.
7. Centrifuge at 1400 × *g* at 15 °C for 20 min.
8. Pipet out interface cells with a plugged Pasteur pipet into 50 mL conical tubes. Dilute cells at least twofold with cold PBS. Spin cells down at 200 × *g* at 4 °C for 10 min.
9. Suction off supernatant. Pool all the cells into one 50 mL conical tube with cold PBS and fill to a final volume of 50 mL. Spin cells down again.
10. Resuspend cells in 5 mL cold PBS. Count a 20× diluted aliquot of cells with a hemocytometer.

3.2 Isolation of $CD14^+$ Monocytes and MDC Derivation (See Note 6)

1. Transfer the washed PBMC to an 8 mL round-bottom tube (Falcon 2027). Wash original tube with 2 mL cold PBS and pool all the cells. Spin cells down at 200 × *g* at 4 °C for 10 min.
2. Resuspend cells in 4 mL cold complete medium. Add 80 μg purified anti-CD14 mAb 63D3. Rotate in the cold for 30 min (*see* **Note** 7).
3. Spin cells down. Wash cells twice in cold PBS.
4. To the cell pellet add 50 μL heat-inactivated plasma, 50 μL PBS/BSA/EDTA, and 80 μL goat-anti-mouse IgG magnetic microbead. Incubate in the refrigerator for 15 min.
5. Mount a LS column on a VarioMACS assembly, and wash with 5 mL cold PBS/BSA/EDTA. Add 0.5 mL cold autologous heat-inactivated plasma to block nonspecific binding (*see* **Note 8**).
6. To the magnetic bead-treated cells, add 1 mL cold PBS/BSA/EDTA and load the cells to the LS column with a plugged Pasteur pipet. Wash tubes and pipet with 0.5 mL PBS/BSA/EDTA solution. Wait until all the cells have drained into the column. Load the wash solution. Collect the flow-through cells with an 8 mL tube. Repeat washing with 2 mL aliquots of PBS/BSA/EDTA solution until the tube is filled.

7. Push the cells out from the bottom of the column with a syringe connected to the column by a sterile three-way stopcock. Use three 2 mL portions of PBS/BSA/EDTA. Pipet cells out from the top of the column with a Pasteur pipet each time and pool the $CD14^+$ cells (*see* **Note 9**).
8. Count cells and culture $CD14^+$ monocytes in complete medium supplemented with 50 ng/mL GM-CSF, 50 ng/mL IL-4 at 1×10^6 cells/mL, and 4 mL/well in 6-well plates (Falcon 3046).
9. At the end of 4 days refeed cells by taking out 2 mL of medium and adding 2 mL of fresh medium containing GM-CSF and IL-4 (*see* **Note 10**).

3.3 T-Cell Purification for Ag-Specific Responses

In this section, Ag-specific response measurements using T cells purified from PBMC from the second donation by negative selection and MDC from the first donation are described.

1. Seven days after the first blood donation, collect another 200 mL blood from the same donor. Process cells and plasma as in the first collection (*see* Subheading 3.1).
2. After the cells are fractionated through the separation column into $CD14^+$ monocytes and $CD14^-$ PBMC (*see* Subheading 3.2), the $CD14^+$ cells are incubated in complete medium with GM-CSF and IL-4 for MDC generation for restimulation in T-cell cytokine production studies (*see* Subheading 3.5).
3. T cells are purified from the $CD14^-$ cell fraction by negative selection. Resuspend the cells in 1 mL complete medium. Add anti-CD19, anti-CD56, anti-CD13, and anti-CD83 mAb to a final concentration of 20 μg/mL. Rotate the cells in the cold room for 30 min.
4. Wash cells twice with PBS/BSA/EDTA and resuspend the cell pellet in 50 μL autologous heat-inactivated plasma, 50 μL PBS/BSA/EDTA, and 80 μL goat-anti-mouse IgG magnetic microbeads. Incubate in the refrigerator for 15 min.
5. Load cells in a LS column and select magnetic microbead-bound cells with a VarioMACS sorting assembly. Collect the flow-through T cells and wash columns as in Subheading 3.2, **step 6**. Count the T cells.

3.4 MDC Ag Presentation in T-Cell Proliferation

1. Detach MDC with a Pasteur pipet. Wash twice with PBS and resuspend in complete medium at 1×10^6 cells/mL (*see* **Note 11**).
2. Resuspend purified T cells at 2×10^6 cells/mL in complete medium. To 96-well plates (Falcon 3072) add 100 μL of T cells into quadruplicate wells.

3. Add graded number of monocyte-derived DC at T:DC ratios of 1000:1, 300:1, 100:1, 30:1, and 10:1 in a final volume of 50 μL complete medium. Add allergen to 10 μg/mL in 50 μL medium.
4. For allergen dose–response studies, use a T:DC ratio of 10:1 and add graded amounts of allergen from 0.1 μg/mL to 10 μg/mL. For the measurement of T-cell responses to overlapping Der p 2 peptides, 4 μL of 1 mM peptides were added to give a final of 20 μM peptide.
5. Include negative and positive controls. Negative control wells contain no Ag. Positive control wells contain 3 μg/mL tetanus toxoid or 20 μg/mL PHA.
6. Incubate the plates for a total of 5 days. At the end of the incubation period, add 50 μL [^{3}H]-thymidine (20 μCi/mL, 6.7 Ci/mmole; New England Nuclear, Boston, MA) and pulse cells for 8 h.
7. Harvest cells by a multi-well cell harvester and count [^{3}H]-thymidine incorporation in a scintillation counter.

3.5 T-Cell Ag-Specific Cytokine Production

1. Resuspend purified T cells at 4 × 10^6/mL. To 16 mm wells in 24-well plates (Falcon 3047), add 250 μL T cells.
2. Add 100 μL of 0.5 × 10^6/mL MDC.
3. To each of the wells add 100 μL graded amounts of allergens (0.3–10 μg/mL final concentration) or 100 μL of 0.1 mM peptide in duplicate and add medium (50 μL) to make the final volume 500 μL. Incubate cells for 7 days.
4. At the end of 7 days, add 1.5 mL of RPMI 1640 to each well to wash. Centrifuge the 24-well plates in microtiter plate carriers at 150 × *g* at 4 °C for 5 min. Pipet out 1.6 mL supernatant carefully with a 1 mL pipetman.
5. Repeat washing and pipet out 1.6 mL supernatant again. Add 100 μL of 0.5 × 10^6/mL fresh DC, 100 μL of fresh Ag, and 10 μL of rIL-2 (2500 U/mL). Incubate cells for 48 h for IL-4 and 72 h for IL-5 and IFN-γ production measurements.

3.6 Assay of Th1 and Th2 Cytokines in Supernatants of Stimulated T Cells by ELISA

1. Coat Nunc Maxisorp plates with 50 μL of 2 μg/mL anti-huIFN-γ, anti-huIL-4, or anti-huIL-5 capture mAb in 0.1 M sodium bicarbonate solution, pH 8.2, at 4 °C overnight.
2. Wash plate three times with PBS/Tween.
3. Add 250 μL of 5% BSA in PBS/Tween to block plates for 2 h at room temperature.
4. Spin down debris in cell supernatants in a microfuge at 12,000 × *g* for 15 min at 4 °C.

5. Dilute supernatants at 3×, 10×, 30×, and 100× for IFN-γ and IL-5 measurements. Use undiluted supernatants for IL-4 measurements.
6. Prepare standard curves for cytokines by making 200 μL for each dilution of 3, 1, 0.3, 0.1, and 0.03 ng/mL of standard cytokine in complete medium.
7. Wash plates three times with PBS/Tween. Add 50 μL supernatants or cytokine standard in duplicates for each dilution. Cover plates with plastic wrap. Incubate at room temperature for 2 h.
8. Discard supernatants and wash plates three times with PBS/Tween.
9. Add 50 μL of 0.2 μg/mL biotinylated detecting anti-huIFN-γ, anti-huIL-4, or anti-huIL-5 mAb. Cover plates with plastic wrap. Incubate at room temperature for 2 h.
10. Wash plates three times with PBS-Tween. Add 1:5000 diluted streptavidin-HRP for 1 h.
11. Wash plates three times, add 100 μL of substrate solution, and incubate for 15 min at room temperature (*see* **Note 12**).
12. Add 50 μL 3 N HCl to stop the reaction. Measure absorbance at 590 nm.

4 Notes

1. T-cell proliferative responses to the presentation of tetanus toxoid or diphtheria toxoid by MDC derived from adherent cells [15] or low-density Percoll-fractionated monocytes [17] are shown in Fig. 1. MDC from adherent cells and Perçoll-purified monocytes comprised only 70% and 85% of the total cell population, respectively. The small contaminating lymphocytes could not be purified from the MDC easily by magnetic depletion. Ag presentation of these MDC is compared with that by E^- cells (Fig. 1), and can be compared with that by MDC from $CD14^+$ monocytes shown in reference [16]. T-cell IFN-γ or IL-5 production in response to MDC presentation of either protein Ag (Der p 2) or Ag peptides is shown in Fig. 2.
2. Human blood monocytes are exquisitely sensitive to endotoxin stimulation. Solutions are prepared from endotoxin-free water and stored in endotoxin-free containers. Glass bottles and heat-resistant caps are baked overnight at 180 °C before use.
3. Avoid repeated freezing and thawing of cytokines and always dilute cytokines in serum-containing solutions to avoid cytokine denaturation.

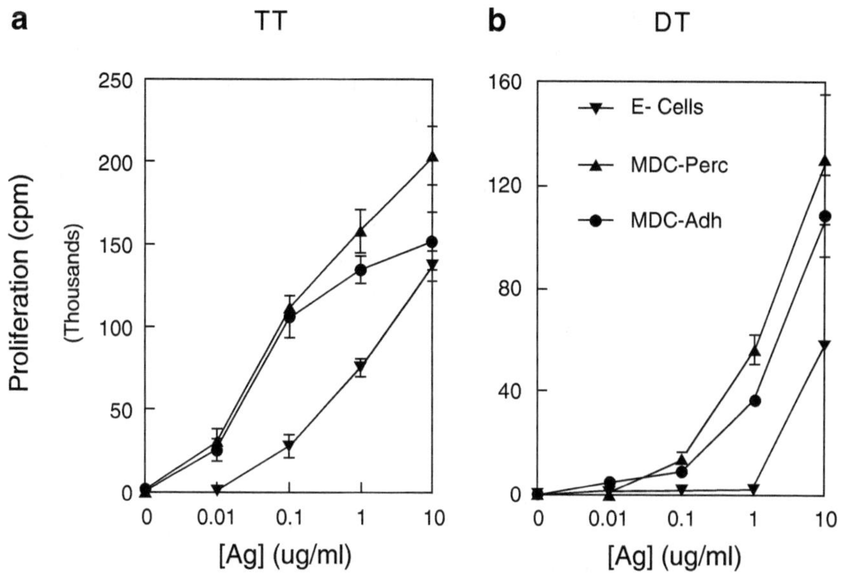

Fig. 1 T-cell proliferation in response to graded doses of Ag presented by MDC. T-cell proliferation was performed as described in Methods. MDC were cultured from Percoll-purified low-density monocytes [17] (MDC-Perc), or from the adherent cells in PBMC [15] (MDC-Adh). The Ag presentation of MDC was also compared with that by sheep erythrocyte-negative non-T cells (E^- cells) added at 6×10^4 cells/well. The Ag used were tetanus toxoid in (**a**) and diphtheria toxoid in (**b**)

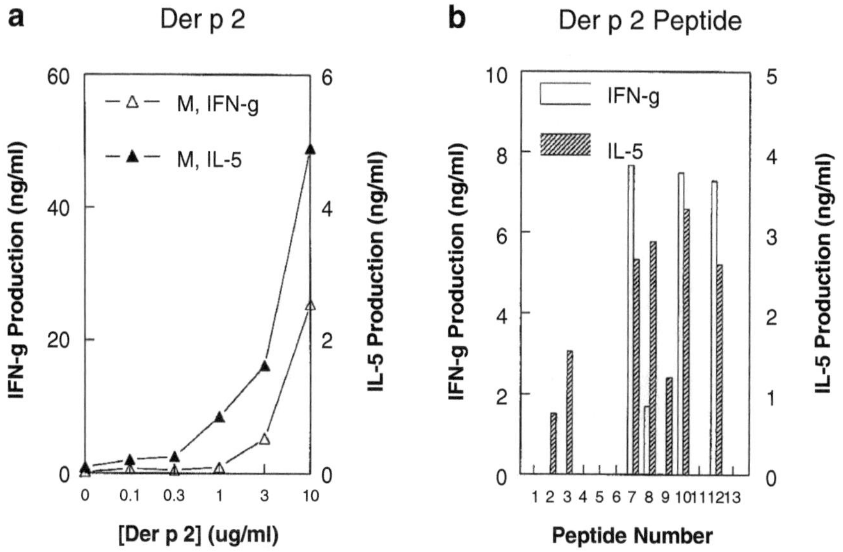

Fig. 2 IFN-γ and IL-5 production by T cells stimulated with house dust mite allergen Der p 2 or Der p 2 peptides. Purified T cells were stimulated with Der p 2 (**a**) or Der p 2 overlapping 20 mer peptides (**b**) as described in Methods. MDC from $CD14^+$ monocytes were used as the APC. The results are representative of four experiments from the same individual

4. The method described is designed for the collection of two blood donations of 200 mL each over a period of 8 days. Volunteers participating in this protocol donate blood for the maximum of eight experiments per year, with 400 mL blood donated per experiment. The method can be scaled down for less blood collected, in which case yellow cap (ACD-A) 8 mL vacutainer tubes (B-D) can be used.
5. Autologous plasma is used for lower background proliferation and cytokine production. The Ca^{2+}-Mg^{2+} solution used to defibrinate the plasma should be kept at minimal amounts. Excessive amount of Ca^{2+} in plasma will lead to the precipitation of $Ca_3(PO_4)_2$ upon culture. Plasma from blood group AB normal volunteers has also been used with good results. CPD-plasma can be obtained from blood banks (e.g., Virginia Blood Service, Richmond, VA). The plasma is defibrinated by the addition of 1 mL of 2 M $CaCl_2$ solution and allowed to coagulate as in autologous plasma. The clot is spun at 1200 × g and the plasma is saved for DC and T-cell cultures.
6. The key to the isolation of pure $CD14^+$ monocytes is to block nonspecific binding on columns with plasma, keep the column washing solution cold and deaerated, and incubate the mAb-coated cells with goat-anti-mouse IgG magnetic microbead at refrigerator temperatures with minimal bead volumes of 20%.
7. Hybridoma supernatants at 1:2 dilution can be used instead of purified mAb.
8. It is important to heat-inactivate the plasma or serum used with magnetic microbead-coated cells. Otherwise the beads which are made of dextran may activate complement by the lectin pathway, resulting in cell killing.
9. It is more efficient to push positively selected cells out from the bottom of the separation column than to allow the cells to drip from the column, especially when the columns are partially clogged.
10. More frequent feeding with cytokines may increase MDC yield.
11. In DC activated with stimulants such as LPS, many DC become adherent. This is minimized by plating the cells in non-treated 6-well plate (BD351146) before activation. After retrieving the nonadherent cells, the adherent cells are incubated in 4 mL of PBS with 10 mM EDTA on ice for 30 min. The cells are detached by pipetting and pooled with the nonadherent cells for subsequent assays.
12. The color development time can be varied so as to obtain the optimal absorbance readings.

References

1. Qu C, Brinck-Jensen NS, Zang M, Chen K (2014) Monocyte-derived dendritic cells: targets as potent antigen-presenting cells for the design of vaccines against infectious diseases. Int J Infect Dis 19:1–5
2. van de Ven R, Lindenberg JJ, Oosterhoff D, de Gruijl TD (2013) Dendritic cell plasticity in tumor-conditioned skin: CD14 cells at the cross-roads of immune activation and suppression. Front Immunol 4:403
3. Steinman RM (2007) Dendritic cells: understanding immunogenicity. Eur J Immunol 37:S53–S60
4. Villadangos JA, Schnorrer P (2007) Intrinsic and cooperative antigen-presenting functions of dendritic-cell subsets in vivo. Nat Rev Immunol 7:543–555. https://doi.org/10.1038/nri2103
5. Dzionek A, Fuchs A, Schmidt P, Cremer S, Zysk M, Miltenyi S et al (2000) BDCA-2, BDCA-3, and BDCA-4: three markers for distinct subsets of dendritic cells in human peripheral blood. J Immunol 165:6037–6046
6. Bachem A, Guttler S, Hartung E, Ebstein F, Schaefer M, Tannert A et al (2010) Superior antigen cross-presentation and XCR1 expression define human CD11c+CD141+ cells as homologues of mouse CD8+ dendritic cells. J Exp Med 207:1273–1281
7. Poulin LF, Salio M, Griessinger E, Anjos-Afonso F, Craciun L, Chen JL et al (2010) Characterization of human DNGR-1+ BDCA3+ leukocytes as putative equivalents of mouse CD8alpha+ dendritic cells. J Exp Med 207:1261–1271
8. Liu K, Nussenzweig MC (2010) Origin and development of dendritic cells. Immunol Rev 234:45–54
9. Shortman K, Sathe P, Vremec D, Naik S, O'Keeffe M (2013) Plasmacytoid dendritic cell development. Adv Immunol 120:105–126
10. Cheong C, Matos I, Choi JH, Dandamudi DB, Shrestha E, Longhi MP et al (2010) Microbial stimulation fully differentiates monocytes to DC-SIGN/CD209(+) dendritic cells for immune T cell areas. Cell 143:416–429
11. Randolph GJ, Beaulieu S, Lebecque S, Steinman RM, Muller WA (1998) Differentiation of monocytes into dendritic cells in a model of transendothelial trafficking. Science 282:480–483
12. Sallusto F, Lanzavecchia A (1994) Efficient presentation of soluble antigen by cultured human dendritic cells is maintained by granulocyte/macrophage colony-stimulating factor plus interleukin 4 and downregulated by tumor necrosis factor alpha. J Exp Med 179:1109–1118
13. Dhodapkar MV, Krasovsky J, Steinman RM, Bhardwaj N (2000) Mature dendritic cells boost functionally superior CD8(+) T-cell in humans without foreign helper epitopes. J Clin Invest 105:R9–R14
14. Thurner B, Haendle I, Roder C, Dieckmann D, Keikavoussi P, Jonuleit H et al (1999) Vaccination with mage-3A1 peptide-pulsed mature, monocyte-derived dendritic cells expands specific cytotoxic T cells and induces regression of some metastases in advanced stage IV melanoma. J Exp Med 190:1669–1678
15. O'Neill DW, Adams S, Bhardwaj N (2004) Manipulating dendritic cell biology for the active immunotherapy of cancer. Blood 104:2235–2246
16. Sung SJ, Taketomi EA, Smith AM, Platts-Mills TA, Fu SM (1999) Efficient presentation of house dust mite allergen Der p 2 by monocyte-derived dendritic cells and the role of beta 2 integrins. Scand J Immunol 49:96–105
17. Rossi M, Young JW (2005) Human dendritic cells: potent antigen-presenting cells at the crossroads of innate and adaptive immunity. J Immunol 175:1373–1381

Chapter 10

The Use of Dual-Cell-Tracker Dye Staining for the Identification and Characterization of Peanut-Specific T-Cell Subsets

Cecilia Dunsterville, Alick C. Stephens, Gideon Lack, and Victor Turcanu

Abstract

Cell-tracker fluorescent dye labeling is widely used for investigating antigen-specific immune responses in vitro and in vivo. Here we describe a development of this technique—the use of dual-cell-tracker dye staining for the identification and characterization of the responses of different T-cell subsets to peanut proteins in vitro.

Key words Allergy, Flow cytometry, Cell-tracking dyes, eFluor670, CFSE, Proliferation

1 Introduction

Identification and characterization of antigen-responding cells by initial labeling with cell-tracker dyes followed by exposure to antigen in vitro or in vivo were originally established in 1990 by Parrish and his collaborators [1]. Out of the 16 fluorochromes tested, carboxyfluorescein succinimidyl ester (CFSE), which binds covalently to cellular components, could be detected up to 8 weeks after injection in mice, which made it ideal for long-term cellular migration studies.

The success of this technique led to its use in many research projects. As found in a PubMed search done on the 23rd March 2018, CFSE has been quoted between May 1990 and March 2018 in 1450 publications. The methodology, advantages, pitfalls, and troubleshooting for using CFSE have therefore been described in great detail in many protocols and methods papers [1–6]. We [7–9] and others [10–14] have applied this technology for the purpose of characterizing specific T-cell responses in a variety of experimental systems in vitro and in vivo.

Here we describe a further refinement of this well-established methodology. We first describe how to perform dual labeling with

Penny Lympany and Meinir G. Jones (eds.), *Allergy: Methods and Protocols*, Methods in Molecular Biology, vol. 2020, https://doi.org/10.1007/978-1-4939-9591-2_10,

eFluor670 and CFSE for the simultaneous characterization of the responses of the CD25+ subset and the CD25− cell subset from peripheral blood mononuclear cell (PBMC) stimulated in vitro with peanut proteins or in a mixed lymphocyte culture (MLR). Briefly, PBMCs were incubated with anti-CD25 MACS beads and then passed through a column to separate the CD25+ and CD25− subsets, respectively. The CD25+ cell subset that comprises the regulatory T cells (Tregs) was labeled with eFluor670 whereas the CD25-depleted cells were labeled with CFSE. The two subsets were then remixed to reconstitute the original PBMC population and set in culture with peanut proteins or an MLR. Thus, the two cell-tracker dyes were used to simultaneously monitor the responses of the populations containing Tregs and effector T cells.

We assessed the loss of fluorescence of dividing cells in order to identify them and measure their proliferative responses as the percentages of CFSElow and eFluor670 low cells, respectively [13–15], corrected for cell death in culture as described below. The ability to simultaneously monitor the allergen-specific responses of T effectors and T regulators in a PBMC culture could be useful for studies of allergen-specific immunotherapy. Indeed specific immunotherapy (SIT) by the administration of allergens was shown to achieve desensitization and/or a level of progression toward immunological tolerance in some allergic patients. The underlying mechanism seems to involve the induction of Tregs, which appear to be very heterogeneous and comprise several phenotypes with different mechanisms of action [16]. Therefore the use of multiple labeling with cell-tracker dyes gives us the ability to identify and monitor the allergen-driven responses of distinct T-cell subsets from the PBMC.

Dual-dye labeling also gives us the possibility to put together two PBMC populations in a culture, e.g., by mixing PBMC isolated from the same donor but collected at different time points (e.g., pre-immunotherapy and post immunotherapy) and then stimulating with allergen in order to monitor the distinct responses of the two populations and the interactions between them.

A significant difficulty in using this system is the high level of apoptosis during culture that affects PBMC from pediatric populations that contain proportionally more naïve T cells than PBMC from older donors [17, 18]. Indeed, in vitro culture of unstimulated PBMC from healthy control children was reported to induce more than 25% apoptosis of CD4+ T cells and more than 30% apoptosis of CD3+ T cells, respectively, within the first 72 h [19]. In order to correct for the level of cell death during the culture, we used Count Standard Beads (Countbright counting beads) as described in the literature [20, 21]. Briefly, as advised by Parish and Walden who originally established the CFSE technique, adding a known number of counting beads to the sample prior to collection on the flow cytometer allows subsequent enumeration of cells in individual CFSE peaks [20]. Adding a set number of internal bead standards (e.g., 25,000 beads per 250 μL of culture) can be used to correct for cell death during the 7-day culture. Thus, acquiring (1) a day-0 sample of 250 μL of culture containing PBMC and 25,000 beads and (2) a day-7 sample of the same volume containing the surviving PBMC and the same number of 25,000 beads allows to correct for the cell death during culture. This is important if the CFSElow population is used to calculate the percentage of cells from the original population that had divided, because in the absence of a correction for cell death of nonspecific T cells the precursor frequency would be overestimated.

In addition to proliferation, intracellular cytokine staining of the CFSE-labeled cells allows for the characterization of their cytokine production phenotype as we show below. Modern multicolor flow cytometers allow for the simultaneous detection of many cytokines in a single tube. This avoids splitting the PBMC into multiple aliquots, which is important in order to collect a relevant minimum number of events specific for the assay [22] especially when working with small cell numbers with low allergen-specific Th counts, such as the case of pediatric studies.

Overall, our results of characterizing peanut allergen-specific responses in vitro are similar to those described in the literature [23, 24] and outline the usefulness of the eFluor670 and/or CFSE labeling approach, for characterizing allergen-specific responses in vitro.

2 Materials

1. Peripheral blood mononuclear cells (PBMCs).
2. Histopaque 1077 (e.g., Hybri-Max #H8889 from Sigma-Aldrich).
3. Fetal calf serum (FCS).
4. Culture medium: RPMI 1640, containing HEPES, penicillin, streptomycin, and 10% fetal calf serum (FCS).
5. Buffer 1: PBS, 1% FCS, and 0.1% NaN_3.
6. Culture plates (24-, 48-, or 96-well plates).
7. Peanut defatted extract 20 mg/mL, dissolved in culture medium.
8. DMSO (e.g., Hybri-Max #D2650 from Sigma-Aldrich).
9. eFluor670 (catalog number 650840 from eBioscience).
10. CFSE (catalog number C1157 from Molecular Probes).
11. Anti-CD4, anti-CD3, anti-CD45RA, anti-CD45RO, anti-annexin V, etc. antibodies for cell surface staining.

12. Anti-interferon gamma, anti-IL-4, IL-5, IL-13, etc. antibodies for intracellular staining and a live/dead fixable dye (e.g., Aqua, L34957 from Thermo Fisher).
13. 50 ng/mL PMA (e.g., #P8139 from Sigma-Aldrich).
14. 1 mg/mL Ionomycin (e.g., #I0634 from Sigma-Aldrich).
15. 10 mg/mL Brefeldin A (e.g., #B6542 from Sigma-Aldrich).
16. Countbright counting beads (e.g., FCSC580 from Serotec, or CaliBRITE or Flow-Count beads as in ref. [20] or TruCount beads as described in ref. [21]).
17. FACS tubes (e.g., BD Falcon 5 mL polystyrene #352054).
18. IntraPrep Permeabilization kit (e.g., from Beckman Coulter, # A07803, containing reagent 1 (fixative) and reagent 2 (permeabilization buffer)).
19. 4% Paraformaldehyde dissolved in PBS, pH 7.4.
20. Phosphate-buffered salt solution without calcium and magnesium (PBS, e.g., Life Technologies #10010-015).
21. FACS Flow buffer (e.g., #342003 from Becton Dickinson).
22. CD25 MicroBeads II for MACS (e.g., #130-092-983 from Miltenyi Biotec).
23. Flow cytometer (e.g., FACS Canto).

3 Methods

3.1 PBMC Culturing, Proliferation Dyes

1. Separate PBMCs from anticoagulated blood using Histopaque 1077 and store the cells frozen in liquid nitrogen or use immediately for culture.
2. Thaw frozen PBMC in a 37 °C water bath. Dilute the freezing medium slowly using PBS+ 20% FCS. Wash the cells by centrifugation (10 min, 300 × *g*).
3. Use whole PBMC or separate into the CD25+ and CD25− populations by MACS (Fig. 1a, b) as detailed below (*see* Subheading 3.5).
4. Resuspend the cell populations (e.g., CD25+ and CD25-depleted PBMC, respectively) in 1 mL PBS at 10^6/mL and label with the cell-tracking dye (eFluor670 or CFSE) at 1 μM final concentration for 10 min in the dark at 37 °C (*see* **Note 1**).
5. After 10-min incubation, dilute unbound eFluor670 or CFSE in 50 mL PBS+ 20% FCS and wash the cells by centrifugation (10 min, 300 × *g*).
6. Resuspend the eFluor670-labeled cells in medium supplemented with 5% autologous plasma. Mix them with the CFSE-labeled cells in order to reconstitute the original PBMC and distribute to cell culture plates.

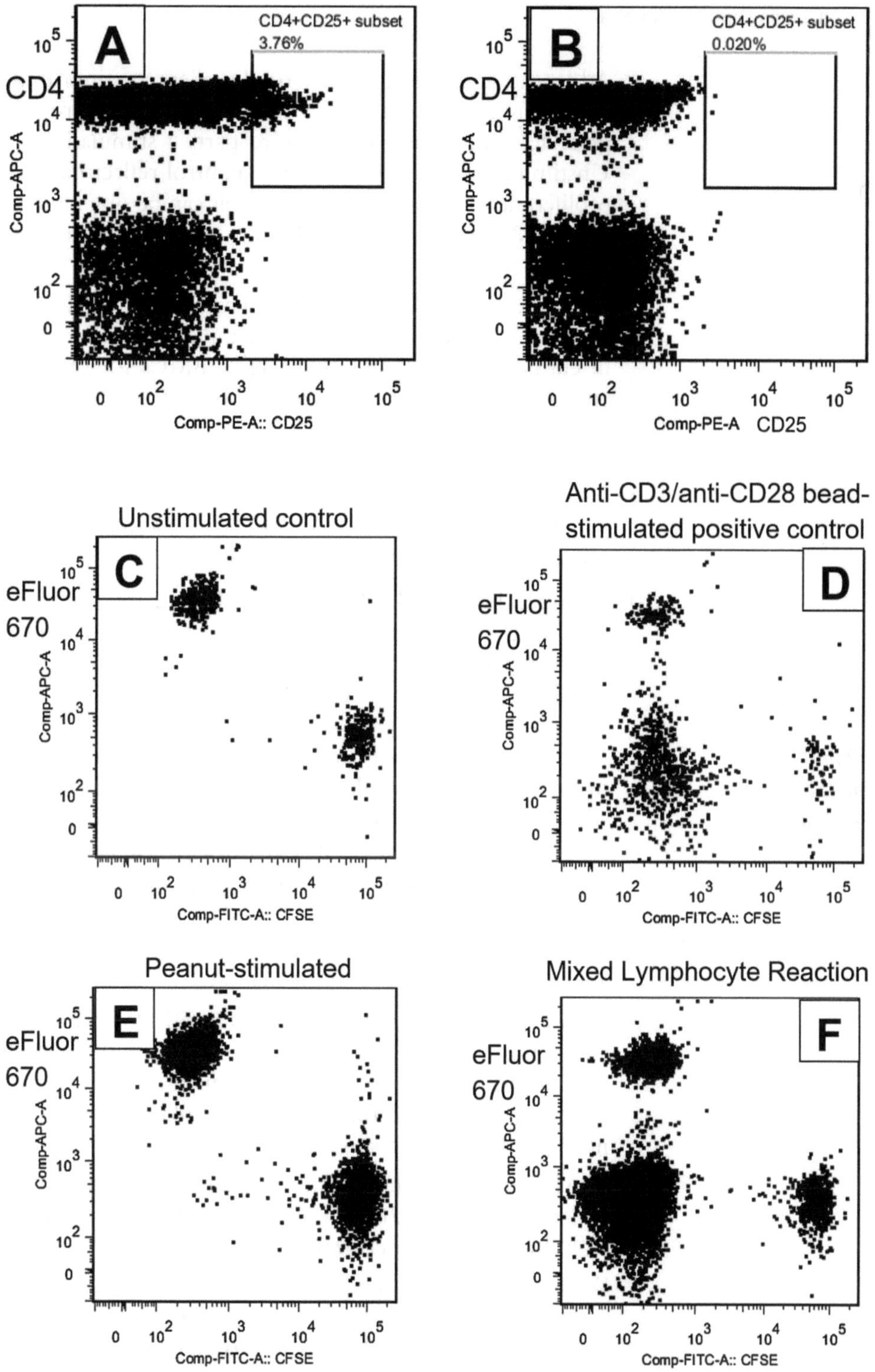

Fig. 1 Using dual-CFSE and -eFluor670 staining to track cell proliferation in vitro. The CD25+ population containing Treg population was separated from PBMC by MACS (**a**, **b**). The CD25+ population was stained with the eFluor670 cell-tracking dye whereas the CD25-depleted PBMCs were stained with CFSE. The initial PBMC population was then reconstituted by mixing the two populations and left unstimulated (**c**), stimulated with anti-CD3/anti-CD28 beads (**d**), cultured in the presence of peanut antigens (**e**), or stimulated in an MLR (**f**). Dual labeling allows for the tracking of different Th cell subsets and analysis of their distinct proliferation profiles

7. Add peanut defatted extract to the allergen-stimulated well (final concentration 200 μg peanut/mL) and set mixed lymphocyte reactions with third-party stimulating cells. Unstimulated PBMCs as negative control reflect background proliferation whereas positive controls can be obtained adding anti-CD3/anti-CD28 stimulating beads or mitogens (*see* **Note 2**).
8. Collect 250 μL PBMC separately when setting up the cultures to assess day-0 eFluor670 labeling and long-term cell viability in culture. Transfer these collected PBMCs to a FACS tube and wash with 4 mL PBS (5 min, 600 × *g*). Resuspend the pellet in 50 μL PBS, stain with 5 μL of anti-CD4 and other antibodies for 30 min, and wash.
9. Resuspend the pellet in 200 μL PBS and then add 200 μL paraformaldehyde (4%) to the tubes. Fix the cells for 20 min at RT and then wash with 3 mL PBS + 2% FCS.
10. Resuspend the fixed cells in 1 mL PBS + 2%FCS and store at 4 °C in the dark until analysis, when 25 μL of Countbright counting beads (from the stock of one million beads/mL) should be added, just before acquisition by FACS.

3.2 PBMC Restimulation and Fixation

1. After 7 days, mix the PBMC cultures well and collect 250 μL from the peanut-stimulated, from the negative (no antigen added) control and the positive control (control antigen or mitogen-stimulated) wells in order to determine proliferation.
2. Transfer the collected PBMC to a FACS tube, wash with 4 mL PBS (5 min, 600 g), and stain with 5 μL of anti-CD4 PE for 1 h. Fix cells with paraformaldehyde (20 min at RT as described above) and store at 4 °C until analysis.
3. Optional: Restimulate the cells for 6 h with PMA (50 ng/mL) and ionomycin (1 μg/mL) in the presence of brefeldin A (10 μg/mL) to induce cytokine production. This step is necessary for the characterization of the cytokine production phenotypes of allergen-responding T cells.
4. PBMC are collected, washed, and resuspended in 50 μL PBS, and then fixed for 20 min at RT with 0.1 mL of reagent 1 from the IntraPrep Permeabilization kit.
5. Wash using 3 mL buffer 1 (5 min, 600 × *g*), then resuspend in 1 mL buffer 1, and store at 4 °C overnight before permeabilization and FACS. 25 μL of Countbright counting beads (from the stock of one million beads/mL) should be added, just before acquisition by FACS, per/250 μL of cell culture volume harvested, in order to normalize the cell counts to account for cell death in the 7-day culture [18, 19].

3.3 PBMC Intracellular Staining and FACS

1. Wash the fixed cells (5 min, 600 × *g*). Resuspend the cells in 0.2 mL permeabilization buffer (Reagent 2 from the IntraPrep Permeabilization kit) for 5 min at RT.
2. Cells are then distributed in the FACS tubes for staining with the different antibody cocktails and incubated for 40 min (final staining volume 65 μL).
3. The cells are washed in 4 mL PBS (5 min, 600 × *g*), resuspended in FACS Flow, and analyzed on the flow cytometer.

3.4 Precursor T Helper Cell Frequency Assessment

The percentage of peanut-responding CD4+ eFluor670low (or CD4+ CFSElow) can be determined by gating the appropriate cell population (Fig. 2c, d). The peanut-specific T helper cell precursor frequency can be further calculated by deconvoluting the eFluor670 low population having undergone at least one division and correcting for the level of cell death that occurred in culture using the cell count beads [5]. Thus, for example, 25 μL of Countbright counting beads can be added and at least 20,000 live PBMCs should be acquired using the flow cytometer on the day of setting the cultures (day 0) and on the day of collecting the allergen-stimulated cultures (usually day 7), but possibly varying for different other allergens that drive earlier proliferation. A small eFluor670 low population may emerge in addition to the Th effectors which have proliferated in the presence of the peanut antigen (Fig. 1e).

3.5 Characterization of Antigen-Specific Responses of Two Distinct Populations

In order to characterize the activity of the allergen-specific T effector cells and, distinctly, of the CD25+ cell population containing the T-regulatory cells (T-reg), we separated the CD25+ cells by MACS from PBMC and stained them with eFluor670. For the MACS separation, the CD25 MicroBeads II should be used according to the manufacturer's protocol (Fig. 1a, b).

1. Stain the separated CD25+ cells with eFluor670 as described above and wash.
2. Label the CD25− MACS column effluent with CFSE, wash, and then mix with the eFluor670-labeled CD25+ cells in order to reconstitute the original PBMC population.
3. Culture in the presence of 200 μg/mL peanut proteins, in an MLR or with anti-CD3/anti-CD28 stimulating beads.
4. Dual labeling allows for the tracking of different cell subsets and analysis of their distinct proliferation profiles. A similar approach can be used to monitor individual responses in MLR or mixed pre/post-SIT lymphocyte reactions if these are used as experimental models in order to investigate immune responses in vitro (Fig. 2c–f).

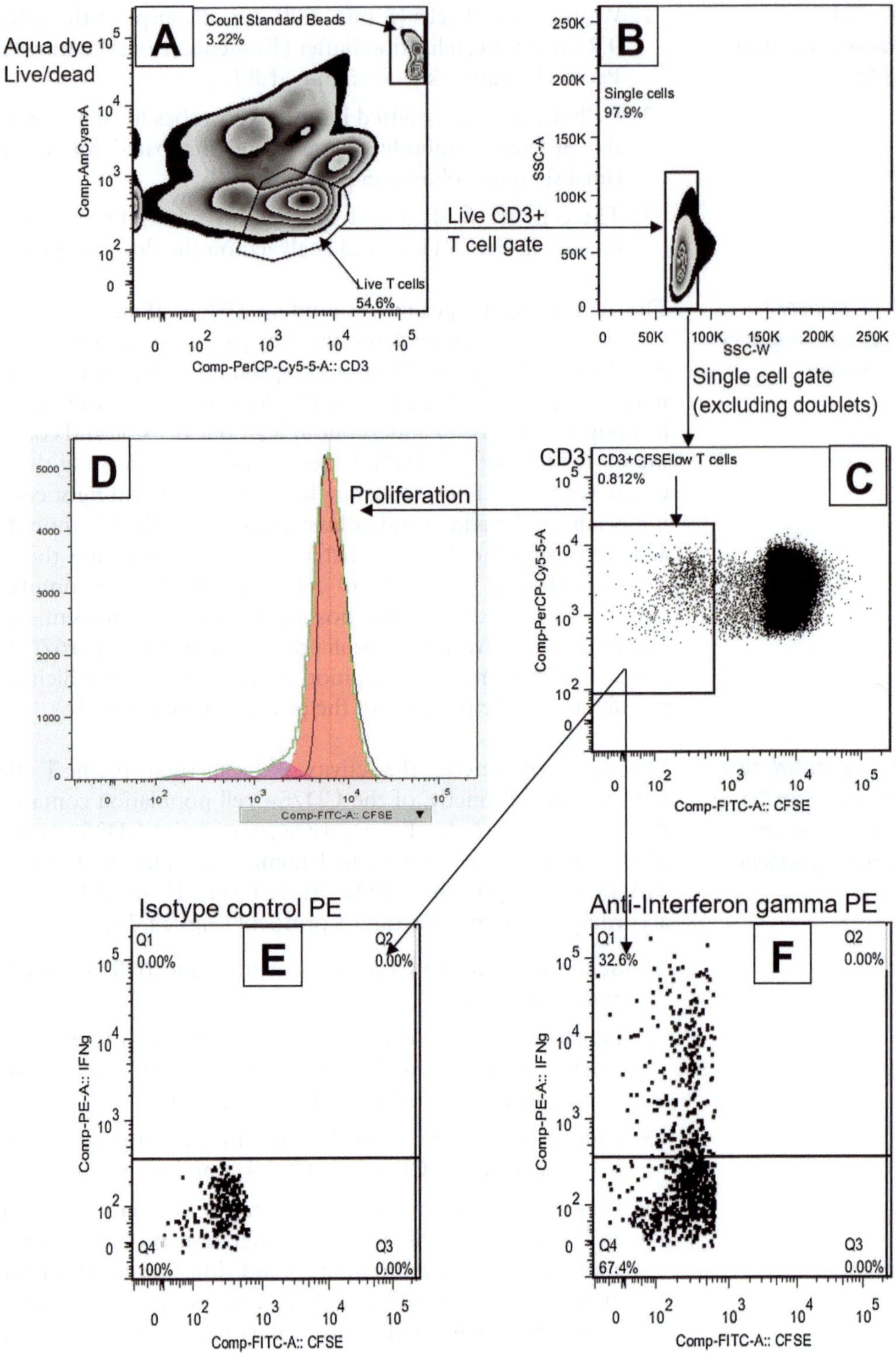

Fig. 2 Characterization of peanut-specific responses in vitro. PBMCs from one donor were stained with CFSE and cultured in the presence of peanut proteins as described. Single, live CD3+ T cells were gated and proliferation as well as cytokine production were determined in the CFSElow population that responded to the allergen stimulation in vitro

4 Notes

1. eFluor670 is dissolved in DMSO to obtain a stock solution with a final concentration of 1 mM. 10 μL of the stock solution is distributed per aliquot into 1 mL Eppendorf tubes that should be stored at −20 °C. Just before labeling, the eFluor670 is removed from the freezer and the stock solution is diluted by adding 990 μL PBS. 10 μL of this fluorochrome working solution is then transferred to the 1 mL PBMC preparation to be labeled in order to achieve a 1 μM final concentration. Working solutions should be discarded after staining. Depending upon the expected intensity of proliferation, higher or lower concentrations may be used, as determined by titration.
2. PBMC can be separated from anticoagulated blood or leukocyte concentrates. For the experiments shown here, blood was collected in accordance with the REC approvals 10/H0802/45 or 11/LO/0123. Peanut allergy was diagnosed as previously described [25]. Positive controls (mitogens or control antigens such as tetanus toxoid or PPD) can be used to prove the proliferative potential of the PBMC. Indeed, the absence of allergen-specific proliferation in the peanut-stimulated cultures and/or high levels of spontaneous cell death in culture (as described for PBMC isolated from children in references [17–19]) may reflect the absence of a memory allergen-specific response rather than poor cell responsiveness.

Acknowledgments

This work was supported by the National Peanut Board, USA. The authors acknowledge financial support from the Department of Health via the National Institute for Health Research (NIHR) comprehensive Biomedical Research Centre award to Guy's & St Thomas' NHS Foundation Trust in partnership with King's College London and King's College Hospital NHS Foundation Trust.

References

1. Weston SA, Parish CR (1990) New fluorescent dyes for lymphocyte migration studies. Analysis by flow cytometry and fluorescence microscopy. J Immunol Methods 133:87–97
2. Lyons AB, Parish CR (1994) Determination of lymphocyte division by flow cytometry. J Immunol Methods 171:131–137
3. Hawkins ED, Hommel M, Turner ML et al (2007) Measuring lymphocyte proliferation, survival and differentiation using CFSE time-series data. Nat Protoc 2:2057–2067
4. Quah BJC, Warren HS, Parish CR (2007) Monitoring lymphocyte proliferation in vitro and in vivo with the intracellular fluorescent dye carboxyfluorescein diacetate succinimidyl ester. Nat Protoc 2:2049–2056
5. Parish CR, Glidden MH, Quah BJ et al (2009) Use of the intracellular fluorescent dye CFSE

to monitor lymphocyte migration and proliferation. Curr Protoc Immunol 84:1–4.9.13

6. Quah BJ, Parish CR (2012) New and improved methods for measuring lymphocyte proliferation in vitro and in vivo using CFSE-like fluorescent dyes. J Immunol Methods 379:1–14
7. Turcanu V, Maleki SJ, Lack G (2003) Characterization of lymphocyte responses to peanuts in normal children, peanut-allergic children, and allergic children who acquired tolerance to peanuts. J Clin Investig 111: 1065–1072
8. Turcanu V, Winterbotham M, Kelleher P et al (2008) Peanut-specific B and T cell responses are correlated in peanut-allergic but not in non-allergic individuals. Clin Exp Allergy 38:1132–1139
9. Turcanu V, Stephens AC, Chan SM et al (2010) IgE-mediated facilitated antigen presentation underlies higher immune responses in peanut allergy. Allergy 65:1274–1281
10. Tsuge I, Kondo Y, Tokuda R et al (2006) Allergen-specific helper T cell response in patients with cow's milk allergy: Simultaneous analysis of proliferation and cytokine production by carboxyfluorescein succinimidyl ester dilution assay. Clin Exp Allergy 36:1538–1545
11. Bosco A, McKenna KL, Devitt CJ et al (2006) Identification of novel Th2-associated genes in T memory responses to allergens. J Immunol 176:4766–4777
12. Yates A, Chan C, Strid J et al (2007) Reconstruction of cell population dynamics using CFSE. BMC Bioinformatics 8:196
13. Semmrich M, Plantinga M, Svensson-Frej M et al (2012) Directed antigen targeting in vivo identifies a role for CD103 + dendritic cells in both tolerogenic and immunogenic T-cell responses. Mucosal Immunol 5:150–160
14. Cerovic V, Houston SA, Scott CL et al (2013) Intestinal CD103—dendritic cells migrate in lymph and prime effector T cells. Mucosal Immunol 6:104–113
15. Sicherer SH, Munoz-Furlong A, Godbold JH et al (2010) US prevalence of self-reported peanut, tree nut, and sesame allergy: 11-year follow-up. J Allergy Clin Immunol 125: 1322–1326
16. Duhen T, Duhen R, Lanzavecchia A et al (2012) Functionally distinct subsets of human FOXP3+ Treg cells that phenotypically mirror effector Th cells. Blood 119:4430–4440
17. Thornton CA, Upham JW, Wikstrom ME et al (2004) Functional maturation of CD4_CD25_ CTLA4_CD45RA_ T regulatory cells in human neonatal T cell responses to environmental antigens/allergens. J Immunol 173:3084–3092
18. Law HKW, Tu W, Liu E et al (2008) Insulin-like growth factor I promotes cord blood T cell maturation through monocytes and inhibits their apoptosis in part through interleukin-6. BMC Immunol 9:74
19. Di Carlo P, Casuccio A, Romano A et al (2011) Lymphocyte apoptosis in children with central nervous system tuberculosis: a case control study. BMC Pediatr 11:108
20. Parris CR, Warren HS (2001) Use of the intracellular fluorescent dye CFSE to monitor lymphocyte migration and proliferation. Curr Protoc Immunol 4:4.9.1–4.9.10
21. Roederer M (2008) How many events is enough? Are you positive? Cytometry A 73A: 384–385
22. Fiebig EW, Johnson DK, Hirschkorn DF et al (1997) Lymphocyte subset analysis on frozen whole blood. Cytometry 29:340–350
23. Higgins JA, Lamb JR, Lake RA et al (1995) Polyclonal and clonal analysis of human CD4+ T-lymphocyte responses to nut extracts. Immunology 84:91–97
24. Flinterman AE, Pasmans SG, Den Hartog Jager CF et al (2010) T cell responses to major peanut allergens in children with and without peanut allergy. Clin Exp Allergy 40:590–597
25. Roberts G, Lack G (2005) Diagnosing peanut allergy with skin prick and specific IgE testing. J Allergy Clin Immunol 115:1291–1296

Chapter 11

The Use of pMHCII Tetramer Technology for the Identification and Characterization of CD4+ T Cells

Erik Wambre

Abstract

Understanding the mechanism underlying allergic disease is dependent upon definition of the heterogeneity and complexity of the cellular immune response toward allergens both in the context of disease and clinical intervention. Among all components of the immune system, CD4+ T cells play a key role in the orchestration of immune response toward allergen and have become a dynamic area of research. Because of their unique ability to identify antigen-specific CD4+ T cells irrespective of functional outputs, fluorescently labeled peptide–MHC class II (pMHCII) tetramers in combination with multiparameter flow cytometry have now provided an unprecedented opportunity to track and subsequently quantify and characterize rare allergen-specific CD4+ T cells at single-cell level. This chapter describes methods to use pMHCII tetramer technology for the direct visualization and characterization of antigen-specific CD4+ T cells in the allergy context.

Key words pMHCII tetramer, Magnetic cell enrichment, Allergen-specific CD4+ T cells

1 Introduction

The central role of CD4+ T cells in the orchestration of the allergic immune response provides an attractive and clinically relevant target for immunomodulation and therapy. Following activation, reactive CD4+ T cells can differentiate in many distinct T-cell subsets with distinct maturation states and function that can be identified based on the cell-surface markers expressed and/or the effector molecules they produced. Although it is well established that allergen-specific TH2 cells are key component of allergic disease, little is known about the specific nature of allergen-specific T-cell responses in the generation of a protective immune response during allergen-specific immunotherapy. In this context, there is a growing need for more precise phenotypic and functional distinction of these specialized T-cell subsets to better understand the contribution of these cells to allergic disease.

Penny Lympany and Meinir G. Jones (eds.), *Allergy: Methods and Protocols*, Methods in Molecular Biology, vol. 2020,
https://doi.org/10.1007/978-1-4939-9591-2_11,

The antigen specificity of T lymphocytes is based on recognition through the T-cell receptor (TCR) of unique antigenic peptides (epitopes) presented by MHC molecules on antigen-presenting cells (APC). Growing access to allergen T-cell epitope data through the Immune Epitope Database (IEDB) (http://www.iedb.org) [1, 2] in conjunction with recent advancement in fluorescently labeled peptide MHC class II (pMHCII) tetramer technology has now provided an adequately sensitive approach to identify and subsequently recover and characterize allergen-specific T cells at a single-cell level [3, 4]. This method relies on the highly specific interaction between peptide-loaded MHC and the corresponding T-cell receptor to directly label antigen-specific CD4+ T cells. While restricted to frequently expressed HLA class II molecules and prior knowledge of immunodominant epitopes, pMHCII tetramer has become the gold standard to assess allergen-specific CD4+ T-cell responses both in allergic and nonatopic individuals [5–8]. However, a major challenge for routine use of such antigen-specific cell-tracking dye remains the low frequency of CD4+ T cells recognizing immunodominant epitopes in peripheral blood. Two different methods of pMHCII tetramer staining are described in this chapter, the choice of which depends on the availability of starting materials and type of analysis. One method relies on an in vitro amplification step to increase the number of these rare cells prior to pMHCII tetramer staining and facilitate the analysis. This allows the investigator to recover and further study a large amount of tetramer-positive T cells with limited sample access. However, a major problem with this pre-amplification process is the potential for phenotypic changes introduced by in vitro manipulation. The alternative method relies on combining the use of pMHCII tetramers with magnetic cell enrichment technology. With this technique, cells that are labeled with the antigen-specific cell-tracking dye are enriched by magnetic beads in a magnetic field allowing direct ex vivo visualization and quantification of these cells along with confident characterization in a setting closer to their natural physiological state.

2 Materials

2.1 Patient's PBMCs

Due to polymorphisms of the immune system, patient's HLA class II restrictions must be determined before bleeding to ensure an appropriate use of the pMHCII tetramer reagent of interest. HLA class II tetramers for 30 of the most common genotypes are now available (http://www.benaroyaresearch.org/our-research/core-resources/tetramer-core-laboratory). Following study approval by the local ethics committee and written informed consent from each donor, fresh peripheral blood is taken into EDTA (typically 2 mL of 2.5% EDTA for 40–50 mL blood) or heparinized tubes (20 mL heparinized blood for 2–3 × 10^7 cells) by venipuncture. For ex vivo pMHCII/peptide tetramer procedure, the amount of blood taken from donor should be a minimum of 30 mL for allergic individuals (IgE level >3.5 kU/L) and of 50 mL for nonallergic subject (*see* **Note 1**).

2.2 Allergen-Specific T-Cell Amplification

- Antigen: In general we find that any antigen that elicits an allergen-specific CD4+ T-cell response in primary culture also elicits pMHCII tetramer staining. Relevant antigen we have used include allergen-derived peptide (13–20 amino acids), natural/recombinant allergen, and purified natural extract.
- Complete culture medium: RPMI supplemented with 2 mM L-glutamine, 100 U/mL penicillin, and 100 μg/mL streptomycin (all Life Technologies, Paisley, UK) and 10% heat-inactivated human AB serum (Sigma). The prepared medium is stored at 4 °C until use. The shelf life is 4 weeks.
- Cell incubator (37 °C, 5% CO_2, humidified atmosphere).
- Centrifuge with tube and microtiter plate carriers.
- Microscope.
- Laminar flow hood.
- Sterile repeater pipet (Jencons).
- 48-Well flat-bottom culture plates (Nunc, Fisher Scientific, Loughborough, UK).
- Recombinant IL-2 (R&D Systems, Abingdon; PeproTech, London).

2.3 Labeling with pMHCII Tetramers

- Purchase or assemble fluorescently labeled pMHCII tetramer reagent to match the peptide/MHC combinations of interest (*see* **Note 2**). Tetramers should be ~0.5 mg/mL solution (*see* **Note 3**). The pMHCII tetramers we routinely used were produced by the Tetramer Core Laboratory at the Benaroya Research Institute using insect cell culture [9].
- 5 mL Polystyrene FACS tube
- Centrifuge with tube carriers.
- Cell incubator (37 °C, 5% CO_2, humidified atmosphere).
- Dasatinib (Sigma).
- pMHCII tetramer-based enrichment,
- Anti-PE Microbeads (Miltenyi Biotec, Surrey, UK, MACS® 130-048-801).
- Running buffer (degassed): 100 mL Dulbecco's PBS (Sigma) containing 0.5% BSA and 2 mM EDTA.

- MACS separator (OctoMACS™ and MiniMACS™ separation unit).
- MACS MS columns.

2.4 Dual-Cell-Surface Abs and pMHCII Tetramer Staining for Flow Cytometry

- Dead cell exclusion Dye (e.g., Viaprobe).
- 5 mL Polystyrene FACS tubes (BD Biosciences).
- Running buffer (degassed): 100 mL Dulbecco's PBS (Sigma) containing 0.5% BSA and 2 mM EDTA.
- Fluorochrome-conjugated human antibodies suitable for use in flow cytometry.
- Isotype control antibodies.

2.5 Flow Cytometer Acquisition and Analysis

- Flow cytometer (Becton Dickinson, Cowley, Oxford, UK).
- FlowJo software (Treestar, Inc., Ashland, Ore).

3 Methods

3.1 Amplification of Allergen-Specific T Cells for In Vitro pMHCII Tetramer Analysis

Because of the intrinsic low clonal precursor frequencies, allergen-specific CD4+ T cells can be difficult to be detected on isolated PBMC. One method relies on an in vitro amplification step with either synthesized peptides or whole allergen to increase the number of these rare cells prior to pMHCII tetramer staining. This method is preferred to determine relevant peptide antigens and when HLA class II restrictions of the studied individuals are not readily available.

- Using sterile technique, plate four million live isolated PBMCs per well in a total volume of 1 mL culture media in a 48-well flat-bottom culture plate.
- Add desired antigen to each well. We recommend using the same peptide as the one loaded on pMHCII tetramer. The typical concentration for peptide stimulation is 5–10 μg/mL and for whole allergen is 50 μg/mL. For allergen extract stimulation we recommend 1–2 μL of standardized allergen extract per mL.
- Incubate plate at 37 °C, 5% CO_2. Allergen-stimulated cells develop to form clusters of proliferation.
- After 7 days, exchange half of the media with fresh medium containing 10 IU IL-2/mL. On each subsequent day, monitor cell growth using a microscope. Feed wells that are not yet confluent by removing half of the media, adding fresh media containing 10 IU IL-2/mL. Split confluent wells by resuspending the cells, moving half of the cells to an empty well,

adding fresh media containing 10 IU IL-2/mL. Return cells to incubator.

- Fourteen days (±2 days) after setting up the culture, the expanding cells are ready for tetramer staining as described under Subheading 3.2 (*see* **Note 4**).

3.2 pMHCII Tetramer Staining Procedure in T-Cell Line

- Remove the expanding cells (*see* Subheading 3.1) from incubator.
- Carefully resuspend cells in culture and collect an aliquot of cells from each well per staining—typically 150–200 μL—into a 5 mL polystyrene FACS tube.
- Add one test of appropriate fluorescently labeled pMHCII tetramer per staining—typically 1 μL per 50 μL total volume (*see* **Notes 5** and **6**).
- Gently mix the tube and incubate at 37 °C for extended periods of time (30–120 min) (*see* **Note 7**).
- Label cells with optimally titrated amount of anti-CD3, anti-CD4, anti-CD19, and anti-CD14 antibodies—typically 2 μL of each antibody. This analysis can be combined with large panels of surface or functional markers which now allow more biological meaning to be extracted (*see* **Notes 8** and **9**).
- Incubate at 4 °C for 10–15 min in the dark.
- Wash cells in running buffer by centrifugation at 300 × *g* for 5 min.
- Decant supernatant, add 1 μL of the dead cell exclusion dye, and resuspend the pellet in 200–400 μL of running buffer.
- The cells are now ready for subsequent flow cytometric analysis (*see* Subheading 3.7 and **Note 10**).

3.3 pMHCII Tetramer Staining Procedure for Direct Ex Vivo Analysis

Combination of the use of pMHCII tetramers and magnetic cell enrichment technology (Subheading 3.4) can allow reliable and direct ex vivo visualization of rare allergen-specific CD4+ T cells, enabling quantification and characterization of these cells in a setting closer to their natural physiological state.

- Resuspend 20–50 × 10^6 live PBMC in 250 μL of culture media into a 5 mL polystyrene FACS tube. We recommend to use 10–30 × 10^6 PBMC from allergic individuals and 25–50 × 10^6 PBMC from nonallergic individuals (*see* **Note 1**).
- Add 50 mM dasatinib to the cells and incubate for 10 min at 37 °C (*see* **Note 11**).
- Add one test of appropriate PE-labeled pMHCII tetramer reagent per staining—typically 6–8 μL per tube (*see* **Notes 5**, **6**, and **12**).

- Incubate at room temperature for 2 h in the dark. If possible, gently agitate occasionally during staining (*see* **Note 13** and Subheading 3.4).

3.4 pMHCII Tetramer-Based Enrichment of Allergen-Specific T Cells

- Wash PE-conjugated pMHCII tetramer-labeled cells with 2 mL running by centrifugation of the cell suspension for 5 min at 300 × *g* at room temperature.
- Remove supernatant completely and resuspend cell pellet with 150 μL cold running buffer.
- Add 50 μL of Miltenyi anti-PE microbeads.
- Gently mix and incubate for 15 min at 4 °C.
- Resuspend cells with 2 mL cold running buffer and centrifuge the tube for 5 min at 300 × *g*.
- Place a Miltenyi MS magnetic column on a suitable MACS Separator. Position a 5 mL polystyrene FACS tube on a rack directly underneath the column.
- Prepare Miltenyi separation columns by priming with 500 μL running buffer allowing it to drain into the 5 mL FACS tube.
- When cells have finished the washing procedure, carefully aspirate the supernatant and resuspend the cell pellet in 1 mL of running buffer. For optimal enrichment, we recommend to pass cells through 30 μM nylon mesh to obtain a single-cell suspension before magnetic separation.
- Transfer the cell suspension onto the column allowing it to drain completely into the 5 mL FACS tube. This tube collects the PE-labeled pMHCII tetramer-depleted cell fraction (unbound fraction).
- Rinse the column by adding 1 mL of running buffer onto the column allowing it to drain completely into the collecting 5 mL FACS tube.
- Remove the column from the magnet and place over a new 5 mL polystyrene FACS tube. This tube collects the PE-labeled pMHCII tetramer-enriched cell fraction (bound fraction).
- Add 1 mL of running buffer and immediately flush the magnetically labeled cells out of the column by firmly pushing the plunger into the column.
- Centrifuge the tubes containing the bound fraction and the unbound fraction for 5 min at 300 × *g*.
- Carefully aspirate the supernatant of the bound fraction and resuspend pellet with 150 μL cold running buffer.
- Carefully aspirate the supernatant of the unbound fraction and resuspend pellet to a final volume of 3 mL. This fraction will be used for estimating the precursor frequency of allergen-specific T cells tracked by pMHCII tetramer (*see* Subheading 3.6) and

to set up a panel of single-color compensation controls to calibrate the flow cytometer (*see* Subheading 3.7).

3.5 Dual-Cell-Surface Antibodies and pMHCII Tetramer Staining for Flow Cytometry

- Prepare a master mix of appropriate titer-conjugated antibodies to stain surface markers on the cells. This should include at least anti-CD3, anti-CD4, anti-CD19, and anti-CD14 antibodies—typically 2 μL of each antibody. This analysis can be combined with large panels of surface or functional markers which will allow more biological meaning to be extracted from such rare allergen-specific CD4+ T cells (*see* **Notes 8**, **9**, and **14**).
- Label cells in the bound fraction by adding a dose of antibody cocktail.
- Gently mix and incubate cells for 30 min at room temperature in the dark.
- Wash cells in running buffer by centrifugation at 300 × *g* for 5 min and decant supernatant (*see* **Note 15**).
- Add 1 μL of the dead cell exclusion dye and resuspend the pellet in 200–400 μL of running buffer (*see* **Note 10**).

3.6 Estimation of the Ex Vivo Frequencies of Allergen-Specific CD4+ T Cells

- Transfer 1% (30 μL) of the resuspended tetramer-unbound fraction *see* Subheading 3.4) into a new 5 mL polystyrene FACS tube.
- Label cells by adding a dose of antibody cocktail (*see* Subheading 3.5).
- Incubate at room temperature for 15–30 min in the dark.
- Wash cells in running buffer by centrifugation at 300 × *g* for 5 min.
- Decant supernatant, add 1 μL of the dead cell dye exclusion, and resuspend the pellet in 200–400 μL of running buffer (*see* **Note 10**).
- Determine the number of CD4+ T cells by flow cytometry analysis (*see* Subheading 3.7).

Estimation of the absolute numbers of epitope-specific T cells in a sample is simply calculated by dividing the number of total tetramer-positive T cells determined in the bound fraction with 100 times the number of CD4+ cells determined in the 1% tetramer-unbound fraction (Fig. 1). The estimated frequency is usually expressed as the number of tetramer-positive T cells per million CD4+ T cells according to the formula:

$$\text{Frequency} = \frac{\text{Number tetramer} - \text{positive T cells in bound fraction} \times 10^6}{100 \times \text{Number of CD4} + \text{T cells in } 1\% \text{ of depleted fraction}}$$

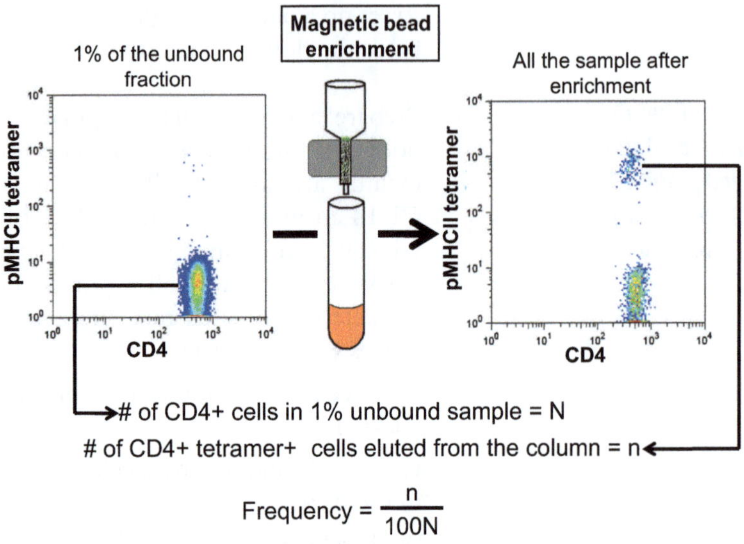

Fig. 1 Calculation of the ex vivo frequency of allergen-specific CD4+ T cells

3.7 Flow Cytometer Acquisition and Data Analysis

Proper exclusion and/or inclusion of gating strategies during FACS data analysis can dramatically enhance the resolution of the pMHCII tetramer-positive events by distinguishing true cell events from background. Figure 2 gives an example of experimental data generated by pMHCII tetramer reagents and FACS data analysis of tetramer-positive cells.

- Set up a panel of single-color compensation controls to calibrate the flow cytometer. For each fluorochrome to be calibrated, transfer 50 μL of the resuspended unbound fraction cells (*see* Subheading 3.4) in a 5 mL FACS tube and add 1 μL of anti-CD4 antibody conjugated to the corresponding fluorochrome. Include an unstained control to the panel as well to adjust the location of the viable lymphocyte gate (FSC vs. SSC).
- Gently mix and incubate cells for 30 min at room temperature in the dark.
- Wash cells in running buffer by centrifugation at 300 × *g* for 5 min.
- Decant supernatant and resuspend the pellet in 200 μL of running buffer (*see* **Note 10**).
- Calibrate the flow cytometer using the single-color compensation controls.
- Acquire data for each stained sample. For estimation of ex vivo frequencies of allergen-specific CD4+ T cells (*see* Subheading 3.6) collect as many cells as possible for both the bound and corresponding 1% unbound fraction. Keep the acquisition rate at or below 3000 events per second.

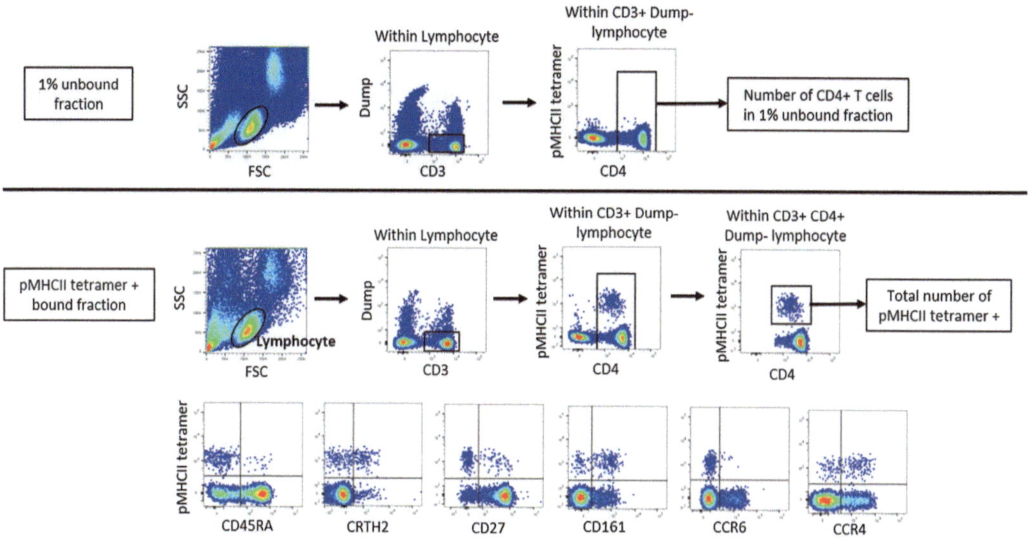

Fig. 2 Representative ex vivo pMHCII tetramer staining results in peanut allergic individual using ten-color flow cytometry approach. The tetramer positive appears as a distinct CD4+ population on the anti-CD4 versus tetramer panel

- Save and transfer all data as FCS files.
- Analyze FCS data into FACS analysis software using a sequence of successive inclusion/exclusion gates to identify live CD4+ T lymphocytes as illustrated in Fig. 2.
- Plot FSC versus SSC and draw a gate around the live lymphocytes.
- Plot CD3 versus dump channel (CD14, CD19, dead cell exclusion dye) and draw a gate around the CD3+ and dump population (*see* **Note 8**).
- Plot CD4 versus pMHCII tetramer and draw a gate around the CD4+ including tetramer+ and tetramer– population (*see* **Note 16**). For estimation of ex vivo frequencies of allergen-specific CD4+ T cells, determine at that step the number of CD4+ cells detected in the 1% tetramer-unbound fraction. Multiply the number of CD4+ cells in the sample by 100 to define the total number of CD4+ cells (*see* Subheading 3.6).
- Plot any other marker of interest versus pMHCII tetramer and draw quadrant.
- Plot CD45RO (or CD45RA) versus pMHCII tetramer and draw a gate around the tetramer+ including memory (CD45RO+ or CD45RA–) and naive population (CD45RO– or CD45RA+). For estimation of ex vivo frequencies of allergen-specific CD4+ T cells (*see* Subheading 3.6) determine the total number of tetramer-positive cells detected in each sample.

4 Notes

1. It is easier to get a higher frequency of pMHCII tetramer-positive T cells from patients with clinically severe forms of allergy. Therefore, patients' reactivity to the allergen to be studied should be verified by skin prick tests and/or by measuring allergen-specific IgE.
2. In order to use pMHCII tetramers in HLA-matched samples, several requirements have to be met. Immunodominant epitopes derived from the allergen of interest must have been defined and mapped to a certain HLA allele. pMHCII tetramer reagent can be obtained from several sources and can be designated as tetramers, pentamers, octamers, dextramers, oligomers, and multimers [10].
3. Conjugated pMHCII tetramer can be stored at 4 °C for 6–18 months and should never be frozen.
4. For weak antigen or low-frequency T cells you may need to triplicate the sample and 2–3 rounds of antigen stimulation.
5. Before adding tetramer, quickly spin the stock vial in a microfuge to remove any large aggregates.
6. To evaluate the nonspecific binding, it is also advisable to run in parallel a negative control with a mismatched pMHCII tetramer or matched tetramer loaded with nonsense peptide. The negative control reagent should have the same fluorescent label.
7. Except for ex vivo tetramer staining (Subheading 3.3), optimal staining of CD4+ T cells with fluorescently labeled pMHCII tetramer is obtained upon incubations at 37 °C [11, 12]. Under these conditions, bounded pMHCII tetramer is internalized and accumulated over time.
8. To exclude undesired monocyte (CD14+), B cells (CD19+), and dead cells that may increase background staining, we recommend to use viability dye (e.g., Viaprobe) and a fluorochrome (e.g., PercP) for your exclusion antibodies that would all fall in the same channel (dump channel).
9. pMHCII tetramer staining is compatible with cell fixation and permeabilization, and we have successfully analyzed intracellular cytokine and transcription factor expression in pMHCII-positive cells [8, 13]. However, the extra steps involved contribute to additional cell losses in the samples.
10. Keep the cells in the dark at 4 °C in a fridge until your scheduled time for flow cytometric analysis. For best results, we recommend flow cytometer analysis on the same day. For extended storage (>18 h), resuspend cells in 1–4% paraformaldehyde to prevent deterioration.

11. Protein kinase inhibitors such as dasatinib improve physical interaction between pMHCII tetramer and CD4+ T cells [14]. Similar increase in pMHCII tetramer staining can be obtained upon pretreatment of the cells with neuraminidase (Roche Ltd., Basel, Switzerland; 0.03 μ/mL for 30 min at 37 °C).
12. Due to the brightness of PE fluorochrome, we recommend the use of PE-conjugated pMHCII tetramer during the ex vivo staining procedure. However, other fluorochromes can also be used as long as corresponding magnetic microbeads are available.
13. It is critical to incubate cells at room temperature for the ex vivo tetramer staining. In contrast to incubation at physiological temperature, pMHCII tetramers are not efficiently internalized at low temperatures and therefore allow efficient enrichment process of non-internalized pMHC multimers with anti-PE magnetic beads.
14. T-cell activation can be determined by measuring activation markers such as CD38, Ki-67, and CD69 expression on tetramer-positive T cells [13]. The expression of these special markers is time dependent; for example CD69 is an early proliferation marker.
15. If an unconjugated primary antibody was used, incubation with an appropriate secondary antibody should occur now. Incubate for 20–30 min in the dark and wash cells.
16. The CD3+ CD4– T-cell population serves as a useful internal negative control for pMHCII tetramer staining of CD4+ T cells (Fig. 2). Like CD3+ CD4– T cell, CD8+ T-cell populations can be used as an internal negative control, since they should not bind to pMHCII ligands.

References

1. Vita R, Vasilevsky N, Bandrowski A et al (2016) Reproducibility and conflicts in immune epitope data. Immunology 147:349–354
2. Novak AE, Liu JW, Gebe JA et al (2001) Tetramer-guided epitope mapping: rapid identification and characterization of immunodominant CD4+ T cell epitopes from complex antigens. J Immunol 166:6665–6670
3. Wambre E, Van Overtvelt L, Maillere B et al (2008) Single cell assessment of allergen-specific T cell responses with MHC class II peptide tetramers: methodological aspects. Int Arch Allergy Immunol 146:99–112
4. Kwok WW, Roti M, Delong JH et al (2010) Direct ex vivo analysis of allergen-specific CD4+ T cells. J Allergy Clin Immunol 125:1407–1409.e1401
5. Bonvalet M, Wambre E, Moussu H et al (2011) Comparison between major histocompatibility complex class II tetramer staining and surface expression of activation markers for the detection of allergen-specific CD4(+) T cells. Clin Exp Allergy 41:821–829
6. Wambre E, DeLong JH, James EA et al (2014) Specific immunotherapy modifies allergen-specific CD4(+) T-cell responses in an epitope-dependent manner. J Allergy Clin Immunol 133:872–879.e877
7. Van Hemelen D, Mahler V, Fischer G et al (2015) HLA class II peptide tetramers vs.

allergen-induced proliferation for identification of allergen-specific CD4 T cells. Allergy 70:49–58

8. Van Overtvelt L, Wambre E, Maillere B et al (2008) Assessment of Bet v 1-specific CD4+ T cell responses in allergic and nonallergic individuals using MHC class II peptide tetramers. J Immunol 180:4514–4522
9. Novak EJ, Liu AW, Nepom GT et al (1999) MHC class II tetramers identify peptide-specific human CD4(+) T cells proliferating in response to influenza A antigen. J Clin Invest 104:R63–R67
10. Dolton G, Lissina A, Skowera A et al (2014) Comparison of peptide-major histocompatibility complex tetramers and dextramers for the identification of antigen-specific T cells. Clin Exp Immunol 177:47–63
11. Scriba TJ, Purbhoo M, Day CL et al (2005) Ultrasensitive detection and phenotyping of CD4+ T cells with optimized HLA class II tetramer staining. J Immunol 175:6334–6343
12. Cameron TO, Cochran JR, Yassine-Diab B et al (2001) Cutting edge: detection of antigen-specific CD4+ T cells by HLA-DR1 oligomers is dependent on the T cell activation state. J Immunol 166:741–745
13. Wambre E, DeLong JH, James EA et al (2012) Differentiation stage determines pathologic and protective allergen-specific CD4+ T-cell outcomes during specific immunotherapy. J Allergy Clin Immunol 129:544–551, 551.e1–7
14. Lissina A, Ladell K, Skowera A et al (2009) Protein kinase inhibitors substantially improve the physical detection of T-cells with peptide-MHC tetramers. J Immunol Methods 340:11–24

Chapter 12

Isolation and Characterization of Lymphocytes from Human Mucosal Biopsies

Nadine E. G. Upton, Thomas S. Hayday, and Louisa K. James

Abstract

The important role of the local mucosal environment in both the initiation and progression of allergic disease is well established. Analysis of tissue-resident lymphocyte subsets by flow cytometry requires isolation of viable cells from mucosal samples.

Here we describe an advanced method to dissociate lymphocytes from human mucosal (e.g., nasal, bronchial) biopsies. Single-cell suspensions are obtained through a combination of gentle mechanical disruption and incubation of tissue with proteolytic enzymes. This method fully utilizes limited clinical samples and is amenable to a variety of downstream applications for phenotypic, single-cell analysis of tissue lymphocytes or pooled lymphocyte subsets.

Key words Biopsy, Flow cytometry, Mucosa, Lymphocytes, Lung, Tissue dissociation, Cell isolation, Tissue-resident lymphocytes

1 Introduction

Human nasal and bronchial biopsies can vary in size from 1 to 5 mm^2, weighing a few micrograms, and may be obtained from highly heterogeneous sites within the airways. Furthermore, analysis of mucosal biopsies by immunohistochemistry highlights the significant variation in both numbers and phenotype of cells within individual biopsies [1–3]. This variation can limit the assessment of lymphocyte populations within the human airways in health and disease [4]. Single-cell analysis of lymphocytes by polychromatic flow cytometry provides a means to analyze multiple cell types in parallel using extensive combinations of fluorophore-labeled antibodies [5]. Flow cytometers equipped with cell sorting capabilities expand the potential for analysis of pooled cell subsets or even single lymphocytes for further downstream analysis (e.g., gene expression or cell culture). Flow cytometry requires the preparation of a homogenous single-cell suspension, which in turn requires

Penny Lympany and Meinir G. Jones (eds.), *Allergy: Methods and Protocols*, Methods in Molecular Biology, vol. 2020, https://doi.org/10.1007/978-1-4939-9591-2_12,

the prior dissociation of resident lymphocytes from tissue matrices. Depending on the sampling location of the biopsy, tissue-resident lymphocytes can be embedded within an extracellular matrix of varying complexity. Enzymatic dissociation of cells from tissue is a well-established method for use in large tissue samples and whole organs obtained from animal models [6–8], but there are few reports on the use of small human mucosal biopsies in similar approaches [9, 10]. We have developed and optimized an efficient technique for the preparation of single-cell suspensions from human bronchial and nasal biopsies, using commercially available blends of proteolytic enzymes (Fig. 1).

This chapter provides a detailed protocol for dissociation of cells from intact tissue and gives examples of flow cytometry staining of airway lymphocytes and other downstream applications. We have also isolated lymphocytes from nasal polyps, skin biopsies, and tonsillar tissue using minor modifications of this protocol. Given the invasive nature of biopsy collection, our methods have been developed to ensure that clinical samples are fully utilized and generate informative and reproducible data.

Effective cell dissociation is obtained by gentle mechanical disruption followed by incubation of tissue with proteolytic enzymes for 1 h at 37 °C. Dissociated cells are filtered and prepared as a single-cell suspension for polychromatic flow cytometry. Downstream applications include but are not limited to:

(a) Immunophenotyping of lymphocyte subsets by polychromatic flow cytometry.

(b) FACS sorting of pooled lymphocyte subsets (e.g., memory B/T cells) for gene expression analysis or cell culture.

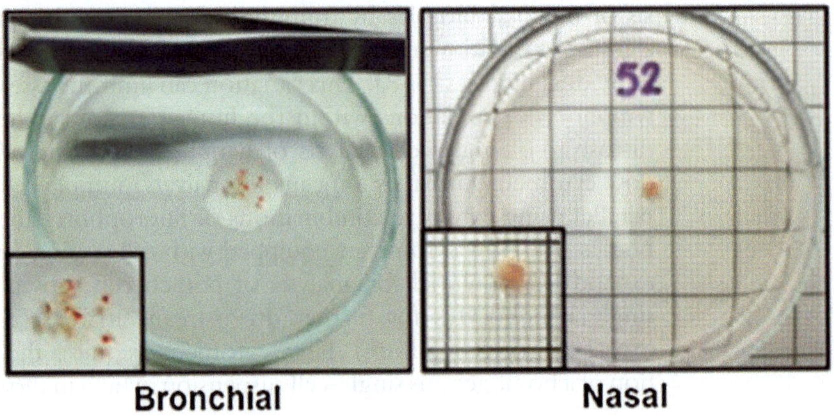

Fig. 1 Intact human bronchial and nasal biopsies. Small (1–2 mm^2) bronchial biopsies were pooled prior to dissociation with proteolytic enzymes. A larger (3 mm^2), thawed nasal biopsy was first chopped into smaller pieces before enzymatic dissociation

(c) FACS sorting of single cells for single-cell gene expression analysis or cloning.

Together this range of downstream techniques allows extensive characterization of human tissue-resident lymphocytes from mucosal biopsies. The protocol provided below details the dissociation conditions for nasal and bronchial biopsies followed by flow cytometric analysis of T- and B-cell populations.

2 Materials

All buffers and reagents should be sterile and cell culture grade. Store all reagents at 4 °C unless otherwise stated.

2.1 Cell Dissociation

Buffers should be warmed to 37 °C prior to use.

Hanks' balanced salt solution (HBSS).

Proteolytic enzymes (*see* **Note 1**).

Nasal biopsies	5 mg/mL Liberase TM (Roche) 10 mg/mL Hyaluronidase (Sigma) 10 mg/mL DNase I (Roche)
Bronchial biopsies	2.5 mg/mL Liberase TL (Roche)

Disposable scalpels (size 11 or equivalent).

Sterile glass petri dishes (*see* **Note 2**).

Sterile 96-well round-bottomed tissue culture plates.

BD Falcon with cell strainer tube (12 × 75 mm tube with 35 μM cell strainer, BD Biosciences).

2.2 Flow Cytometry

Buffers should be ice cold.

FACS buffer: Phosphate-buffered saline (PBS) supplemented with 10% FBS and 2 mM EDTA.

Compensation Beads (Anti-mouse Ig k/Negative Control, BD Biosciences).

FcR blocking Reagent (Miltenyi Biotech) (*see* **Note 3**).

Anti-Human CD19-APC-Cy7 (Clone HIB19, Biolegend).

Anti-Human CD3-PE (Clone UCHT1, Biolegend).

Anti-Human CD38-PE-Cy7 (Clone HB-7, Biolegend).

Anti-Human IgD-PerCP-Cy5.5 (Clone IA6-2, Biolegend).

LIVE/DEAD® Fixable Aqua Dead Cell Stain Kit (Invitrogen).

RNaseZap™ (Sigma-Aldrich).

3 Methods

Local regulations concerning safety and ethics of working with human tissues should be consulted prior to experimental work, and all procedures should be performed within a Class II safety hood as a minimum.

3.1 Dissociation of Biopsy Tissue

1. Using sterilized forceps, transfer intact tissue (*see* **Note 4**) to either a sterilized glass petri dish (samples <2 mm^2) containing 150 μL HBSS or a sterile 96-well round-bottomed plate (samples >2mm^2) containing 150 μL HBSS (*see* **Note 5**).
2. Using a pipette, transfer any remaining storage buffer to a 15 mL Falcon tube and centrifuge for 5 min at 300 × *g*.
3. Carefully decant the supernatant, resuspend pellet in 50 μL of HBSS (*see* **Note 6**), and add to the dish/well containing the biopsy.
4. Using two sterile scalpels gently cut the tissue into 1–2 mm pieces using a chopping action (*see* **Note 7**).
5. Add enzymes according to tissue type:
   (a) Bronchial biopsies: 500 μg/mL Liberase TL in a final volume of 250 μL (i.e., 50 μL of 2.5 mg/mL stock).
   (b) Nasal biopsies: 250 μg/mL Liberase TM (100 μL), 50 μg/mL hyaluronidase (10 μL), 50 μg/mL DNase I (10 μL) in a final volume of 2 mL.
6. Cover the petri dish and place on a rocking platform in a 37 °C CO_2 incubator for 1 h.
7. Using a sterile 1 mL syringe slowly pass the entire sample through a sterile 18 gauge needle a maximum of two times to further dissociate the tissue (*see* **Note 8**).
8. Using the sterile 1 mL syringe, pass the entire sample through a 35 μM filter lid placed directly onto a 5 mL FACS tube.
9. Wash the filter with 2.5 mL of ice-cold HBSS; the total volume in the tube should be approximately 3–5 mL (*see* **Note 9**).
10. Centrifuge the cells for 10 min at 300 × *g* and carefully decant the supernatant.

3.2 Labeling Cells for Analysis of B- and T-Cell Populations

All labeling steps should be performed on ice and shielded from light.

1. Prepare a suspension of 2 × 10^6 control cells (e.g., peripheral blood mononuclear cells, PBMC) at 1 × 10^6 cells/mL (*see* **Note 10**).
2. Label 12 FACS tubes according to Table 1 and add:

Table 1
Volumes of antibodies and buffer for FACS tubes

Tube	Purpose	Antibody volume (μL)				
		CD19-APC-Cy7	CD3-PE	CD38-PE-Cy7	IgD-PerCP-Cy5.5	Buffer volume (μL)
1	Unstained	–	–	–	–	50
2	CD19-APC-Cy7 compensation	2	–	–	–	48
3	CD3-PE compensation	–	2	–	–	48
4	CD38-PE-Cy7 compensation	–	–	2	–	48
5	IgD-PerCP-Cy5.5 compensation	–	–	–	2	48
6	Live/dead aqua compensation	–	–	–	–	50
7	CD19-APC-Cy7FMO	–	2	2	2	44
8	CD3-PE FMO	2	–	2	2	44
9	CD38-PE-Cy7 FMO	2	2	–	2	44
10	IgD-PerCP-Cy5.5 FMO	2	2	2	–	44
11	Live/dead aqua (Amcyan) FMO	2	2	2	2	42
12	Gating control	2	2	2	2	42
13	Sample	2	2	2	2	42

(a) Compensation controls (*see* **Note 11**): 1 drop of each compensation bead per tube to tubes 2–5 and 50 μL PBMC to tubes 1–6 (*see* **Note 12**).

(b) Fluorescence minus one (FMO) controls (*see* **Note 13**): Add 50 μL PBMC to tubes 7–11.

(c) Gating control (*see* **Note 14**): Add 1 mL PBMC to tube 12.

3. Add 4 mL FACS buffer tubes 6–12, and centrifuge for 5 min at 300 × *g* at 4 °C.
4. Carefully decant the supernatant and resuspend the cell pellet by gently flicking the bottom of the tube.
5. Add 50 μL of FcR block to each tube and incubate for 15 min on ice.
6. Add fluorophore-labeled antibodies/FACS buffer directly to tubes according to the volumes in Table 1 (*see* **Note 15**).

7. Incubate for 30 min on ice, shielded from light.
8. Add 4 mL FACS buffer to each tube, and centrifuge for 5 min at 300 × *g* at 4 °C.
9. Carefully decant the supernatant and resuspend the cell pellet by gently flicking the bottom of the tube.
10. Add 1 mL PBS containing 1 μL of live dead/aqua to tubes 6–10, 12, and 13.
11. Incubate for 10 min on ice in the dark.
12. Add 4 mL FACS buffer to the live/dead aqua-stained cells, and centrifuge for 5 min at 300 × *g* at 4 °C.
13. Carefully decant the supernatant and resuspend the cell pellets by gently flicking the bottom of the tube.
14. Add 200 μL of FACS buffer to each tube and keep cells on ice prior to acquisition (*see* **Note 16**).

3.3 Flow Cytometry and Gating Strategy

1. Set up the flow cytometer with a 70 μM nozzle at ~70 psi.
2. Rinse out the flow cell with RNaseZap™ and then with RNase-free water.
3. Maintain the sample chamber temperature at 4 °C and keep the sample agitator running at 300 rpm.
4. Ensure that samples are strained before passing through the cytometer.
5. To avoid cross-sample contamination, clean the single flow cell between samples with FACSClean and then rinse with deionized water.
6. Use single-stained compensation control tubes to determine the PMT voltages and compensation matrix (*see* **Note 17**).
7. Create an FSC-A versus SSC-A plot (Fig. 2a) and using unstained PBMC (tube 1) define the lymphocyte gate (*see* **Note 18**).
8. Create an FSC-H versus SSC-W plot (Fig. 2b) and using unstained PBMC gate on singlets (*see* **Note 19**).
9. Create an SSC-A versus live/dead aqua plot (Fig. 2c) and using the live/dead aqua FMO (tube 11) gate on live cells.
10. Create a CD19-APC-Cy7 versus CD3-PE plot (Fig. 2d) and use the respective FMOs (tubes 7 and 8) to gate on $CD19^{+}CD3^{-}$ and $CD3^{+}CD19^{-}$ populations, identifying B cells and T cells, respectively.
11. Create a CD38-PE-Cy7 versus IgD-PerCP-Cy5.5 plot and use the respective FMOs (tubes 9 and 10) to gate on B-cell subpopulations of interest (Fig. 3).
12. Verify the staining using a fully stained PBMC sample (tube 12) and then acquire the sample (*see* **Note 20**).

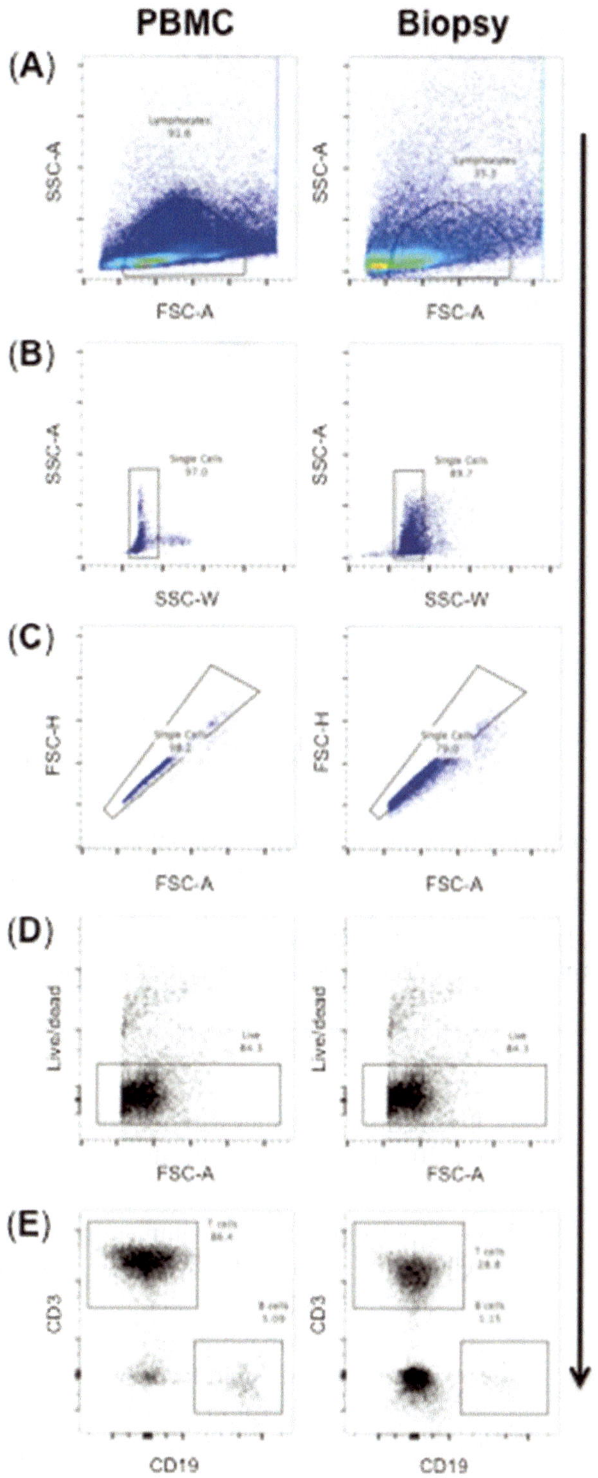

Fig. 2 Flow cytometry analysis of lymphocytes isolated from human PBMC (left panel) or bronchial biopsies (right panel). Lymphocyte gates are defined by cell granularity (SSC-A) and size (FSC-A) (**a**). Duplet cells and cell debris are excluded by gating single cells using area (SSC-A) vs. width (SSC-W) (**b**) and then area (FSC-A) vs. height (FSC-H) (**c**). Dead cells are excluded from analysis using a live/dead marker (**d**). T- and B-cell populations are identified by gating on CD3+ cells and CD19+ cells, respectively (**e**)

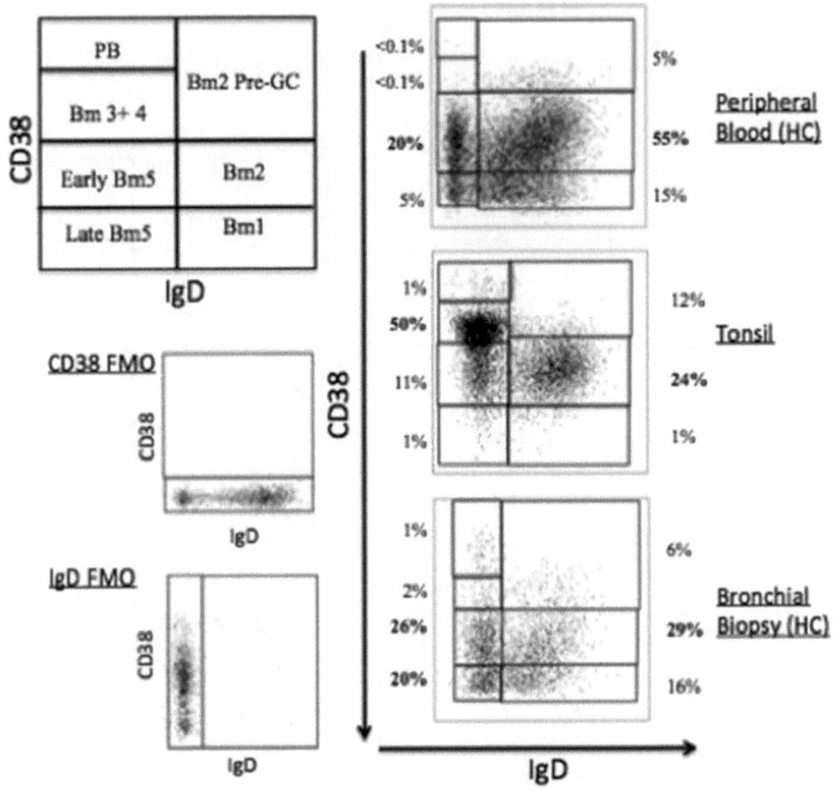

Fig. 3 Flow cytometry analysis of B-cell subsets in human mucosal biopsies. Proportions of B-cell subset populations are defined using CD38 and IgD expression ("Bm classification" of B cells [11]) in PBMC (**a**), tonsil cells (**b**), and bronchial biopsy cells (**c**) from healthy control subjects (HC). CD38- and IgD-positive cells were determined by CD38 and IgD FMO controls, respectively (bottom left). Clear populations are visible by dot plots (**a**–**c**) where proportions of each B-cell subset are presented as percentage of total $CD19^+$ B cells

4 Notes

1. Reconstitute enzymes with ice-cold sterile HBSS, place on ice for 30 min, gently agitate the vial until dissolved, and store aliquots at −20 °C.
2. Glass petri dishes are recommended to prevent adherence of cells to the surface; dishes can be decontaminated and autoclaved for subsequent reuse.
3. Alternative blocking buffers can be used depending on the species of antibody used for labeling.
4. Fresh tissue is preferable; however we have successfully isolated single cells from biopsies that had been stored frozen in cryopreservation medium (CryoSFM, PromoCell) and thawed prior to dissociation. Cryopreservation can have a detrimental effect on cell viability and yields so care should be taken when freezing and thawing whole tissue.

5. To reduce heterogeneity, when multiple biopsies are obtained from a single individual, we pool biopsies along with any cells harvested from storage buffer. We also make a note of the approximate size of the biopsies to inform assessment of cell yield variations between samples.
6. Following centrifugation it is common that the cell pellet is not visible by eye.
7. It is not necessary to chop biopsies smaller than 2 mm^2.
8. For biopsies smaller than 1 mm^2, we break up the tissue using the tip of a needle (size 10G) and then pipette up and down in a 100 μL pipette; this avoids loss of tissue that may occur using a syringe and needle.
9. At this stage we may harvest a fraction of the cell suspension for RNA/DNA isolation.
10. In order to calibrate the flow cytometer a series of control samples will be required comprising cells stained with the antibodies of interest. For this purpose we obtain peripheral blood mononuclear cells from anonymous healthy donors, which are stored frozen in liquid nitrogen. We thaw an aliquot prior to each experiment.
11. Single-stained controls are essential for proper compensation and should be prepared and run at each experiment.
12. For accurate compensation it is useful to have clear negatively and positively stained populations within a given sample. We subject our single-stained compensation tube (tube 6) to high temperature (65 °C for 10 min) using a heat block; this kills some of the cells, thus generating a distinct live/dead aqua-positive population for gating.
13. FMO controls are used to accurately determine the fluorescence of the negative population and are essential to establish the correct gating in an experiment. These controls are particularly important given the low abundance of cells within mucosal tissue biopsies.
14. A fully stained PBMC sample is a useful quality control to check that the expected proportions of lymphocytes are observed, thus verifying the staining procedure.
15. Take particular care when pipetting small volumes, and change tips each time to avoid cross-contamination of antibody stocks. If multiple samples are being processed in one experiment, we would typically prepare a "mastermix" cocktail of antibodies.
16. We prepare the samples so that they can be acquired immediately.
17. Using compensation control tubes 1–6 (Table 1), ensure that the positive fluorescence in each channel is contained within

the scale of the FACS plots. PMT voltages may need to be reduced or increased to achieve this.

18. Determine the lymphocyte population gate using the unstained PBMC sample (tube 1), as the biopsy sample (tube 13) will have large populations of debris and potential red blood cell contamination that can obscure the lymphocyte population.
19. Doublet discrimination is essential when working with dissociated tissue samples that may contain residual debris. Doublets have double the width of singlets but the same length so can be excluded by plotting width versus height.
20. Set sort purity mode to four-way purity (0 yield, 32 purity, 0 phase). Run samples at an appropriate flow rate, with an aim to have event rate at no more than 2000 evt/s to improve sort efficiency of small populations.

References

1. Walker RA (2006) Quantification of immunohistochemistry-issues concerning methods, utility and semiquantitative assessment II. Histopathology 49:406–410
2. Taylor CR, Levenson RM (2006) Quantification of immunohistochemistry-issues concerning methods, utility and semiquantitative assessment II. Histopathology 49:411–424
3. Dunstan RW, Wharton KA, Quigley C et al (2011) The use of immunohistochemistry for biomarker assessment-can it compete with other technologies? Toxicol Pathol 39:988–1002
4. Pawankar R, Ra C (1996) Heterogeneity of mast cells and T cells in the nasal mucosa. J Allergy Clin Immunol 98:S248–S262
5. Baumgarth N, Roederer M (2000) A practical approach to multicolor flow cytometry for immunophenotyping. J Immunol Methods 243:77–97
6. Freeman CM, Curtis JL, Chensue SW (2007) CC chemokine receptor 5 and CXC chemokine receptor 6 expression by lung CD8+ cells correlates with chronic obstructive pulmonary disease severity. Am J Pathol 171:767–776
7. Havenith CE, Breedijk AJ, Verdaasdonk MA et al (1992) An improved and rapid method for the isolation of rat lymph node or spleen T lymphocytes for T cell proliferation assays. J Immunol Methods 153:73–79
8. https://lifescience.roche.com/shop/en/es/overviews/brand/tissue-dissociation-overview
9. Lethbridge MW, Kemeny DM, Ratoff JC et al (2010) A novel technique to explore the functions of bronchial mucosal T cells in chronic obstructive pulmonary disease: application to cytotoxicity and cytokine immunoreactivity. Clin Exp Immunol 161:560–569
10. Vijayanand P, Seumois G, Pickard C et al (2007) Invariant natural killer T cells in asthma and chronic obstructive pulmonary disease. N Engl J Med 356:1410–1422
11. Bohnhorst JØ, Bjørgan MB, Thoen JE et al (2001) Bm1–Bm5 classification of peripheral blood B cells reveals circulating germinal center founder cells in healthy individuals and disturbance in the B cell subpopulations in patients with primary Sjögren's syndrome. J Immunol 167:3610–3618

Chapter 13

Development of a Dipstick Assay for Soy Allergens: Inexpensive Detection to Control Allergen Exposure

Daniel Álvarez-Simón and Susana Gómez-Ollés

Abstract

Allergen measurements are use in the food industry and are also routinely performed as part of indoor air quality investigations and occupational health monitoring. In this chapter we describe how to develop a simple, convenient, rapid test to analyze soy allergens that can be used in production environments by non-skilled staff to facilitate immediate corrective action and minimize risk and that can be produced in laboratories not equipped with sophisticated instruments.

The strip assay described consists of a membrane that is bonded to an adhesive support where an absorbent pad is also attached to absorb excess reagents. The membrane is stripped with specific antibodies against soy allergens in this case (test line) and a goat anti-rabbit IgG antibody (control line). The strip is exposed to a mix of sample and gold-conjugated specific antibody. Colored bands are read out visually or by densitometry.

Key words Lateral flow assay, Strip assay, Rapid test, Allergen, Monitoring

1 Introduction

Allergen measurements are used in the food industry and are also routinely performed as part of indoor air quality investigations and occupational health monitoring [1, 2], and for standardization of allergenic products.

There are several different screening methods available for allergen testing and each has its advantages and disadvantages. Traditionally food and environmental allergen analysis relies on immunological methods such as enzyme-linked immunosorbent assay (ELISA). ELISA has the advantage of being relatively quick and simple to perform and can be used to detect many known allergens; however, it can only detect one allergen at a time, is susceptible to cross-reactivity, and can lead to the generation of false-positive and false-negative results [3]. In food allergen analysis also polymerase chain reaction (PCR) approaches have been used

Penny Lympany and Meinir G. Jones (eds.), *Allergy: Methods and Protocols*, Methods in Molecular Biology, vol. 2020, https://doi.org/10.1007/978-1-4939-9591-2_13,

traditionally. PCR methods are complementary to ELISA methods, and are used to amplify and detect the DNA of an allergen. PCR approaches are highly specific, sensitive to very low levels of allergen, and can be used to detect more than two allergens at once. However, the PCR is limited because some food processing methods can destroy detectable DNA, causing false-negative results. PCR methods are also highly susceptible to food matrix interferences. In addition, DNA methods are not suitable for the detection of certain allergens, such as egg [3].

More sophisticate methods are liquid chromatography–tandem mass spectrometry (LC–MS–MS) and fluorescent multiplex array technology. LC–MS–MS is an alternative method for allergen detection that is highly specific and sensitive, and has the ability to directly analyze multiple allergens in a single analysis [3]. Fluorescent multiplex array technology has also been developed that allows the simultaneous detection of multiple allergens in a single reaction well, with significantly increased sensitivity [4], which is increasingly being used for allergen detection in homes, schools, and occupational health settings [5, 6].

All these techniques described for food allergen analysis or environmental monitoring require the use of a specialized laboratory staffed by skilled personnel. In this chapter we would like to provide tools and tips to develop a simple, convenient, rapid test to analyzed allergens that can be used in production environments by non-skilled staff to facilitate immediate corrective action and minimize risk and that can be produced in laboratories not equipped with sophisticated instruments.

Here, we describe a simple strip assay where a membrane is bonded to a support structure such as a plastic strip for ease of handling the membrane for exposure to the test sample and readout. In this assay, differently than the traditional concept of a lateral flow device, the conjugate is not set in a dry format on a separate pad along the membrane flow path, but the conjugate is added in a liquid format mixed with the sample in an ELISA plate well. Typical components of a traditional lateral flow immunoassay device are a plastic backing card, membrane, sample pad, absorbent pad, conjugate pad, and possibility a wick and/or cover tape. Reagents are dispensed or coated; each material is kept in place in the backing card. Finally card is cut into individual test strips. Manufacturing can be done from completely manual to completely automated. In this chapter we want to explain step by step how to be able to prepare a prototype of a strip test in a common research laboratory housing basic laboratory equipment, but no sophisticated instruments (e.g., dispense platform, laminator, sheet slitters). When we want to jump from research to product development and scaled up to manufacturing, manual procedures should be avoided and automatic equipment should be used in place. There are several companies that can help you in the way through to full-scale automated manufacture.

2 Materials

2.1 Diluents and Buffers

1. Phosphate-buffered saline (PBS): To 1200 mL of physiological saline (0.9% NaCl) add 216 mL of Na_2HPO_4 solution (9.4 g/L) and 72 mL of KH_2PO_4 solution (8.9 g/L). Adjust pH to 7.4.
2. Soy hull low-molecular-weight extract (SHLMWE), in house extract (*see* Ref. [7]).
3. Elution buffer: PBS containing 0.2% bovine serum albumin (BSA) (A7030-100G; Sigma Aldrich) and 0.5% Tween-20 (Sigma Aldrich).
4. Dilution buffer: PBS containing 1% BSA and 0.5% Tween-20 (*see* **Note 1**).

2.2 Strip Components

1. Direct cast-backed nitrocellulose nitrate membrane (UniSart CN95 19,910 Sartorius Stedim Biotech, Goettingen, Germany) (*see* **Note 2**).
2. Capture antibody test line: Rabbit anti-soy hull low-molecular-weight extract (SHLMWE) polyclonal antibodies (*see* Ref. [7]).
3. Capture antibody control line: Goat anti-rabbit IgG antibody (Southern Biotechnology Associates, Inc., Birmingham, AL, USA).
4. Adhesive support: Sealing tape for multiwell plates (polyolefin sealing tape, acrylate adhesive) (Nunc®).
5. Absorbent pad: Filter paper grade 470, pore size 20–30 μm (Schleicher & Schuell, Dassel, Germany).

2.3 Assay Assembly Components

Airborne sample collection, extract production, and antibody conjugation are out of the scope of this chapter.

1. Samples: Collect airborne samples in glass microfiber filters and elute them in elution buffer overnight at 4 °C as previously reported [7]. Store eluates at −20 °C. Dilute eluates to be tested in the strip assay at 1:100 in dilution buffer (*see* **Note 3**).
2. Standards: Prepare three solutions of SHLMWE at the following concentrations: 1.56, 6.25, and 25 ng/mL in dilution buffer.
3. Ninety-six-well microplate (Costar®; Corning, NY).

4. Gold-conjugated antibody: Conjugate a portion of rabbit anti-SHLMWE polyclonal antibody to 40 nm colloidal gold particles using passive adsorption (*see* **Note 4**). Check optical density (OD) of the concentrated conjugate. Store conjugate at 4 °C. Make up daily conjugate working solution with a final OD of 2 by diluting concentrated conjugated antibody in dilution buffer.

3 Methods

Wear gloves. Diligently follow all waste disposal regulations when disposing waste materials. Carry out all procedures at room temperature unless otherwise stated.

3.1 Strip Assembly

1. Cut a rectangular piece of nitrocellulose membrane of 10 × 1.3 (W × H cm) (*see* **Notes 5** and **6**).
2. Prepare capture antibody solution for **test line**: Prepare rabbit anti-SHLMWE polyclonal antibodies at a final concentration of 1 mg/mL in PBS, pH 7.2 (*see* **Notes** 7 and **8**).
3. Prepare capture antibody solution for **control line**: Prepare goat anti-rabbit IgG antibody at a final concentration of 500 μg/mL in PBS, pH 7.2.
4. Perform hand stripping of the test line by pipetting 30 μL of the capture antibody solution for test line following an imaginary straight line at 0.3 cm from the membrane origin (*see* Fig. 1, **Note 9**).
5. Perform hand stripping of the control line by pipetting 30 μL of the capture antibody solution for control line following an imaginary straight line at 0.6 cm from the membrane origin (*see* Fig. 1, **Note 10**).
6. Dry membranes for 1 h at 37 °C in an oven (*see* **Note 11**).

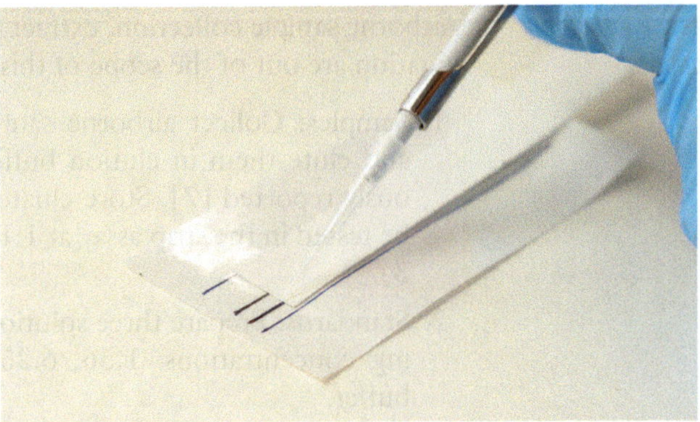

Fig. 1 Manual stripping process. Test line positioned at 0.3 cm from the membrane origin and control line at 0.6 cm from the membrane origin

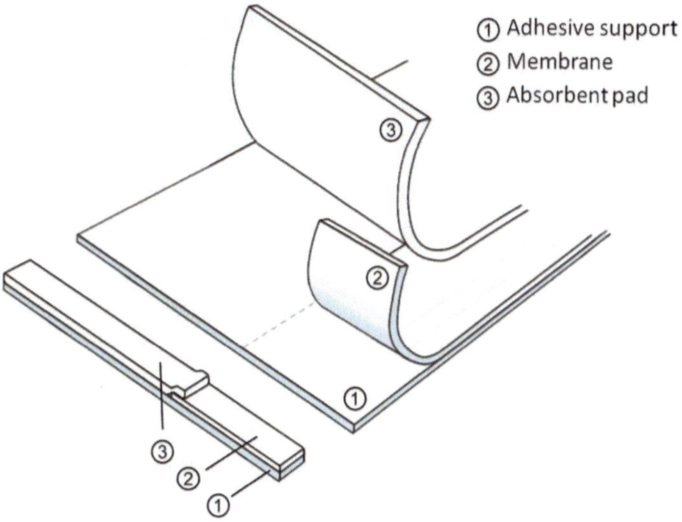

Fig. 2 Scheme of strip assembly

7. Cut an adhesive support of the following dimensions: 10 × 3.6 (W × H cm).
8. Put membrane on top of the adhesive support starting at the origin, as shown in Fig. 2 (*see* Fig. 2, **Note 6**).
9. Cut an absorbent pad of the following dimensions: 10 × 2.5 (W × H cm) (*see* **Notes 5** and **12**).
10. Place absorbent pad on top of the adhesive support and overlapping the membrane by 2 mm as shown in Fig. 2 (*see* Fig. 2).
11. Cut vertically in strips of 4 mm of width by a guillotine (*see* **Notes 13** and **14**).
12. Store strips in a zipped bag with a silica gel pouch (desiccant to absorb moisture) at 4 °C.

3.2 Assay Assembly

1. Add 20 μL of the three standard solutions of SHLMWE or diluted samples to the corresponding well.
2. Add on top 20 μL of conjugate working solution (diluted rabbit anti-SHLMWE polyclonal antibody gold-conjugated solution; OD 2).
3. Mix gently by repeatedly pipetting up and down.
4. Insert a test strip in each well to allow allergen-antibody complexes to diffuse across the membrane and react with the antibodies immobilized on the test and control lines. If allergen-antibody complexes react with the immobilized antibodies a red-purple line appears.
5. Remove the test strips from the well after 30 min.
6. Read them **immediately** by naked eye and/or by densitometry (Fig. 3).

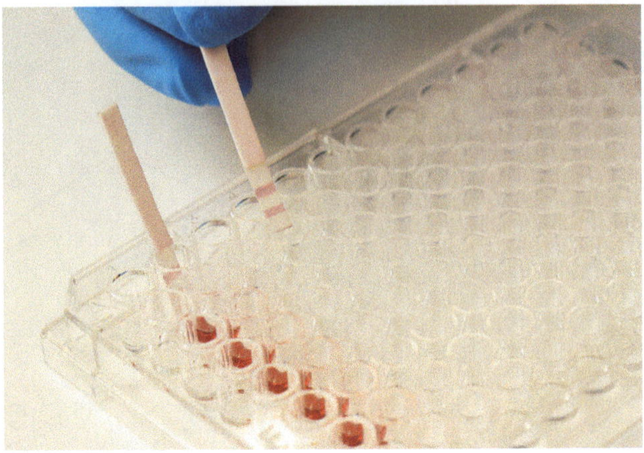

Fig. 3 A positive test with the test and control line colored after having been inserted in the well

3.3 Result Analysis by Naked Eye

After the liquid reagent flows through the test and control lines a colored line could be observed with naked eye.

1. Results should be read on the side of the membrane to which capture reagents are applied.
2. A visible red-purple line has to appear at the control line for the test to be valid.
3. Reader can rank sample results as negative (−), positive (+), or double positive (++) by comparing the intensity of the test line appeared with the intensity of the line obtained with a three-point standard curve of known concentrations (1.56, 6.25, and 25 ng/mL) of SHLMWE.

3.4 Result Analysis by Densitometry

1. A visible red-purple line has to appear at the control line for the test to be valid (Fig. 3).
2. Scan the side of the membrane to which capture reagents are applied with a flatbed scanner (Epson Expression 1600).
3. Analyze line intensity by densitometry with Image J 1.45 s (NIH, USA) (*see* **Note 15**) or a similar software.

3.5 Densitometry with Image J 1.45 s

1. Open the image file using File>Open in ImageJ.
2. The analysis requires the image to be a grayscale image. The simplest method to convert to grayscale is to go to Image>Type>8-bit.
3. Choose the Rectangular Selection tool from the toolbar. Draw a rectangle around the first strip. ImageJ assumes that your

lanes run vertically (so individual bands are horizontal), so your rectangle should be tall and narrow to enclose a single strip.

4. After drawing the rectangle over your first strip, press the 1 key (command +1 on Mac) or go to Analyze>Gels>Select First Lane to set the rectangle in place. The selection will now be highlighted and have a 1 in the middle of it.
5. Use your mouse to click and hold the rectangle on the first strip and drag it over to the next strip. Press 2 or go to Analyze>Gels>Select Next Lane.
6. Repeat **step 5** for each strip to set the rectangle in place.
7. After you have set the rectangle on the last strip press 3 or go to Analyze>Gels>Plot Lanes to draw a profile plot of each membrane.
8. The profile plot represents the relative density of the contents of the rectangle over each membrane. The rectangles are arranged top to bottom on the profile plot. Higher peaks represent darker bands.
9. Images of immunoassays always have some background signal, so the peaks do not reach down to the baseline of the profile plot. It will be necessary to close the peak so that we can measure its size. Choose the Straight Line tool and draw a line across the base of the peak. This step requires some subjective judgment to decide where the peak ends and the background noise begins.
10. When each peak has been closed off at the base, select the Wand tool and click inside the first peak. Repeat this for each peak and measurements should pop up in the Results window.
11. The values from the Results window can be moved to a spreadsheet program by selecting Edit>Copy All in the Results window (*see* **Note 16**).

4 Notes

1. Conjugate diluent/antigen diluent contains Tween-20. Detergent is required for uniform capillary flow. The addition of a nonspecific protein such as bovine serum albumins (BSA) can be used to stabilize the capture reagent.
2. Choosing a membrane is one of the most critical steps of the strip development. Membrane characteristics will determine in a great extent the strip performance (i.e., response time, background, sensitivity). The UniSart® CN 95 is a large-pore-size (around 15 μm pore size) cellulose nitrate membrane with a

capillary speed of around 100 s/4 cm that is directly cast onto a 100 μm clear polyester backing and with a binding capacity for proteins of 28 μg IgG/cm^2. Choosing a fast lateral speed membrane, like the UniSart® CN 95, generates less background and gives a shorter time to signal on the test strip, but gives lower sensitivities. Choosing a backed membrane offers two advantages: they are easier to handle and the polyester film acts as a barrier to chemical contamination from adhesives used to stick membranes to cards during strip assembly.

3. Optimal dilution was chosen in order to minimize the "hook effect" throughout the range of concentrations likely to be encountered in environmental samples. The hook effect, also known as prozone effect, describes an artifact seen when the analyte is in very high concentration, beyond the dynamic range of the method. This excess amount cannot be measured accurately and yields lower signal than expected in the assay (*see* Ref. [8]).
4. You can perform conjugation by yourself or alternatively contract this service. There are several companies that offer gold colloidal conjugation and assure a good-quality conjugate.
5. Be very careful with strip and all its component dimensions (i.e., nitrocellulose membrane; absorbent pad). They are crucial in the strip performance. Strip performance can also be modified by the test line and control line position from origin.
6. Always manipulate membrane and absorbent pad gently. Do not exert pressure on them in order to avoid damaging their structure. Wear gloves at all times and do not handle them with tweezers as it would leave marks on it. If tweezers are required choose a blunt flat-tip tweezers.
7. **Capture reagent diluent** should be always buffered to achieve consistency and pH must be around 7.0–7.5 as most antibodies have their isoelectric points between 5.5 and 7.5. Detergents (i.e., Tween® 20, Triton™ X-100) should be avoided or used at concentrations <0.01% in capture buffers. These chaotropic agents may interfere the molecular interaction between the protein and the nitrocellulose membrane. We will observe that the signal may start to develop, but as soon as the capture reagent will start to detach, signal will start to disappear.
8. The reagent dispensing rate (μL/cm) and the concentration of capture reagent to be dispensed should be optimized.
9. For **stripping reagents** onto the membrane by hand there are several tips that can be handy. We recommend using low-volume pipettes (i.e., P10) even though you have to pipette several times to cover all the membrane width. That would help you to have a narrower line as the width of the protein

line is mainly determined by the contact zone between the dispensed liquid and the membrane. If capture reagent is applied with a higher volume pipette (i.e., P20, P100) the reagent is spread out over a wider area, resulting in a broader line with less color intensity and potentially achieving a lower sensitivity. In order to dispense antibody following a straight line we found it useful to create a template on a paper with the test and control lines drawn with a permanent pen at 0.3–0.6 cm from the origin, respectively. To start stripping reagents place your membrane on top of your template (*see* Fig. 1) and guide your dispensing by looking at the drawn lines that show through. Avoid using a ruler to dispense as you can damage the membrane structure by exerting too much pressure. It is also advisable to avoid drawing lines at the backing film of the membrane. Ink may smear when getting wet even if a permanent ink is used.

10. To prevent you from touching the already dispensed test line rotate the membrane 180° before dispensing the control line. Before rotating the membrane do a little mark on one corner to know the membrane orientation.
11. **Blocking**: Normally it is not necessary to block the membrane after applying the capture reagent. The presence of nonspecific proteins such as BSA in the sample and conjugate diluents is frequently sufficient to prevent the detector reagent and analyte from nonspecific binding.
12. Absorbent pad's bed volume will control the volume of sample analyzed and depends on absorbent pad characteristics and dimensions.
13. Avoid exerting pressure on the strip while cutting with the guillotine.
14. Discard one-half of strip at each side border as stripping could be less homogenous near the borders.
15. ImageJ is a public-domain, Java-based image-processing program developed at the National Institutes of Health that can be used to compare the density (or intensity) of bands on an immune test strip. You have to obtain a digital image of your strips in .tif, .jpg, .png, or other image formats. You can use a flatbed scanner, and the appropriate scanner software to save a well-exposed good-quality image.
16. The values calculated by ImageJ are essentially arbitrary numbers; they only have meaning within the context of the set of peaks that you selected on the image you have been working on. They do not have units. The usual procedure is to express the density of the selected bands relative to some standard band that you also selected during this process.

Acknowledgments

SGO is a postdoctoral fellow supported by the Beatriu de Pinós programme from El Comissionat per a Universitats i Recerca del Departament d'Innovació, Universitats i Empresa, Generalitat de Catalunya.

References

1. Curtin-Brosnan J, Paigen B, Hagberg KA et al (2010) Occupational mouse allergen exposure among non-mouse handlers. J Occup Environ Hyg 7(12):726–734
2. Olmedo O, Goldstein IF, Acosta L et al (2011) Neighborhood differences in exposure and sensitization to cockroach, mouse, dust mite, cat, and dog allergens in New York City. J Allergy Clin Immunol 128(2):284–292
3. Sage A (2015) Food allergen analysis using LC–MS–MS. The Column 10(7). http://www.chromatographyonline.com/food-allergen-analysis-using-lc-ms-ms. Accessed 3 Nov 2015
4. Earle CD, King EM, Tsay A et al (2007) High-throughput fluorescent multiplex array for indoor allergen exposure assessment. J Allergy Clin Immunol 119(2):428–433
5. Permaul P, Hoffman E, Fu C et al (2012) Allergens in urban schools and homes of children with asthma. Pediatr Allergy Immunol 23(6):543–549
6. Samadi S, Heederik DJ, Krop EJ et al (2010) Allergen and endotoxin exposure in a companion animal hospital. Occup Environ Med 67(7):486–492
7. Álvarez-Simón D, Cruz MJ, Untoria MD et al (2014) A rapid test for soy aeroallergens exposure assessment. PLoS One 9(2):e88676
8. Mire-Sluis AR, Barrett YC, Devanarayan V et al (2004) Recommendations for the design and optimization of immunoassays used in the detection of host antibodies against biotechnology products. J Immunol Methods 289(1–2):1–16

Chapter 14

Novel Method for the Purification of House Dust Mite Allergen Der p 1 and Its Use in Structure-Based Chemical Design of Novel Inhibitors

Jihui Zhang and Clive Robinson

Abstract

House dust mites are globally significant triggers of allergic disease. Notable among their extensive repertoire of allergens are the Group 1 cysteine peptidase allergens which function as digestive enzymes in house dust mites. Compelling evidence suggests that the proteolytic activity of these molecules plays a key role in the development and maintenance of allergic diseases through the activation of innate immune mechanisms which exploit genetic predispositions to allergy. Growing interest in this area creates a requirement for high-quality purified protein, whether natural or recombinantly expressed. It has also identified these allergens as therapeutic targets for a novel approach to allergy treatment through modulation of innate immune responses. The purpose of this chapter is to describe a new method for the purification of Der p 1 and use of the protein produced in a screening assay designed for the discovery of novel inhibitors of Group 1 house dust mite allergens.

Key words House dust mite, Der p 1 purification, Allergen delivery inhibitors, Innate immunity, Structure-based drug design, Protein purification, Protease assay

1 Introduction

In 1921 the American physician Richard Kern postulated that house dust was a cause of allergic disease because many patients with asthma or rhinitis had positive skin responses to extracts of dust from their dwellings. This concept was developed further by Willem Storm van Leeuwen whose work led him to believe that house dust mites (HDM) were key components of this house dust allergy. However, formal proof of this idea was elusive and it was not until the work of Voorhorst and Spieksma in 1967 that the involvement of HDM was eventually acknowledged by most allergists. Under environmental conditions which enable HDM to thrive, they elicit the production of allergen-specific IgE and form a notable allergen source strongly associated with asthma. Many species of mite are found in house dust, with the Pyroglyphid

Penny Lympany and Meinir G. Jones (eds.), *Allergy: Methods and Protocols*, Methods in Molecular Biology, vol. 2020, https://doi.org/10.1007/978-1-4939-9591-2_14,

family (e.g., *Dermatophagoides pteronyssinus, D. farinae,* and *Euroglyphus maynei*) dominating in most parts of the world. The unusually extensive allergen repertoire of HDM includes proteins of several classes [1]. Of these, the Group 1 allergens have attracted particular scrutiny because of their strong association with sensitization and disease. In studying Group 1 HDM allergens, Der p 1 has frequently been used as a meaningful archetype for Group 1 allergens from other mite species. This approach is reasonable because Group 1 allergens from different HDM species show a high degree of sequence identity, giving encouragement that their immunological, and other, behavior should be similar if not the same.

In HDM, Group 1 allergens function as digestive enzymes belonging to the cysteine protease family. In fact, they represent a novel subfamily of 25 kDa cysteine proteases based on the length, structure, and behavior of the propiece which regulates latency of these enzymes [2]. The recognition that Group 1 allergens were cysteine proteases prompted interest into the possible relevance of this bioactivity to the mechanisms of allergy, in particular fundamental questions surrounding the molecular basis of allergenicity [1]. It is clear from exploration of this topic that proteolytic activity of Group 1 HDM allergens is significant for the development of sensitization to themselves, other mite allergens, and allergens from unrelated sources. Proteolytic activity acts as a means of facilitating allergen delivery to antigen-presenting cells, as an adjuvant to stimulate a vigorous immune response which exhibits Th2 polarization, and contributes to mechanisms which have chronic pathophysiological consequences [3]. These biophysical and innate immune mechanisms are summarized in Table 1. A recent, and unexpected, finding was the discovery that Der p 1 is a prothrombinase capable of triggering interstitial thrombin formation in the absence of coagulation pathway activation [4]. This triggering of thrombin formation initiates a complex signaling cycle in which the intracellular generation of ROS eventuates, and whose operation forms a nexus with inflammatory signaling from Toll-like receptors 3 and 7 which act as sensors for viral RNA [4, 5].

The realization that these events are relevant to allergic sensitization and, significantly, exert a collateral priming effect for the sensitization to other allergens has prompted interest in Group 1 HDM allergens as novel therapeutic targets for asthma and other allergic conditions. Conveniently, amino acid sequence similarities between Group 1 allergens from different species of HDM mean that they represent a single target for drug design purposes. This is pleasingly helpful compared to their epitopes which, although showing many similarities, are sufficiently different to be immunologically distinguishable.

Provisioning a drug discovery campaign requires a supply of purified target protein for screening, and generally recombinantly

Table 1
Actions of Der p 1 mediated through pathways central to innate immunity

Biosignature	Notes
Cleavage of tight-junction adhesion molecules/allergen delivery	Demonstrated for Der p 1. Molecular targets are occludin and claudins. Reversible increase in epithelial permeability eventuates. Prevented by ADI drugs
Prothrombinase activity	Intrinsic property of Der p 1. Prevented by ADIs
Activation of protease activated receptor (PAR) 1 and 4	Due to formation of thrombin by prothrombinase action. Prevented by ADIs
Activation of protease-activated receptor 2	Direct cleavage of receptor by Der p 1
Breakdown of immune tolerance—development of allergic sensitization	Der p 1 promotes sensitization to itself and unrelated allergens. Prevented by ADIs
Cleavage of low-affinity IgE receptor (CD23)	Regulates IgE biosynthesis in B cells
Cleavage of DC-SIGN/R	Regulate recruitment of dendritic antigen-presenting cells
Cleavage of IL-2R (CD25)	Promotes Th2 polarization of immune responses
Inactivation of surfactant proteins A and D	Demonstrated for Der p 1 and Der f 1. Predicted to promote allergy development
Inactivation of airway antiproteases, e.g., α_1-antitrypsin	Der p 1 impairs natural defense against other proteases
IgE-independent mast cell stimulation	Demonstrated for Der p 1
Cytokine and chemokine release (e.g., IL-6, IL-8, GM-CSF, CCL-5, CCL-11 from epithelial cells)	Demonstrated for Der p 1. Possibly mediated through PAR activation
Activation of epidermal growth factor receptor (EGFR) signaling	Dependent on Der p 1. Thought to be cross talk from PAR activation. Requires activation of a disintegrin and metalloprotease (ADAM) 17. Prevented by ADIs
Pannexon gating in airway epithelial cells	ATP release and signaling through P_2X_7 receptors eventuate. Dependent on Der p 1 and thought to be downstream of EGFR signaling. Prevented by ADIs
Activation of ADAM 10	Downstream signaling consequence of ATP release by Der p 1. Exerts significant control over IgE biosynthesis (as a CD23 sheddase) and involved in stem cell factor-dependent recruitment of mast cells. Prevented by ADIs
Thrombin formation	Endogenously formed from prothrombin by ADAM 10-dependent mechanism activated as above. Prevented by ADIs
Intracellular reactive oxidant formation in airway epithelial cells	Downstream consequence of Der p 1. Mechanism involves PAR, EGFR signaling, ATP, and ADAM 10 components as described above. Provides fundamental redox-dependent transcriptional control of cytokine expression. Prevented by ADIs
Inflammatory cell recruitment in vivo	Innate mechanisms activated by Der p 1 and prevented by ADIs

expressed protein is used for this purpose. However, in the case of Der p 1 inhibitor design this was not an immediately available option. Although recombinant Der p 1 had been expressed prior to drug discovery work, this was produced by prokaryotic expression and lacked catalytic competence due to the absence of correct protein folding. Purified protein is also the basis of structure-based drug discovery approaches because the availability of high-resolution target structures facilitates rational decision-making in chemical design. In the initial absence of definitive structural data for Der p 1 itself, we generated its likely structure by homology modeling using high-quality crystallographic data for the cysteine peptidases cathepsin K, papain, and actinidin. Subsequently, high-resolution crystal structures became available for Der p 1 and Der f 1 from *D. farinae* and, with only few notable differences, these are generally consistent with our homology models [6, 7]. In its monomeric form, Der p 1 comprises a pair of globular domains between which is located a substrate-binding groove whose composition, as predicted by empirical examinations of substrate and inhibitor kinetics, is highly conserved at both the isoallergen and homologous species levels. This substrate-binding groove contains the Cys, His, and Asn catalytic triad typical of the C1 family of CA clan cysteine peptidases. The availability of high-quality structural data, together with information gathered during screening using highly purified Der p 1, corrects an erroneous report that Der p 1 allergens (and by implication other Group 1 HDM allergens) are mechanistically bifunctional enzymes with both cysteine and serine protease activity [8]. No credible evidence exists to support this suggestion, which most likely originates from inadequacies in protein purification based on immunoaffinity chromatography which has been a commonly employed method of obtaining Der p 1 for research studies. Der p 1 prepared as described herein will not degrade *N*-succinyl-Ala-Ala-Pro-Phe-*p*-nitroanilide, which is an effective substrate for chymotrypsin, and while trypsin and Der p 1 are both able to utilize *N*-Bz-Phe-Val-Arg-*p*-nitroanilide as substrate, the latter enzyme's behavior is not affected by the broad-spectrum serine peptidase inhibitor 4-(2-aminoethyl)benzene sulfonyl fluoride (AEBSF), whereas it is blocked by the thiol-reactive Der p 1 inhibitor ADZ 50,000 [3]. Indeed, structural inspection of Der p 1 reveals that none of the serine residues it contains are located in a proximity to His or Asp residues for the creation of a catalytic triad.

Examination of protease substrate specificity provides an efficient means of identifying target motifs which may be useful as scaffolds in structure-based drug design. Screening a library of fluorescence resonance energy transfer (FRET) substrates of general formula Abz-B-C-D-E-Tyr(NO_2)-Asp-NH_2 revealed preferences as follows: B: Val > Ala, Gln, Leu, Phe; C: Ala>> Gln or Lys; D: Leu, Nle or Ala>Ser; E: Ser. This information was employed in the elaboration of substrates into inhibitors such as acyloxymethyl ketones based around the scaffold Val-Ala-Nle-Ser (Fig. 1).

An unfortunate corollary of this otherwise valuable approach is that while initial inhibitor "hits" may exhibit exquisite potency, they lack significant drug-likeness [3, 9]. Thus, progress toward developable candidate drugs requires careful optimization of necessary credentials (potency, selectivity, pharmacokinetic properties, physical form, etc.). An additional concern in the case of the acyloxymethyl ketone derivatives is that their mechanism of Der p 1 inhibition is irreversible, creating the potential for hapten generation. This negates the optimization of this particular series for the intended therapeutic indications where the intended patient population has a genetic predisposition to allergy. However, considerable success was achieved in optimization of a lead series based around a pyruvamide motif [9]. These inhibitors have a reversible mechanism on the target enzyme and through a structure-based design campaign around this series we obtained a range of develop-

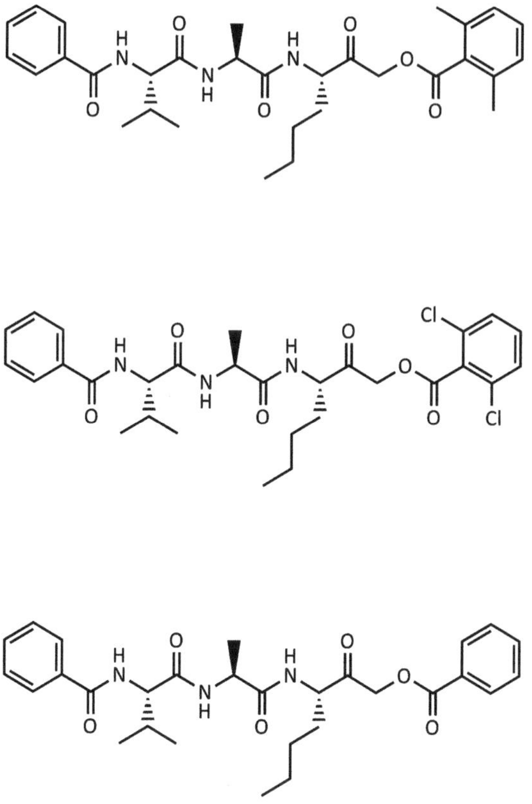

irreversible
1.6×10^{7} $M^{-1}s^{-1}$

irreversible
6.8×10^{7} $M^{-1}s^{-1}$

irreversible
3.7×10^{5} $M^{-1}s^{-1}$

Fig. 1 Exemplification of acyloxymethyl ketone inhibitors of the proteolytic activity of Group 1 HDM allergens. Inhibitory activity is expressed as second-order inhibitor rate constant for each compound when evaluated against Der p 1. These compounds were identified by making systematic variations to a peptide sequence identified from peptide library screening

Table 2
Structure-activity relationships for simple modifications to a pyruvamide scaffold and their effects on the ability to inhibit the proteolytic activity of Der p 1 and cathepsin B

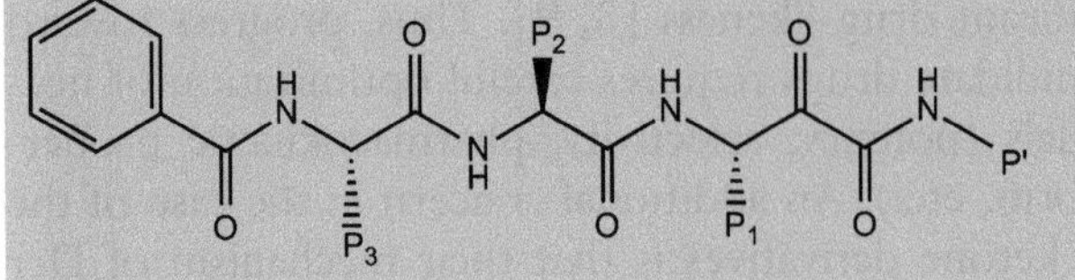

P_1	P_2	P_3	P'	Der p 1 IC_{50} (nM)	Cathepsin B IC_{50} (nM)
n-Bu	Me	Benzyl	Cyclohexyl	8 ± 1	17 ± 2
i-Pr	Me	Benzyl	Cyclohexyl	18 ± 2	52 ± 5
i-Pr	Me	Benzyl	Benzyl	12 ± 2	50 ± 5
t-Bu	Me	Benzyl	Cyclohexyl	9167 ± 880	*Not Determined*
i-Pr	Me	*t*-Bu	Cyclohexyl	14 ± 3	378 ± 27
i-Pr	Me	$C(Me)_2Ph$	Benzyl	42 ± 6	446 ± 11
i-Pr	*n*-Pr	benzyl	Cyclohexyl	164 ± 24	67 ± 1

Cathepsin B inhibition was measured using enzyme from human liver preactivated by 2.5 mM 1,4 dithioerythritol at 37 °C for 10 min. Substrate was ABz-Gly-Ile-Val-Arg-Ala-Lys-DNP-OH. Progress curves were measured at 30 °C by detection of fluorescence (excitation/emission 320/420 nm)

able compounds with the required combination of properties for delivery by inhalation in dry powder form [9]. Arrival at this position required iterative rounds of screening and counter-screening of compounds in which structure variations at key positions in the basic pyruvamide scaffold were introduced systematically. An illustration of one small aspect of this, made using the screening method described herein for Der p 1 purified as described, is shown in Table 2. Comprehensive details of structure-activity relationships for the Der p 1 target are available elsewhere [9]. We call this new class of drugs "allergen delivery inhibitors" (ADIs) because of their ability to inhibit the transepithelial delivery of allergens to subepithelial dendritic antigen-presenting cells. However, their efficacy profile extends considerably beyond this action given the wide-ranging effects of the target's proteolytic activity on innate immune responses.

2 Materials

2.1 Reagents for Der p 1 Extraction and Purification

1. House dust mites (*Dermatophagoides pteronyssinus*) are maintained in continuous solid-phase culture with controlled temperature and relative humidity (25 °C, 75%) in a custom-built containment system. Mite growth medium comprises 50%

(w/w) of Brewer's Yeast (*Saccharomyces cerevisiae*) and 50% desiccated liver that has been ground in a Waring blender and hot air sterilized at 80 °C for 3–4 h in a Stericell oven. Cultures grown for 1.5–3 months provide a suitable feedstock for Der p 1 purification.

2. Dulbecco's phosphate-buffered saline, without calcium chloride and magnesium chloride (D-PBS).
3. Ethylenediaminetetraacetic acid disodium salt (EDTA) 100 mM in H_2O: Dissolve 18.6 g EDTA into 500 mL deionized water to make up 100 mM EDTA solution.
4. Elution buffer for Sephacryl S200 column (EB):
   (a) Add 98 mL 0.2 M Na_2HPO_4, 10 mL 100 mM EDTA, and 890 mL double-deionized water into a 1000 mL beaker.
   (b) Weigh out 29.22 g NaCl and dissolve in the above solution.
   (c) Carefully adjust the pH to 7.4 with 0.2 M NaH_2PO_4.
   (d) Add double-deionized water to a total volume 1000 mL.
   (e) Vacuum filter through 0.2 μm porosity membrane. The filter device can be of any type having a suitable pore size. For routine batch preparations a filter device of 500 mL volume is adequate.
5. Buffer A (20 mM Tris–HCl buffer, pH 8.0):
   (a) Dissolve 60.5 g Trizma base in 900 mL deionized water, and adjust to pH 8.0 using 50% (v/v) HCl.
   (b) Add deionized water to a total volume of 1000 mL to produce 0.5 M Tris–HCl buffer, pH 8.0.
   (c) Add 20 mL 0.5 M Tris–HCl buffer, pH 8.0, to 480 mL deionized water to yield buffer A.
6. Buffer B (20 mM Tris–HCl buffer, pH 8.0, containing 2 M NaCl): Dissolve 58.4 g NaCl into 500 mL buffer A.
7. 0.1 M Glycine-HCl buffer, pH 2.8 (GB):
   (a) Dissolve 7.5 g glycine in 995 mL deionized water, and adjust the pH to 2.8 using 50% (v/v) HCl.
   (b) Adjust volume to 1000 mL using deionized water.

2.2 Reagents for SBTI (Trypsin Inhibitor from Soybean) Affinity Column

1. SBTI (from Sigma-Aldrich, UK).
2. CNBr-activated Sepharose 4 Fast Flow (from Sigma-Aldrich, UK).
3. 0.1 M $NaHCO_3$ pH 8.3 containing 0.5 M NaCl.
4. 1 mM HCl.

5. 0.5 M Tris–HCl, pH 8.0 buffer: Dissolve 60.5 g Trizma base in 900 mL deionized water, and adjust to pH 8.0 with 50% (v/v) HCl. Then adjust to a final volume of 1000 mL with deionized water to produce 0.5 M Tris–HCl, pH 8.0. Add 100 mL of this solution to 400 mL deionized water to produce 0.1 M Tris–HCl buffer, pH 8.0
6. 0.1 M acetate buffer pH 3–4 containing 0.5 M NaCl: Dissolve 8.2 g sodium acetate in 500 mL deionized water to produce a 0.2 M solution. Mix 10 mL glacial acetic acid with 865 mL deionized to produce a 0.2 M solution. Take 410 mL of the acetic acid solution and adjust to pH 4.0 using 0.2 M sodium acetate (requires about 90 mL). Dilute twofold with deionized water to produce 0.1 M acetate buffer and dissolve 14.6 g NaCl into 500 mL of this.
7. 0.1 M Tris–HCl buffer pH 8–9 containing 0.5 M NaCl.
8. Binding buffer: EB.

2.3 Reagents for Der p1 Identification by Matrix-Assisted Laser Desorption/Ionization Time-of-Flight (MALDI-TOF) Mass Spectrometry

1. 50 mM Ammonium bicarbonate solution.
2. Ammonium bicarbonate, 40 mM, pH 8.9, containing 9% v:v acetonitrile.
3. 50% v:v Acetonitrile.
4. 1 mM Hydrochloric acid (HCl): Add 1 mL concentrated HCl to 11 mL deionized water yielding 1 M HCl which should then be diluted 1000-fold with deionized water to provide, finally, 1 mM HCI.
5. Trypsin solution: 20 μg Trypsin (Sigma Aldrich, UK) is supplied lyophilized in vials. Reconstitute the lyophilized trypsin in 100 μL 1 mM HCl and mix the vial briefly until completely dissolved. Add 900 μL ammonium bicarbonate, 40 mM, pH 8.9, containing 9% v:v acetonitrile to the vial and mix. The final concentration of trypsin is 20 μg/mL. Aliquot and store at −20 °C (*see* **Note 1**).
6. Matrix: α-Cyano-4-hydroxycinnamic acid (CHCA) for peptides with molecular weight <10 kDa. Weigh out 10 mg CHCA and add 700 μL acetonitrile and 300 μL 0.1% v:v trifluoroacetic acid (TFA) in deionized water. Vortex mix to dissolve completely.

2.4 Reagents for Der p 1 Activity Test with or Without ADZ 50,000

1. 50 mM Potassium phosphate buffer containing 1 mM EDTA, pH 8.29 (PPE) (*see* **Note 2**):
   (a) Mix 97.4 mL, 0.5 M K_2HPO_4 with 10 mL, 100 mM EDTA, and 890 mL deionized water.
   (b) Adjust pH to 8.29 with 0.5 M KH_2PO_4 (about 2.6 mL).
   (c) Adjust to 1000 mL using deionized water.

2. Substrate solution (125 μM substrate in buffer PPE, reagent I): Weigh out 10 mg Der p 1 substrate ((3S,6S,9S,12S,15S,18S)-1-(2-aminophenyl)-9-butyl-18- carbamoyl-1 5-(4-hydroxy-3 -nitrobenzyl)-12-(hydroxymethyl)-3-isopropyl- 6-methyl-1,4,7,10,13,16-hexaoxo-2,5,8,11,14,17-hexaazaicosan-20-oic acid), and dissolve in dry dimethyl sulfoxide (DMSO) to make a 10 mM stock solution. Aliquot as 50 μL/vial and store frozen at 4 °C or lower. Before use, add 987.5 μL buffer PPE into 12.5 μL 10 mM substrate solution. Vortex mix immediately and thoroughly.
3. 10 mM DL-dithiothreitol (DTT) (reagent II):
   (a) 1 M DTT stock solution: Dissolve 1.55 g DTT in 8 mL water and adjust the final volume to 10 mL. Aliquot as 50 μL/vial and store frozen at −20 °C.
   (b) Make up 10 mM DTT from the stock solution by adding 10 μL 1 M DTT stock solution into 990 μL buffer PPE.
4. 9 mM DTT (reagent II*): Make up 9 mM DTT by adding 9 μL 1 M DTT stock solution into 991 μL buffer PPE.
5. Reagent III (2.5 μg/mL Der p 1 in PPE): Add 7.5 μL 1 mg/mL Der p 1 into 2992.5 μL PPE. Mix well. For pre-activation: Add Der p 1 (7.5 μL × 1 mg/mL) to 2989.5 μL PPE and 3 μL 1 M DTT. Mix well and leave at room temperature for 5 min (*see* **Note 3**).
6. Inhibitor preparation: Dissolve inhibitors in dry DMSO to make 100 mM stock solutions if they can be dissolved; otherwise the stock solutions could be 50 mM or 10 mM (the default inhibitor stock concentration). Prior to use, dilute the stock solution to 10 mM with DMSO.

2.5 Apparatus and Columns

1. Amicon Stirred Cell 50 mL (Merck Millipore, UK).
2. Ultracel membrane with 10 kDa cutoff (Merck Millipore, UK).
3. Cylinder of oxygen-free, compressed nitrogen (or nitrogen line from an infrastructure "boil off" supply).
4. Magnetic stirrer.
5. Balances, analytical and general laboratory.
6. pH meter.
7. pH paper.
8. Sephacryl S-200 column, Hiprep, 16/60 (GE Healthcare, UK).
9. Resource Q column, 1 mL (GE Healthcare, UK).
10. Refrigerated centrifuges with fixed-angle rotors: The *g* force needs to be 23,500 × *g* or above for 30 mL tubes and 10,000 × *g* for 15 mL microcentrifuge tubes.

11. Microplate reader equipped with fluorescence reading modes and heated plate carrier.
12. ÄKTA Purifier or similar equipment for protein chromatography.
13. MALDI-TOF mass spectrometer.

3 Methods

All Der p 1 purification steps are carried out at 4 °C. This may be achieved by working in a cold room or, more comfortably, in a suitably equipped laboratory cold cabinet.

3.1 Preparation of the SBTI Affinity Column

1. Dissolve 400 mg SBTI in 40 mL coupling buffer (0.1 M $NaHCO_3$, pH 8.3, containing 0.5 M NaCl) to make up 10 mg/mL SBTI as coupling solution.
2. Add 20 mL of cold 1 mM HCl to 2 g dried CNBr-activated Sepharose 4 Fast Flow. Wait until all the powder is wet, then pack the matrix into a 25 mL syringe, and wash with 10–15 column volumes of cold 1 mM HCl.
3. Cycle load 40 mL of 10 mg/mL SBTI in coupling buffer and allow to react for 4 h (or overnight) at 4 °C (*see* **Note 4**).
4. Wash away excess ligand with at least five column volumes of coupling buffer.
5. After coupling, non-reacted groups on the matrix should be blocked. To do this, run 100 mL 0.1 M Tris–HCl pH 8.0 buffer through the column and allow to stand for at least 2 h (*see* **Note 5**).
6. Wash the coupled matrix using alternate low- and high-pH buffers. Recommended buffers are 0.1 M acetate buffer pH 3–4 containing 0.5 M NaCl and 0.1 M Tris–HCl buffer pH 8–9 containing 0.5 M NaCl. A suitable procedure is three column volumes of Tris–HCl buffer followed by three column volumes of acetate buffer. Repeat this cycle 3–6 times.
7. The coupled matrix is now ready for use. To prevent microbial growth, store in 20% v:v ethanol.
8. Equilibrate the column with binding buffer before applying samples.

3.2 Preparation of PBS Extracts and 50% Ammonium Sulfate Fraction

1. Der p 1 PBS extracts from house dust mite medium.
   (a) Add 200 mL D-PBS to 50 g spent medium from house dust mite cultures in a 500 mL beaker.
   (b) Cover with parafilm and stir at 4 °C for 4 h to overnight. Ensure that the stirrer is operating satisfactorily in order to achieve efficient extraction.

(c) Transfer the mixture into suitable centrifuge tubes (e.g., 30 mL for a Sorvall RC-5B centrifuge). Weigh the tubes to make sure that each pair of tubes has the same weight so that the rotor can be balanced.

(d) Put a pre-cooled fixed-angle rotor in the centrifuge, and ensure that it is correctly located on the spindle.

(e) Put the tubes into the rotor in a balanced (symmetrical) position.

(f) Centrifuge at 23,500 × *g* and 4 °C for 30 min.

(g) Remove the tubes gently to avoid disturbing the pellets and carefully transfer the supernatants to a 250 mL measuring cylinder to measure the volume. Then transfer the combined supernatants to a 500 mL beaker. This combined supernatant is called the PBS extract (PBSE).

(h) Clean the rotor with water and wipe dry with tissues. Return the rotor to cool storage.

2. 50% Ammonium sulfate precipitates.

(a) Add 100 mM EDTA (stock solution in H_2O) to PBSE so the final concentration for EDTA is 1 mM.

(b) Calculate the amount of solid ammonium sulfate (ammonium sulfate (grams) = (supernatant volume/100) × 30) required for the supernatant to make up 50% saturation.

(c) Add the required solid ammonium sulfate to PBSE gradually, and stir at 4 °C for 4 h or overnight.

(d) Centrifuge at 23,500 × *g* and 4 °C for 30 min.

(e) Discard the supernatants. Gently raise the pellets with D-PBS to remove excess ammonium sulfate (*see* **Note 6**).

(f) Add 3 mL D-PBS to each tube, and redissolve the precipitates.

(g) Centrifuge again, as above, and collect the supernatants.

(h) Transfer the supernatants carefully to an Amicon filtration cell equipped with a 10 kDa cutoff membrane for concentration with stirring at 4 °C under compressed nitrogen (*see* **Note 7**).

(i) After concentration, wash the 50% ammonium sulfate fraction into 1–3 mL Sephacryl S200 EB buffer (**Note 7**).

(j) Centrifuge at 23,500 × *g* and 4 °C for 10 min and transfer the supernatant into a clean vial for chromatography. This supernatant is called the concentrated 50% ammonium sulfate fraction.

3.3 Isolation of Der p 1 by Chromatography

1. Equilibrate a Sephacryl S-200 column (16/60, Hiprep) on an ÄKTA Purifier system using three column volumes (CV) of buffer EB.
2. Apply 2–3 mL (*see* **Note 8**) of the concentrated 50% ammonium sulfate fraction to the column and elute with EB. Collect the fraction with a retention volume of 90–120 mL (RT90) (Fig. 2).
3. Equilibrate the SBTI affinity column with EB before applying samples.
4. Load the sample RT90 on the SBTI affinity column by cycle loading for 4 h to overnight using a flow rate of 0.1 mL/min.
5. Collect the flow-through solution and concentrate it under pressurized nitrogen in an Amicon cell equipped with 10 kDa cutoff ultrafiltration membrane.

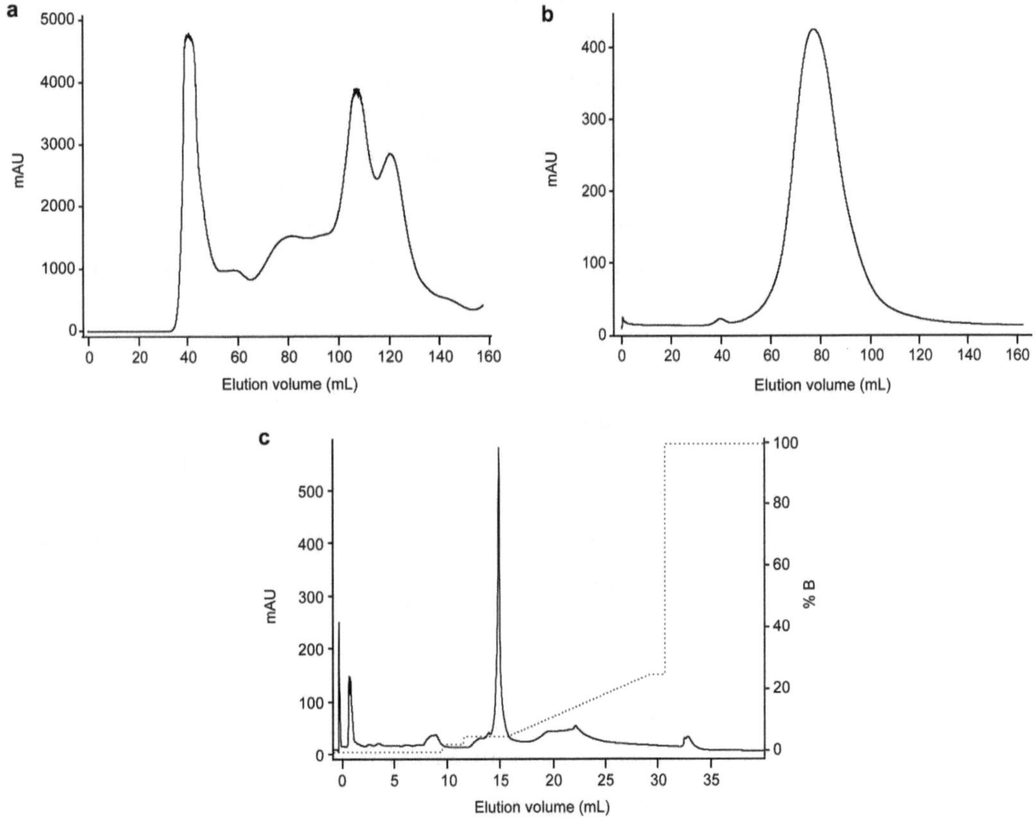

Fig. 2 Purification of Der p 1. (**a**) Initial chromatography of HDM allergen extract on Sephacryl S200 with monitoring of absorbance at 280 nm. (**b**) Rechromatography of HDM allergen extract on Sephacryl S200. (**c**) Resource Q chromatography of Der p 1 monitored by absorbance at 280 nm. The peak pattern is dependent on sample purity, and indicates various forms of Der p 1 caused by different degrees of glycosylation, autolysis, or cleavage of the propiece from pro-Der p 1 at different cleavage sites. More than one peak containing Der p 1 is not unusual at this stage. The dotted line shows the gradient profile

6. After each run, regenerate the SBTI affinity column by washing it with 5 CV 0.1 M glycine-HCl buffer, pH 2.8, and re-equilibrate it with 5 CV of EB for the next run.
7. Add elution buffer for Sephacryl S200 chromatograph, transfer the concentrated sample into 1.5 mL vials, and then centrifuge at 13,400 × *g*, for 10 min at 4 °C, to get rid of any insoluble precipitates. Then repeat **steps 2–5** (Fig. 2).
8. Concentrate and desalt the samples obtained from **step** 7 (*see* **Note 9**) and then redissolve them in 20 mM Tris–HCl, pH 8.0 buffer, followed by centrifugation at 23,400 × *g*, for 10 min at 4 °C with fixed-angle-head rotor. Collect the supernatant for Resource Q chromatography.

3.4 Chromatography on Resource Q

1. Equilibrate a Resource Q column with 5 CV of pH 8.0, 20 mM Tris–HCl buffer before use. Then load the samples.
2. Gradient elution from 0.05–0.5 M NaCl is done with buffer A and buffer B (Fig. 2c) (*see* **Note 10**). It is possible to modify the gradient to improve the resolution if samples show complex behavior. Table 3 illustrates one possible alternative.
3. Collect each peak and concentrate and desalt them using an Amicon cell as above. Then transfer into D-PBS for quality assurance.
4. Determine the concentration of the fractions from the Resource Q column by measuring A_{280} in a quartz cell or microplate. The concentration of Der p 1 is calculated using the equation (Der p 1 concentration (mg/mL) = absorption $A_{280nm}/1.8$).
5. Run the Der p 1 activity assay with or without inhibitor ADZ 50,000 to confirm the purity from a proteolytic class activity perspective.
6. Determine the purity of purified Der p 1 by 15% sodium dodecyl sulfate-polyacrylamide gel electrophoresis (SDS-PAGE) (ref. Molecular Cloning: A Laboratory Manual, by Sambrook, Fritsch, and Maniatis) (*see* **Note 11**).
7. Identify Der p 1 in each eluted fraction by MALDI-TOF mass spectrometry.
8. Combine the Der p 1 fractions which combine high purity on SDS-PAGE with good proteolytic activity (*see* **Note 12**).
9. Redetermine the concentration of the combined Der p 1 sample and its activity.
10. Aliquot and store at −20 °C or lower.

In a typical run, about 0.4 mg (measured by A_{280nm}) purified Der p 1 is obtained from 50 g spent house dust mite culture medium (*see* **Note 13**). The purity of Der p 1 is ≥90% on SDS-PAGE by Coomassie blue staining (Fig. 3). Fractions eluted from Resource Q column were characterized by mass spectrometry, and

Table 3
Fine gradient elution program for Resource Q chromatography using an ÄKTA Purifier system with Buffer A and Buffer B containing 1 M NaCl

Start_Conc_B	Start_ConcB {%B}	0
Column_Equilibration	Equilibrate_with {CV}	1
Sample_Injection	Empty_loop_with {ml}	5
Wash_Out_Unbound_Sample	Wash_column_with {CV}	2
Gradient_Segment_1	Target_ConcB_1 {%B}	5
	Length_of_Gradient_1 {CV}	0
Gradient_Segment_2	Target_ConcB_2 {%B}	5
	Length_of_Gradient_2 {CV}	5
Gradient_Segment_3	Target_ConcB_3 {%B}	10
	Length_of_Gradient_3 {CV}	5
Gradient_Segment_4	Target_ConcB_4 {%B}	10
	Length_of_Gradient_4 {CV}	5
Gradient_Segment_5	Target_ConcB_5 {%B}	17.5
	Length_of_Gradient_5 {CV}	20
Gradient_Segment_6	Target_ConcB_6 {%B}	20
	Length_of_Gradient_6 {CV}	10
Gradient_Segment_7	Target_ConcB_7 {%B}	50
	Length_of_Gradient_7 {CV}	5
Gradient_Segment_8	Target_ConcB_8 {%B}	50
	Length_of_Gradient_8 {CV}	5
Gradient_Segment_9	Target_ConcB_9 {%B}	100
	Length_of_Gradient_9 {CV}	5
Gradient_Delay	Gradient_Delay {ml}	5
Clean_after_Elution	Clean_with {CV}	10
Length_of_Reequilibration	Reequilibrate_with {CV}	10

combined for activity testing. The enzymatic activity of purified Der p 1 was confirmed by assay with the specific substrate which incorporates a FRET fluorescor-quencher pair.

3.5 Der p 1 Confirmation by MALDI-TOF Mass Spectrometry

1. Carefully excise the band of interest from the SDS-PAGE gel and transfer to a 1.5 mL microcentrifuge vial.
2. Cut the excised band into smaller pieces and wash with 50 mM ammonium bicarbonate followed by 50% acetonitrile in water (500 μL). Then dehydrate the gel with 100% acetonitrile.

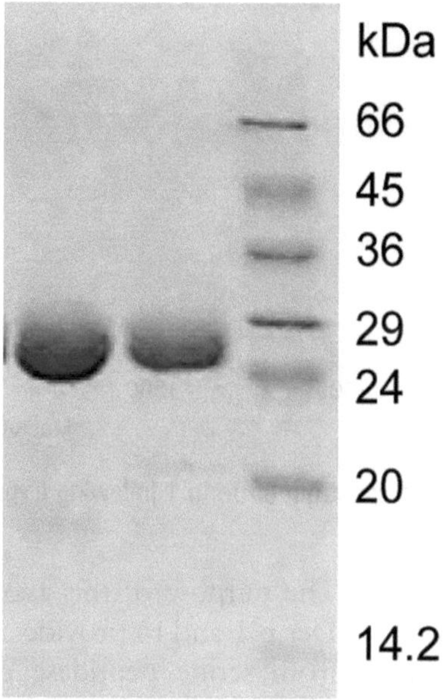

Fig. 3 SDS-PAGE of purified Der p 1

3. Remove acetonitrile and cover the vial with pierced parafilm. Vacuum dry the gel for 20 min in a freeze dryer.
4. Add 20 μL (0.4 μg of trypsin) of the trypsin solution prepared for in-gel digests to the sample and rehydrate for 15 min.
5. Add sufficient 9% v:v acetonitrile in 40 mM ammonium bicarbonate to cover the gel and incubate for 4 h to overnight at room temperature.
6. After incubation, pipette 1 μL solution onto a MALDI-TOF target and mix with 1 μL matrix α-cyano-4-hydroxycinnamic acid. Air-dry the samples before running.
   (a) MALDI-TOF mass spectrometry can be performed using any suitable instrument. Details are given here for work performed using a Kratos Axima instrument operated in positive reflectron mode at an accelerating voltage of 100 kV. The calibrant contained peptides with m/z^+ from 700 to 2000.
   (b) The ions obtained by MALDI-TOF mass spectrometry of trypsin-digested Der p 1 (m/z^+: 622.49, 647.51, 741.66, 1830.83, 1734, 1759, 2056.57, 2585.88, 3214.87) can be observed on the sample mass spectrum (Fig. 4) and match to the calculated data of the Der p 1 sequence (*see* **Note 14**). Among them, m/z^+ 1830.83 is the variant of fragment ^{209}FGISNYCQIYPPN<u>V</u>NK, in which V^{222} was changed to A^{222} FGISNYCQIYPPN<u>A</u>NK, as reported in UniProtKB/Swiss-Prot.

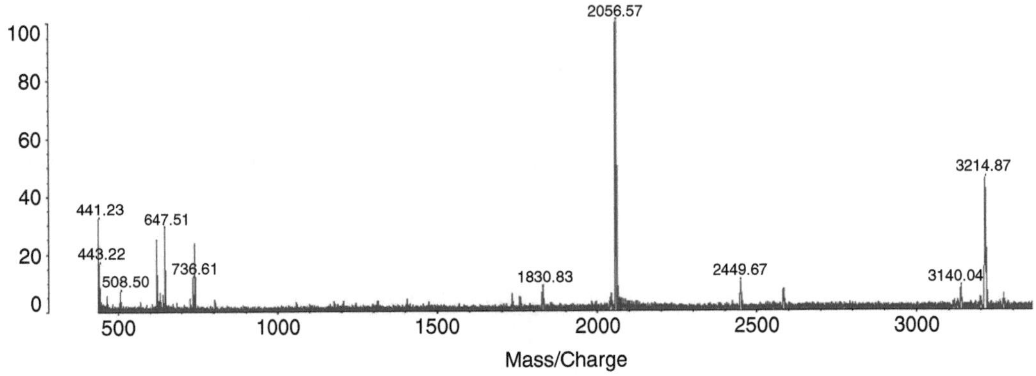

Fig. 4 MALDI-TOF mass spectrum of Der p 1 following trypsin digestion as described in these methods

3.6 Der p 1 Proteolytic Activity Measurement with or Without ADZ 50,000

The purpose of this assay is to measure the enzymatic activity of Der p 1 and to provide assurance that the measured activity is free from serine peptidase contamination. This is achieved using a potent and selective inhibitor, ADZ 50,000. The proteolytic activity assay is performed on a black 96-well plate (Optiplate, Perkin Elmer, Buckinghamshire, UK) by adding reagent I (10 μL), PPE (70 μL), and reagent II (10 μL) into each well, and then adding 10 μL reagent III to initiate the reaction. The plate is read in a kinetic assay mode for 33 min at 30 °C using excitation/emission at 330/420 nm immediately after adding reagent III. Our preference has been to perform these assays using Perkin Elmer Fusion or Envision microplate readers, but recognized alternatives are available. The ADZ 50,000 inhibition component of the assay is performed as described above except for the addition of 10 μL/well of ADZ 50,000 at a range of concentrations into wells before adding substrate. To accommodate this, the volume of PPE is reduced to 60 μL in these wells. This modification is also used in the screening of inhibitors, e.g., in the evaluation of novel compounds synthesized in a drug discovery campaign directed against the enzymatic activity of Group 1 house dust mite allergens (*see* description below). Example progress curves for Der p 1 activity assays are shown in Fig. 5.

3.7 $K_{obs}/[I]$ Measurement of Irreversible Inhibitors

The assay is set up on a 96-well plate containing different concentrations of inhibitors according to the format shown in Table 4. Examples of progress curves for determining inhibitor constant $K_{obs}/[I]$ are presented in Fig. 6. $[I]$ is the inhibitor concentration. The reproducibility was measured by determining $K_{obs}/[I]$ of ADZ 50,000 on Der p 1. K_{obs} is calculated as shown below:

$$[P]_t = V_z / K_{obs}\left(1 - e^{-Kobs.t}\right).$$

In this equation, $[P]_t$ is the product concentration at time t (RFU in this case).

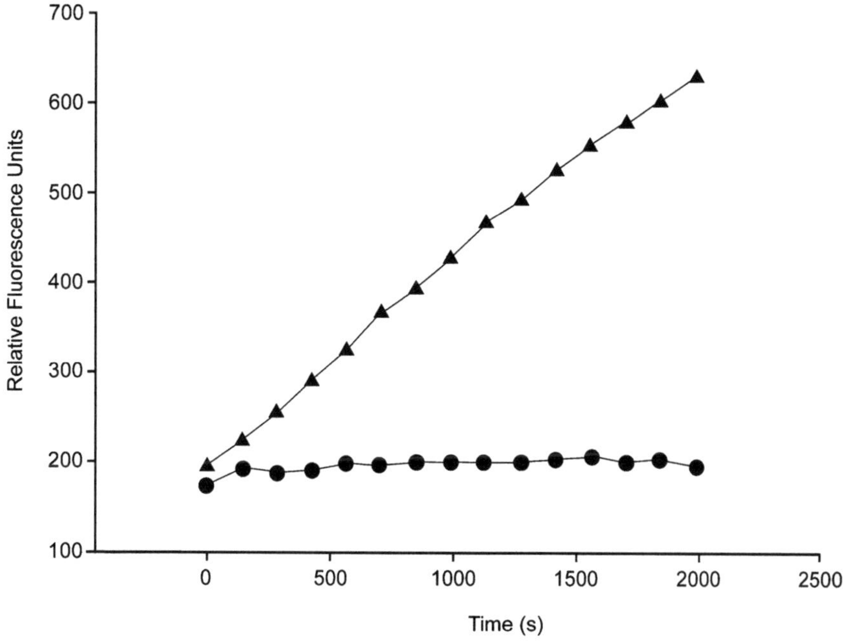

Fig. 5 Measurement of Der p 1 enzymatic activity by FRET assay performed as described herein using (3S,6S,9S,12S,15S,18S)-1-(2-aminophenyl)-9-butyl-18-carbamoyl-15-(4-hydroxy-3 -nitrobenzyl)-12-(hydroxymethyl)-3-isopropyl-6-methyl-1,4,7,10,13,16-hexaoxo-2,5,8,11,14,17-hexaazaicosan-20-oic acid as substrate. Triangles show activity in the absence of any inhibitor. Circles depict reaction progress in the presence of 25 nM of the acyloxymethyl ketone derivative ADZ 50,000

Table 4
Map for screening Der p 1 inhibitors using a 96-well format

C1	50	25	12.5	6.25	3.125	1.56	0.78	0.39	0.195	0.0975	0.0488	NC
C1	50	25	12.5	6.25	3.125	1.56	0.78	0.39	0.195	0.0975	0.0488	NC
C2	50	25	12.5	6.25	3.125	1.56	0.78	0.39	0.195	0.0975	0.0488	NC
C2	50	25	12.5	6.25	3.125	1.56	0.78	0.39	0.195	0.0975	0.0488	NC
C3	50	25	12.5	6.25	3.125	1.56	0.78	0.39	0.195	0.0975	0.0488	PC
C3	50	25	12.5	6.25	3.125	1.56	0.78	0.39	0.195	0.0975	0.0488	PC
C4	50	25	12.5	6.25	3.125	1.56	0.78	0.39	0.195	0.0975	0.0488	PC
C4	50	25	12.5	6.25	3.125	1.56	0.78	0.39	0.195	0.0975	0.0488	PC

C1–C4: Compound identifier
The unit of concentration for the inhibitors is μM
PC: Positive control (Der p 1 without inhibitors)
NC: Blank without Der p 1

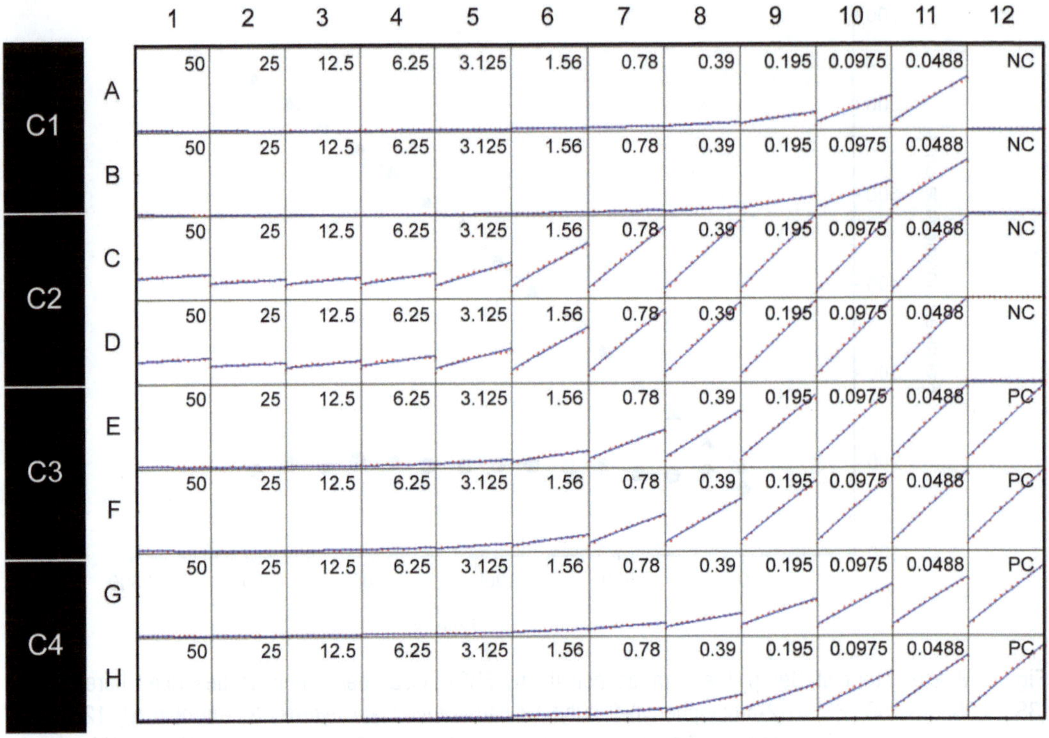

Fig. 6 Annotated screenshot of sample progress curves showing the activity of Der p 1 in the absence or presence of various experimental inhibitors from an experiment to determine inhibition constants

Table 5
Second-order rate determinations for acyloxymethyl ketone derivative ADZ 50,000 vs. Der p 1 showing example assay standard deviation (SD)

K_{obs}/I (× 10[8] M[−1] s[−1])	Assay 1	Assay 2	Assay 3	Assay 4	SD inter-daily
Plate 1a	1.42	1.74	1.48	1.33	0.1761
Plate 1b	1.52	1.33	1.15	1.35	0.1513
Plate 2a	0.97	1.0	0.93[a]	0.83[a]	0.0741
Plate 2b	1.18	1.29	0.95[a]	0.99[a]	0.1603
Within-day SD	0.2470	0.3045	0.2551	0.2568	/

K_{obs}/I was measured in five replicates except where indicated [a] when $n = 4$

V_z is the velocity of uninhibited reaction (mRFU/min).

K_{obs} is a pseudo first-order rate constant.

$K_{obs}/[I]$ unit is s^{-1} M^{-1} and calculated with SigmaPlot (*see* **Note 13**).

The inter-daily standard deviation and within-daily standard deviation of $K_{obs}/[I]$ are below 0.3 (Table 5), suggesting that the assays display good reproducibility and reliability.

3.8 Measurement of IC_{50} for Reversible Inhibitors

For reversible inhibitors, the screening assays are constructed similarly, except a 20-min preincubation is required prior to initiating the reaction by substrate addition. Inhibitory activity is analyzed from progress curves of reactions in the presence of a range of inhibitor concentrations. Initial reaction velocities are calculated by computational nonlinear regression and degree of inhibition produced by compounds determined, from which the concentration required to inhibit the reaction by 50% (IC_{50}) is calculated according to the scheme below:

Initial velocity in each well is converted to fractional activity by Eq. 1:

$$\text{Fractional activity} = \left(V_t / \mathrm{V}_0\right) \times 100 \tag{1}$$

where

V_t: Initial rate at inhibitor concentration [X].

V_0: Initial rate at inhibitor concentration zero.

Then, IC_{50} is determined by fitting the data of fractional activity and inhibitor concentration to a four-parameter logistic curve, using Eq. 2:

$$V = V_{\min} + \left[V_{\max} - V_{\min}\right] / \left[1 + \left(X / \mathrm{IC}_{50}\right)^{\text{Hillslope}}\right] \tag{2}$$

where

V is the fractional activity of the enzyme in the presence of inhibitor at concentration $[X]$.

$[X]$ is the inhibitor concentration.

$V_{\min}$ is the minimum of V observed at high inhibitor concentration.

$V_{\max}$ is the maximum of V observed at zero inhibitor concentration.

Hill slope is the slope of the dose-response (inhibition) curve.

4 Notes

1. Trypsin solution can be stored at −20 °C. Minimize the aliquot volumes so it can be used with little wastage because the activity will drop significantly if the enzyme is refrozen and thawed.
2. The pH will drop slightly after adding DTT, so the working pH would be very close to 8.25. If >2.6 mL NaH_2PO_4 is required to adjust the pH to 8.29, the total volume will be slightly over 1000 mL, but the buffer can still be used as normal.

3. Der p 1 is a cysteine peptidase and the active site contains reduced cysteine residues. When the catalytic cysteine is oxidized, the activity of Der p 1 drops. During purification, the cysteine residues in Der p 1 might have been oxidized, so pre-activation of Der p prior to use is very necessary. Therefore, reducing reagents such as DTT need to be added in the reaction to ensure maximal activation of the enzyme. Activation of Der p 1 by DTT is fast so this step should be done immediately prior to use. Der p 1 should not be stored in DTT to minimize the risk of autolysis.
4. The coupling process can be done as cycle loading to increase the coupling efficiency.
5. For good blocking efficiency, more blocking buffer can be used and the blocking time of non-reacted groups on the medium can be longer up to overnight.
6. When raising the pellets with D-PBS, be quick and gentle to avoid D-PBS dissolving the pellets.
7. Make sure that the membrane is intact. An Ultracel membrane with 10 kDa cutoff is used. Carefully pipette EB buffer into the cell, try to dissolve all materials in the cell, and divide the mixture into 2 × 1.5 mL Eppendorf vials for centrifugation. To avoid damaging the filtration membrane, do not touch it with pipette tips. The membrane can be reused after washing thoroughly with buffer and stored in water at 4 °C.
8. For the first chromatography on Sephacryl S200 the sample volume can be up to 5 mL.
9. For concentration of **step 7** samples using Amicon cell ultrafiltration, try to filter all liquid through the membrane to remove salt as much as possible. Residual salt may affect the binding efficiency of samples on Resource Q columns.
10. For the elution gradient on Resource Q, the gradient change from 0.05 to 0.5 M NaCl can be adjusted according to different purposes. For example, to polish samples the gradient could be set as a linear change from 0.05 to 0.5 M. For complex samples, the gradient can be finely tuned using a lower NaCl concentration in buffer B (e.g., 1 M can be used instead of 2 M to achieve a small gradient change). Table 3 is an example of this application.
11. On SDS-PAGE, there will be more than one fraction containing Der p 1 eluted by the NaCl gradient. This is due to different isoforms of Der p 1 in the mite medium. Although these contain Der p 1 they may also contain significant impurities and therefore should not be used for experimental purposes where purity is paramount. Der p 1 appearing in different frac-

tions of Resource Q column indicates the different forms of Der p 1.

12. In activity tests, Der p 1 in different eluted peaks displays different activities due to autolysis and/or Der p 1 isoforms. The fractions with significantly lower activity should not be combined in the purification workup.
13. The yield of purified Der p 1 is highly dependent on the initial production in the mite medium and this should be borne in mind when comparing different batches purely according to gross yield.
14. SigmaPlot is our preferred data-processing software, but suitable alternatives are available (e.g., Prism or WorkOut).

References

1. Stewart GA, Richardson JP, Zhang J et al (2014) The structure and function of allergens. In: Adkinson NF, Bochner BS, Burks AW, Busse WW, Holgate ST, Lemanske RF et al (eds) Middleton's allergy—Principles and practice. Elsevier, Philadelphia, pp 398–429
2. Zhang J, Hamilton JM, Garrod DR et al (2007) Interactions between mature Der p 1 and its free prodomain indicate membership of a new family of C1 peptidases. Allergy 62: 1302–1309
3. Robinson C, Zhang J, Newton GK et al (2013) Nonhuman targets in allergic lung conditions. Future Med Chem 5:147–161
4. Zhang J, Chen J, Allen-Philbey K et al (2016) Innate generation of thrombin and intracellular oxidants in airway epithelium by allergen Der p 1. J Allergy Clin Immunol 138:1224–1227
5. Chen J, Zhang J, Tachie-Menson T et al (2017) Allergen-dependent oxidant formation requires purinoceptor activation of ADAM 10 and prothrombin. J Allergy Clin Immunol 139: 2023–2026
6. Meno K, Thorsted PB, Ipsen H et al (2005) The crystal structure of recombinant pro Der p 1, a major house dust mite proteolytic allergen. J Immunol 175:3835–3845
7. de Halleux S, Stura E, VanderElst L et al (2006) Three-dimensional structure and IgE-binding properties of mature fully active Der p 1, a clinically relevant major allergen. J Allergy Clin Immunol 117:571–576
8. Hewitt CR, Horton H, Jones RM et al (1997) Heterogeneous proteolytic specificity and activity of the house dust mite proteinase allergen Der p I. Clin Exp Allergy 27:201–207
9. Newton GK, Perrior TR, Jenkins K et al (2014) The discovery of potent, selective, and reversible inhibitors of the house dust mite peptidase allergen Der p 1: an innovative approach to the treatment of allergic asthma. J Med Chem 57:9447–9462

Chapter 15

Measurement of Specific IgG Anti-Fel d 1 Antibodies

Meinir G. Jones

Abstract

There is currently considerable interest in the role of specific IgG antibodies in allergy. Several studies suggest that specific IgG antibodies may play a protective role in allergy. Successful immunotherapy is associated with increases in allergen-specific IgG antibodies which correlate with clinical outcome. Other studies have identified an inverse relationship between exposure to cat and sensitization, which was associated with high-titer-specific IgG and IgG_4. This immune response was described as a modified Th2 response, since both IgE and IgG_4 require Th2 cytokine IL-4 for their production. A modified Th2 response was described with laboratory animal allergy, where there was almost a twofold reduction in the risk of developing work-related chest symptoms.

In this chapter, we review the major factors to be considered in the development of an ELISA for the determination of specific IgG and IgG_4 antibodies.

Key words IgG antibodies, IgG_4 antibodies, IgE, modified Th2 response, Blocking antibodies

1 Introduction

There has been considerable interest in the role of IgG in allergy: recent evidence suggests that it may play a protective role. An inverse relationship between exposure to cats and sensitization was described which was associated with high-titer-specific IgG and IgG_4 [1]. This immune response is described as a modified Th2 response, since both IgE and IgG_4 require Th2 cytokine IL-4 for their production. The modified Th2 response is suggestive of clinical tolerance since the shift from specific IgE antibodies to IgG_4 resulted in a decrease in both sensitization and asthma [2].

We have recently established a modified Th2 response in laboratory animal workers. Within our cohort and cross-sectional studies on laboratory animal allergy we observed increasing risks of sensitization and work-related symptoms with increasing exposures to rats, except at highest exposure level where risks of both outcomes were lower [3, 4]. We established a significantly increased ratio of IgG_4:IgE in those workers most heavily exposed. There was

Penny Lympany and Meinir G. Jones (eds.), *Allergy: Methods and Protocols*, Methods in Molecular Biology, vol. 2020,
https://doi.org/10.1007/978-1-4939-9591-2_15,

an almost twofold reduction of symptoms in those who produced both specific IgG_4 and IgE as compared to those producing specific IgE only. The attenuation of sensitization and symptoms at high exposures and the increased ratio of IgG_4:IgE in laboratory animal workers are suggestive of a natural form of immunotherapy.

Ratios of IgE to IgG_4 have been found to change during specific immunotherapy [5]. Specific serum levels of both IgE and IgG_4 increase during the early phase of therapy, but the increase in specific IgG_4 is more pronounced and the ratio of specific IgG_4:IgE is increased 10- to 100-fold, suggesting a protective role for IgG_4 [5]. IL-10 is a potent suppressor of both total and allergen-specific IgE, whereas it simultaneously increases IgG_4 production [6].

Successful immunotherapy is associated with increases in allergen-specific IgG_1 and IgG_4 antibody concentrations occur that correlate with the clinical outcome [7–10]. It is not known whether allergen-specific IgG or IgG_4 antibodies associated with the modified Th2 response exhibit functional activity. It is possible that IgG antibodies may play a protective role by blocking leukocyte histamine release, inhibiting signal transduction and mediator release through the high-affinity IgE receptor (FcεR1) and IgG (FcγRIIB) receptors [11–14] and blocking allergen-induced IgE-dependent histamine release by basophils [15]. IgG antibodies may exert their effect by competitive inhibition of allergen-IgE complexes, which prevents complexes binding to the low-affinity IgE receptor, CD23, and subsequent antigen presentation. Others have suggested that not only quantitative changes occur with the IgG antibody but also the spectrum of the specificity of the IgG is altered [16]. One grass pollen immunotherapy study demonstrated a blunting of seasonal increases in serum allergen-specific IgG and IgG_4. Further examination showed the postimmunotherapy serum to exhibit inhibitory activity, which co-eluted with IgG_4 and blocked IgE-facilitated binding of allergen-IgE complexes to B cells. Increases in IgG and the IgG blocking activity correlated with the patients' overall assessment of improvement [9].

2 Materials

2.1 ELISA

1. Elisa plate.
2. 1× Phosphate-buffered solution (PBS).
3. Allergen at 1 μg/mL Fel d 1 in PBS.
4. Positive control: A pool of serum samples known to have IgG anti-Fel d 1 antibodies.
5. Negative control: A pool of serum samples known to be negative for IgG anti-Fel d 1 antibodies.

6. Test serum samples for the measurement of IgG anti-Fel d 1 antibodies.
7. Coating buffer: 50 mM Carbonate bicarbonate buffer pH 9.6.
8. Blocking buffer: PBS, 1% bovine serum albumin (BSA). Make up fresh on the day of assay.
9. Reagent buffer: PBS, 1% bovine serum albumin (BSA), and 0.05% Tween 20. Make up fresh on the day of assay.
10. Wash buffer: PBS, 0.05% Tween 20. Add sodium azide 0.05% for storage.
11. Biotinylated anti-IgG antibody (Becton Dickinson, Cowley, UK) diluted 1:1000 in reagent buffer: 10 mL is sufficient for 96-well ELISA plate.
12. ExtrAvidin Peroxidase diluted 1:1000 in reagent buffer.
13. Phosphate citrate buffer pH 5.0: 2.48 g Na2HPO4 to 50 mL water—buffer A. 1.92 g citric acid to 50 mL water—buffer B. Add 50 mL of buffer A and B to 100 mL deionized water and bring pH to 5.0. Store at 4 °C.
14. Stock substrate: Dissolve 100 mg 3,3′,5,5′-tetramethylbenzidine (TMB) in 10 mL dimethyl sulfoxide. Store in 200 μL aliquots at −20 °C.
15. Substrate solution: Add 100 μL stock TMB stock solution to 10 mL phosphate citrate pH 5.0 and add 3 μL H_2O_2 (w/w) immediately before use. The substrate solution must be made prior to addition to wells. 10 mL Substrate solution is sufficient for one 96-well ELISA plate.
16. Stop solution: 1.9 M Sulfuric acid. Store at room temperature. N.B.: Always add acid to water in fume cupboard.

2.2 Inhibition Assay

1. In addition to the reagents for the ELISA, a higher concentration of Fel d 1 at 10 μg/mL is required for preincubation with serum.

3 Methods

The method described for the measurement of IgG antibodies specific for Fel d 1 has been optimized. A chequerboard was set up with varying concentrations of allergen, biotinylated antibody, and streptavidin peroxidase (*see* **Note 1**). The optimum concentrations were used for the ELISA. The time and temperature of the incubation periods were also optimized.

We believe that it is essential to subtract the binding of IgG antibodies to the blocking agent BSA. Some sera have much higher binding to BSA than other sera; however it is essential to subtract the background binding for each individual.

We have measured specific IgG antibodies to a panel of allergens. The protocol given for the measurement of IgG-specific antibodies to Fel d 1 can be optimized for each allergen using the chequerboard approach. IgG_4-specific antibodies can also be measured using the same protocol but substituting the biotinylated anti-IgG antibody with biotinylated anti-IgG_4 antibody. The IgG_4 ELISA will need to be optimized as above.

3.1 Protocol for IgG-Specific Antibodies to Fel d 1

1. Coat each well in the upper half of the ELISA plate with 100 μL of 1 μg/mL Fel d 1.
2. Coat each well in the lower half of the ELISA plate with 100 μL of 1% BSA.
3. Store in a polystyrene box with a damp tissue overnight at 4° C.
4. Wash plates ×3 with wash buffer. Plates can be washed by hand using a squeeze bottle or using a dedicated ELISA washer (*see* **Note 2**). The hand method is suitable for a small number of plates. At the end of the third wash bang the plate on a tissue to get most of the remaining buffer out of the wells.
5. Add 200 μL of blocking buffer to each well in the whole plate. Incubate in a damp box for 2 h at 4 °C.
6. Wash plates ×4 with wash buffer.
7. Gently mix serum samples on vortex. Add 100 μL of reagent buffer to wells A1–2 and E1–2. Add 10 μL of positive control and 90 μL reagent buffer to wells A3–4 and E3–4. Add 10 μL negative control and 90 μL reagent buffer to wells A5–6 and E5–6. Add 10 μL of test serum to wells in duplicate to both the upper allergen-coated plate and the BSA-coated plate. Incubate for 2 h at 4 °C.
8. Wash plates ×5 with wash buffer.
9. Add 100 μL of biotinylated anti-human IgG (diluted 1:1000 in reagent buffer) to each well and incubate for 1 h at 4 °C.
10. Wash plates ×6 with wash buffer.
11. Add 100 μL of ExtrAvidin Peroxidase (diluted 1:1000 in reagent buffer) to each well and incubate for 30 min at 4 °C.
12. Wash plates ×7 with wash buffer.
13. Add 100 μL of freshly made substrate solution to each well. Leave for 10 min at room temperature.
14. Add 50 μL of stop solution to each well.
15. Wipe the bottom of ELISA plate with a tissue and ensure that there are no air bubbles in any of the wells. Read ELISA plate at 450 nm absorbance.
16. Calculate the average of duplicates.

17. Subtract the background BSA OD measurement from the allergen OD measurement for each sample. The results are arbitrary values based on OD values.

3.2 Protocol for Determining Specificity of ELISA by Inhibition Assay

1. Coat each well in the upper half of the ELISA plate with 100 μL of 1 μg/mL Fel.
2. Coat each well in the lower half of the ELISA plate with 100 μL of 1% BSA.
3. Store in a polystyrene box with a damp tissue overnight at 4° C.
4. Incubate serum with varying quantities of allergen to set up an inhibition curve. In our Fel d 1 assay we incubated equal volume of serum sample with Fel d 1 solution at 1.0, 0.5, 0.1, and 0 μg/mL final concentration in the well. The serum and allergen were left on a roller at 4 °C overnight.
5. Wash plates ×3 with wash buffer.
6. Add 200 μL of blocking buffer to each well in the whole plate. Incubate in a damp box for 2 h at 4 °C.
7. Wash plates ×4 with wash buffer.
8. Add 10 μL of the preincubated serum and allergen to the wells and incubate for 2 h at 4 °C.
9. Continue with ELISA as for above protocol from **step 8** onwards.
10. The degree of allergen inhibition is taken as (uninhibited − inhibited)/inhibited × 100. An example of our inhibition curve for Fel d 1 is shown in Tables 1 and 2 for two different sera.

3.3 Analysis of ELISA Data

We did not have the appropriate reagents to set up a standard curve for our Fel d 1 assay; we therefore reported our results as arbitrary values based on the optical density. We had to ensure that samples run in different assays were compatible, so we ran a pool of serum

Table 1
Inhibition of IgG anti-Fel d 1antibodies binding with the solid-phase Fel d 1 with inhibitor Fel d 1 allergen

Inhibitor μg/mL	O.D. Feld 1	O.D. HSA	O.D. Fel d 1—HSA	% Inhibition
0	0.947	0.430	0.517	0
0.1	0.761	0.388	0.373	27.8
0.5	0.740	0.369	0.371	28.3
1.0	0.521	0.445	0.076	85.3

Table 2
Inhibition of IgG anti-Fel d 1 antibodies with the solid-phase Fel d 1 with inhibitor Fel d 1 allergen

Inhibitor μg/mL	O.D. Feld 1	O.D. HSA	O.D. Fel d 1—HSA	% Inhibition
0	1.073	0.425	0.648	0
0.1	0.980	0.453	0.527	18.6
0.5	0.849	0.424	0.425	34.4
1.0	0.722	0.789	0	100.0

We were able to get 85–100% inhibition by preincubating two different sera with 1 μg/mL Fel d 1. Less than 1 μg/mL of inhibitor Fel d 1 did not significantly inhibit the binding of specific IgG anti-Fel d 1 antibodies to the solid phase. This demonstrated that the binding to Fel d 1 in the assay was specific to Fel d 1 and was not as a result of nonspecific or low-affinity antibody binding

with low, medium, and high levels of IgG antibody on each plate in every assay run. We ran these samples in ten different assays to establish the coefficient of variance. Our assays would only be accepted if the coefficient of variance of the quality control samples was less than 20%.

4 Notes

1. Optimization of assay.

   Every step within the ELISA needs to be optimized [17]. In particular the following were considered when setting up the IgG assay.

   (a) Concentration of allergen on solid phase—the capacity of microtiter plates to bind proteins is limited. At high concentration of protein, there is a tendency for protein molecules to bind to each other, resulting in dissociation of bound protein during the assay. In practice 1–10 μg/mL is the desired concentration to use for coating your solid-phase ELISA plate. A steep reference curve is desirable since a small change in concentration will give a large color change. In practice we would aim for a 2–3 log range in our dilution curves.

   (b) Choice of coating buffer—the choice of coating buffer should be determined by testing the binding of allergen with pH 9.6 carbonate/bicarbonate buffer, a pH 7.4 phosphate-buffered saline, and a pH 5.0 acetate/citrate buffer. The charge of a protein depends on the buffer it is dissolved in. Therefore the charge of the coating buffer plays an important role in the ability of the allergen to bind to the ELISA plate.

(c) Incubation time for coating plate—1 h is usually sufficient. However it is often desirable to coat the ELISA plate overnight, to allow time to perform the assay the following day. Again it is prudent to optimize the incubation time. It is possible to coat and block ELISA plates and keep frozen until ready for use. Again it is essential to check that this works for your particular assay.

(d) Blocking plates—several blocking reagents can be used ranging among human serum albumin, bovine serum albumin, casein, and gelatine. Again when setting up your assay it is worthwhile comparing the various blocking agents. Typically the blocking agents are used at a concentration of 1–2%.

(e) Volume of reagents—typically we use 100 μL of reagents per well, apart from in the blocking stage where we typically use 200 μL. If the sensitivity of the assay needs to be increased we use 200 μL reagent per well. Anything over 200 μL per well has the potential for crossover of reagent between wells.

(f) Choice of buffer—the concentration and molarity of buffers are generally between 0.05 and 0.1 M. Antibody-antigen reactions normally take place between pH 6.0 and 9.0. Normally the buffers used in the assay will contain blocking buffer. It is essential that the buffers are made fresh on the day since addition of serum albumin can lead to bacterial contamination which will result in erroneous ELISA results.

(g) Incubation times—1 h is usually sufficient for the reaction to be complete. The incubation times can be shortened by placing the ELISA plate on a shaker—the times can typically be cut in half. Again the incubation times will need to be optimized for each assay.

(h) The dilution of the sample will depend on the concentration; low concentration will require high sample volume, whereas high concentration will need to be diluted. At high serum concentrations there is a tendency to get nonspecific binding and binding of low-affinity antibodies. The serum sample needs to be optimized by setting up a dilution curve.

(i) Detecting antibodies—As with other steps in the ELISA these will need to be optimized. It is essential to ensure that the detecting reagent binds only to the sample and not to the other reagents in the ELISA.

2. We normally use a wash bottle to wash our ELISA plate which is perfectly adequate. This is a very simple effective cheap method of washing ELISA plates. It is essential for the user to be very thorough in their washing steps, ensuring that all wells are washed and that the buffer is flicked out of the plate. Some prefer to use an automated plate washer which is useful if running several plates in one assay. The downside of an automated plate washer is the expense; however it is useful if you intend running ELISAs on a regular basis and overcomes user error in the washing process. Others use a bucket of buffer and simply immerse the plate in the bucket of buffer which is a perfectly adequate system of washing.

References

1. Platts-Mills T, Vaughan J, Squillace S, Woodfolk J, Sporik R (2001) Sensitisation, asthma, and a modified Th2 response in children exposed to cat allergen: a population-based cross-sectional study. Lancet 357:752–756
2. Hesselmar B, Aberg B, Eriksson B, Bjorksten B, Aberg N (2003) High-dose exposure to cat is associated with clinical tolerance-a modified Th2 immune response? Clin Exp Allergy 33:1681–1685
3. Akdis CA, Blaser K (1999) IL-10-induced anergy in peripheral T cell and reactivation by microenvironmental cytokines: two key steps in specific immunotherapy. FASEB J 13:603–609
4. Akdis CA, Blesken T, Akdis M, Wuthrich B, Blaser K (1998) Role of interleukin 10 in specific immunotherapy. J Clin Invest 102:98–106
5. Cullinan P, Cook A, Gordon S, Nieuwenhuijsen MJ, Tee RD, Venables KM et al (1999) Allergen exposure, atopy and smoking as determinants of allergy to rats in a cohort of laboratory employees. Eur Respir J 13:1139–1143
6. Jeal H, Draper A, Harris J, Taylor AN, Cullinan P, Jones M (2006) Modified Th2 responses at high dose exposure to allergen; using an occupational model. Am J Respir Crit Care Med 174(1):21–25
7. Gehlhar K, Schlaak M, Becker W, Bufe A (1999) Monitoring allergen immunotherapy of pollen-allergic patients: the ratio of allergen-specific IgG4 to IgG1 correlates with clinical outcome. Clin Exp Allergy 29:497–506
8. Jutel M, Akdis M, Budak F, Aebischer-Casaulta C, Wrzyszcz M, Blaser K et al (2003) IL-10 and TGF-beta cooperate in the regulatory T cell response to mucosal allergens in normal immunity and specific immunotherapy. Eur J Immunol 33:1205–1214
9. Nouri-Aria KT, Wachholz PA, Francis JN, Jacobson MR, Walker SM, Wilcock LK et al (2004) Grass pollen immunotherapy induces mucosal and peripheral IL-10 responses and blocking IgG activity. J Immunol 172:3252–3259
10. Djurup R, Osterballe O (1984) IgG subclass antibody response in grass pollen-allergic patients undergoing specific immunotherapy. Prognostic value of serum IgG subclass antibody levels early in immunotherapy. Allergy 39:433–441
11. Golden DB, Meyers DA, Kagey-Sobotka A, Valentine MD, Lichtenstein LM (1982) Clinical relevance of the venom-specific immunoglobulin G antibody level during immunotherapy. J Allergy Clin Immunol 69:489–493
12. Daeron M, Malbec O, Latour S, Arock M, Fridman WH (1995) Regulation of high affinity IgE receptor-mediated mast cell activation by murine low-affinity IgG receptors. J Clin Invest 95:577–585
13. Daeron M (1997) Negative regulation of mast cell activation by receptors for IgG. Int Arch Allergy Immunol 113:138–141
14. Zhu D, Kepley CL, Zhang M, Zhang K, Saxon A (2002) A novel human immunoglobulin Fc gamma Fc epsilon bifunctional fusion protein inhibits Fc epsilon RI-mediated degranulation. Nat Med 8:518–521
15. Ball T, Sperr WR, Valent P, Lidholm J, Spitzauer S, Ebner C et al (1999) Induction of antibody responses to new B cell epitopes indicates vaccination character of allergen immunotherapy. Eur J Immunol 29:2026–2036
16. Wachholz PA, Durham SR (2003) Induction of 'blocking' IgG antibodies during immunotherapy. Clin Exp Allergy 33:1171–1174
17. Kemeny DM (1991) A practical guide to ELISA. Pergamon Press, Oxford

Chapter 16

Measurement of Specific IgG_4 Anti-mouse Urine Antibodies

Jennifer Canizales

Abstract

IgG_4 and its role in immune tolerance has been investigated widely. Symptom reduction and improved clinical outcomes in immunotherapy trials are associated with significant increases in allergen-specific IgG_4 antibodies. Natural immune tolerance observed in beekeepers and cat owners has also been associated with elevated levels of bee venom and cat allergen-specific IgG_4, respectively. Functionally, allergen-specific IgG_4 has been shown to reduce the binding of IgE-allergen complexes to B cells, a key step in the initiation of the type 1 hypersensitivity allergic response. In laboratory animal allergy, IgG_4 has been described as a "protective/blocking" antibody. However, a consensus on the exact relationship between exposure, IgG_4, and tolerance has yet to be reached. In this chapter, we review the factors that require consideration when developing an ELISA for the quantification of allergen-specific IgG_4.

Key words IgG_4 antibodies, Blocking antibodies, Modified Th2 response, Natural immune tolerance

1 Introduction

Allergy, the type 1 hypersensitivity reaction, is mediated by IgE antibodies. Sensitization first occurs when an individual is exposed to an allergen and their immune cells (B cells) produce specific IgE antibodies to this allergen. These IgE antibodies opsonize/coat immune cells such as mast and basophil cells. Upon re-exposure the allergen can be bound by the specific IgE on the surface of these cells causing "cross-linking," which leads to degranulation of the mast cells and release of histamine and other pro-inflammatory mediators, leading to the common allergic symptoms such as rhinitis.

Those exposed to allergens can also develop allergen-specific IgG and IgG_4 antibodies. There is much interest in these antibodies as they have been implicated in the anti-inflammatory T-regulatory response [1], as well as being shown to block the binding of allergen-IgE complex binding to B cells via the FcεRII receptor [2, 3]. Both IgE and IgG_4 are produced as part of the Th2 response [4]. Cat allergy studies have shown an association between high cat allergen exposures, production of high levels of

Penny Lympany and Meinir G. Jones (eds.), *Allergy: Methods and Protocols*, Methods in Molecular Biology, vol. 2020, https://doi.org/10.1007/978-1-4939-9591-2_16,

allergen-specific IgG_4 (without specific IgE), and clinical tolerance. This suggested switch from the production of specific IgE to specific IgG_4 is known as the "modified Th2 response" [5, 6].

The role of IgG_4 antibodies in tolerance has been widely studied in relation to allergy immunotherapy. It has been established that the administration of allergen immunotherapy leads to a marked increase in the levels of allergen-specific IgG_4 antibody [7–9]. However, it is the level of blocking activity of the IgG_4 antibody (preventing the binding of IgE-allergen complexes to B cells) that directly correlates with immunotherapy treatment efficacy [10]. It may also stand to reason that allergen-specific IgG_4 antibodies also have a role in natural immunotolerance. Studies of beekeepers have demonstrated a positive association between chronic/high exposure (number of stings) and higher levels of bee venom-specific IgG_4, this suggests a role for specific IgG_4 antibodies and natural tolerance [11, 12].

Our work focuses on the role of IgG_4 in natural immunotolerance to laboratory animal allergy (LAA). Many studies have shown a positive correlation between increasing levels of rodent exposure and levels of rodent-specific IgG_4 [13–15]. However, a recent cohort study found no such correlation [16].

Reports vary on whether there is an association between specific IgG_4 and clinical symptoms. A number of studies have shown that increased levels of specific IgG and IgG_4 are positively associated with, or predictive of, sensitization and symptoms [17]. Others suggest that higher levels of specific IgG_4 in fact reduce the risk of symptoms and sensitization [15]. The importance of antibody ratios has also been investigated. Jeal et al. [13] found that increased rat-specific IgG_4 correlated with increased rates of symptoms and sensitization; however, when looking at the ratios of specific IgG_4 to specific IgE, this was reversed (high specific IgG_4/low specific IgE ratio = low symptoms and sensitization). Similarly to immunotherapy trials, the functional role of IgG_4 in LAA has been investigated. It has been shown that increased levels of rat-specific IgG_4 are associated with reduced levels of IgE-allergen complex binding to B cells [13].

2 Materials

2.1 ELISA

1. ELISA plate (Corning EIA/RIA Assay Microplate, Sigma-Aldrich, UK).
2. 1× Phosphate-buffered saline (PBS)
3. In-house mouse urine extract in PBS.
4. Positive control: Pool of serum samples from laboratory animal workers previously identified as having detectable levels of mouse urine-specific IgG_4.

5. Negative control: Pool of serum samples from non-laboratory animal workers, previously identified as being negative for mouse urine-specific IgG_4.
6. Test serum samples for the measurement of mouse urine-specific IgG_4.
7. Reagent/blocking buffer: PBS, 1% bovine serum albumin (BSA), 0.05% Tween-20. Make up fresh on the day of assay.
8. Wash buffer: PBS, 0.05% Tween-20. Make up fresh on the day of assay.
9. Natural Human IgG_4 Protein (Abcam, Cambridge, UK): Aliquot and store at −20 °C.
10. HRP mouse anti-Human IgG_4 (Thermo Fisher Scientific, UK): Add glycerol for a final concentration of 50% and store at −20 °C. To be diluted 1:1000 in reagent/blocking buffer, 12 mL is sufficient for 96-well ELISA plate.
11. Substrate solution: Pierce™ TMB Substrate Kit (Thermo Fisher Scientific, UK): Substrate solution should be made up immediately before use. The two solutions provided in the kit should be mixed in equal parts; 12 mL substrate solution is sufficient for 96-well ELISA plate.
12. Stop solution: 2 M Sulfuric acid. Store at room temperature.
13. Ensure that there are no air bubbles in any of the wells and read plate at 450 nm absorbance.
14. Calculate average OD values of duplicates.
15. Using the average OD values determine the concentration of serum IgG_4 using the standard curve (described below), and express concentrations as arbitrary units (AU).

3 Methods

The method described for the measurement of IgG_4 antibodies specific for mouse urine and the standard curve for the ELISA has been optimized. A checkerboard was set up with varying concentrations of allergen, HRP-labeled antibody, and human IgG_4. The optimum concentrations were used for the ELISA. The time and temperature of the incubation periods were also optimized (*see* **Note 1**).

3.1 Protocol for Human IgG_4 Standard Curve

1. Make up human IgG_4 at a concentration of 125,000 pg/mL in PBS. This will be the highest/first point of the standard curve.
2. From the 125,00 pg/mL human IgG_4, make 11 serial dilutions of 1:2 (doubling dilutions) with PBS, to make the 12-point standard curve.

3. Coat wells A1 and B1 with 200 μL of the first point of the IgG_4 standard curve, followed by 200 μL of the next point in wells A2 and B2 and so on, finishing with the final point of the curve in wells A12 and B12.
4. Seal plate with parafilm and incubate for 1 h at 37 °C.
5. Wash plates 3× with wash buffer by hand using a squeeze bottle. Once third wash is completed, tap plate onto paper towels to remove remaining buffer from the wells and dispel any bubbles.
6. Add 250 μL of blocking buffer to each well.
7. Seal plate with parafilm and incubate for 1 h at 4 °C.
8. Wash plate 3× with wash buffer.
9. Add 250 μL of blocking buffer to each well.
10. Seal plate with parafilm and incubate overnight at 4 °C.
11. Wash plate 4× with wash buffer.
12. Add 200 μL of HRP mouse anti-human IgG_4 (diluted 1:1000 in reagent/blocking buffer) to all wells.
13. Seal plate with parafilm and incubate for 1 h at 4 °C.
14. Wash plate 6× with wash buffer.
15. Add 100 μL of freshly made substrate solution to each well and leave for between 5 and 10 min, until highest point of standard curve is readily visible.
16. Add 100 μL of stop solution to each well.
17. Ensure that no air bubbles are within the wells and read plate at 450 nm absorbance.
18. Calculate average and % CV of duplicates as well as the signal-noise ratio of the positive and negative controls.
19. Plot standard curve and determine arbitrary units (AU) of mouse urine-specific IgG4 in test samples from the standard curve based on optical density (OD) (Fig. 1).

3.2 ELISA protocol for IgG_4-Specific Antibodies to Mouse Urine

1. Coat each well (except the top two rows A1–12, B1–12) of the ELISA plate in 200 μL of 200 μg/mL of mouse urine extract in PBS.
2. Seal plate with parafilm and incubate for 1 h at 37 °C.
3. Wash plates 3× with wash buffer by hand using a squeeze bottle. Once third wash is completed, tap plate onto paper towels to remove remaining buffer from the wells and dispel any bubbles.
4. Add 250 μL of blocking buffer to each well.
5. Seal plate with parafilm and incubate for 1 h at 4 °C.
6. Wash plate 3× with wash buffer.

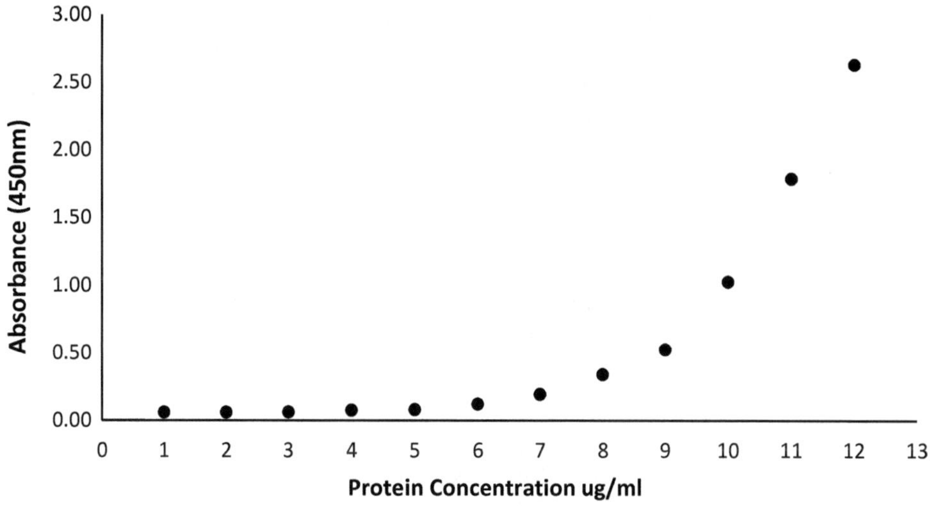

Fig. 1 Example of standard for IgG_4 ELISA. Twelve concentrations of human IgG4 were assayed, absorbance plotted against protein concentration

7. Add 200 μL of reagent/blocking buffer to wells C1–2. Vortex serum samples and add 200 μL of negative control serum to wells G11–12 and positive control serum to wells H11–12. Add test serum samples, in duplicate, to all other wells of the ELISA plate.
8. Continue with ELISA as for above protocol from **step 10** onwards.

3.3 Analysis of ELISA Data

We could not obtain the required amount of analyte (mouse urine-specific IgG_4) for a standard curve. Instead, we developed a curve using human IgG_4. From the standard curve, we could determine quantities of mouse urine-specific IgG_4 and represent the values in arbitrary units (AU).

In addition, we ran a pool of positive serum and negative serum in each assay. The assays would only be accepted if the signal-to-noise ratio was above 20.

The coefficient of variation (CV) was calculated for all duplicates and those with a %CV over 20 were repeated (*see* **Note 2**).

4 Notes

1. Optimization of assay:
   (a) Standard curve: Initial highest point of the curve was 1,000,000 pg/mL. When plotted, the peak of the curve was seen to be at the fourth point (125,000 pg/mL) on the curve; after this point the optical densities plateaued. Thus, for the rest of the experiments the first/highest point on the curve would be 125,000 pg/mL.

(b) Two blocking agents were tested BSA and Chonblock, BSA performed the best of the two.

(c) Checkerboard analysis was performed on the serum and HRP-labeled antihuman IgG_4 to optimize the assay and stop the buildup of precipitate in the wells containing test serum samples with the highest ODs.

(d) To insure less variability between assays, we used a TMB substrate kit. We tested this kit with biotinylated anti-human IgG_4 and ExtrAvidin peroxidase versus HRP-labeled anti-human IgG_4. The HRP-labeled anti-human IgG4 performed better and was therefore used throughout the assay.

(e) It was initially observed that even after optimization there was visible precipitate at the highest points of the standard curve. To prevent this, different blocking times were used. It was found that blocking the curve overnight prevented the formation of precipitate after substrate development.

2. Reducing % coefficient of variance (CV) between duplicates:

(a) After addition of reagents to wells tap plate for 1 min (before incubation) to ensure that all reagents are mixed well.

(b) Pre-wet pipette tips 2–3 times in required solution before pipetting.

(c) Make up new reagent/blocking buffer and wash buffer before every experiment. Make up coating, standard curve, serum, and HRP-labeled anti-human IgG_4 dilutions immediately before use.

(d) Avoid exposing the plate to light during the incubation of the HRP-labeled anti-human IgG_4.

(e) The optical density of the highest point in the curve should be between 2 and 3 OD_{450nm} once developed.

(f) During incubation, ensure that plates are placed on a flat surface and temperature stays constant throughout the experiment (i.e., use fridge and incubator that maintain constant temperatures).

(g) Ensure after each wash step that there are no bubbles left in the wells.

References

1. Satoguina JS, Adjobimey T, Arndts K, Hoch J, Oldenburg J, Layland LE, Hoerauf A (2008) Tr1 and naturally occurring regulatory T cells induce IgG4 in B cells through GITR/GITR-L interaction, IL-10 and TGF-beta. Eur J Immunol 38:3101–3013. https://doi.org/10.1002/eji.200838193
2. Jones M, Jeal H, Schofield S et al (2014) Rat-specific IgG and IgG_4 antibodies associated with inhibition of IgE-allergen complex

binding in laboratory animal workers. Occup Environ Med 71:619–623. https://doi.org/10.1136/oemed-2014-102119
3. Shamji MH, Kappen J, Abubakar-Waziri H et al (2019) Nasal allergen neutralising IgG4 antibodies block IgE-mediated responses: novel biomarker of subcutaneous grass pollen immunotherapy. J Allergy Clin Immunol 143(3):1067–1076. https://doi.org/10.1016/j.jaci.2018.09.039
4. Renand A, Archila LD, McGinty J et al (2015) Chronic cat-allergen exposure induces a TH2 cell-dependent IgG4 response related to low-sensitization. J Allergy Clin Immunol 136:1627–1635. e13. https://doi.org/10.1016/j.jaci.2015.07.031
5. Hesselmar B, Aberg B, Eriksson B et al (2003) High-dose exposure to cat is associated with clinical tolerance—a modified Th2 immune response? Clin Exp Allergy 33:1681–1685
6. Platts-Mills T, Vaughan J, Squillace S et al (2001) Sensitisation, asthma, and a modified Th2 response in children exposed to cat allergen: a population-based cross-sectional study. Lancet 357:752–756
7. Rossi RE, Monasterolo G, Coco G et al (2007) Evaluation of serum IgG4 antibodies specific to grass pollen allergen components in the follow up of allergic patients undergoing subcutaneous and sublingual immunotherapy. Vaccine 25:957–964
8. Subbarayal B, Schiller D, Möbs C et al (2013) Kinetics, cross-reactivity, and specificity of Bet v 1-specific IgG4 antibodies induced by immunotherapy with birch pollen. Allergy 68:1377–1386. https://doi.org/10.1111/all.12236
9. Nouri-Aria KT, Wachholz PA, Francis JN et al (2004) Grass pollen immunotherapy induces mucosal and peripheral IL-10 responses and blocking IgG activity. J Immunol 172:3252–3259
10. James LK, Shamji MH, Walker SM et al (2011) Long-term tolerance after allergen immunotherapy is accompanied by selective persistence of blocking antibodies. J Allergy Clin Immunol 127:509–516.e1-5. https://doi.org/10.1016/j.jaci.2010.12.1080
11. Aalberse RC, Dieges PH, Knul-Bretlova V et al (1983) IgG4 as a blocking antibody. Clin Rev Allergy 1:289
12. Varga EM, Kausar F, Aberer W et al (2013) Tolerant beekeepers display venom-specific functional IgG4 antibodies in the absence of specific IgE. J Allergy Clin Immunol 131:1419–1421. https://doi.org/10.1016/j.jaci.2012.08.037
13. Jeal H, Draper A, Harris J et al (2006) Modified Th2 responses at high-dose exposures to allergen: using an occupational model. Am J Respir Crit Care Med 174:21–25
14. Peng RD, Paigen B, Eggleston PA et al (2011) Both the variability and level of mouse allergen exposure influence the phenotype of the immune response in workers at a mouse facility. J Allergy Clin Immunol 128:390–396. e7. https://doi.org/10.1016/j.jaci.2011.04.050
15. Portengen L, de Meer G, Doekes G et al (2004) Immunoglobulin G4 antibodies to rat urinary allergens, sensitization and symptomatic allergy in laboratory animal workers. Clin Exp Allergy 34:1243–1250
16. Krop EJ, Doekes G, Heederik DJ et al (2011) IgG4 antibodies against rodents in laboratory animal workers do not protect against allergic sensitization. Allergy 66:517–522. https://doi.org/10.1111/j.1398-9995.2010.02508.x
17. Matsui EC, Diette GB, Krop EJ et al (2005) Mouse allergen-specific immunoglobulin G and immunoglobulin G4 and allergic symptoms in immunoglobulin E-sensitized laboratory animal workers. Clin Exp Allergy 35:1347–1353

Chapter 17

Preparation of Samples for a Mass Spectrometry-Based Method to Identify Allergenic Proteins

Mary Brian

Abstract

Western blotting is an immunological technique that has been combined with mass spectrometry analysis, to create a high-throughput method for protein identification. Western blotting using serum allows us to identify a protein within an allergenic extract that specifically binds to a serum antibody, immunoglobulin E. This specific IgE binding protein can then be detected with a highly sensitive chemiluminescence detection substrate.

Proteins detected by western blotting can be analyzed by mass spectrometry following an in-gel digestion protocol. The protein band of interest is excised from the gel and digested with trypsin to form peptides. Mass spectrometry will almost certainly have a pre-chromatographic step in which these peptides are separated before becoming ionized and entering a mass analyzer. It is in the mass analyzer that peptides are identified according to their mass-to-charge ratio, compiled into a mass spectrum which is compared to mass spectra held within online protein databases.

Key words Allergen, Mass spectrometry, Gel electrophoresis, Western blotting

1 Introduction

Mass spectrometry (MS) is a powerful analytical technique used to measure the mass of ionic species within a sample. It has become an invaluable tool within many scientific disciplines, including the field of proteomics. In the last two decades, MS-based proteomics has seen significant advancements and is now the method of choice to identify and characterize biological proteins [1]. This method is now used in the identification of allergens as well as their isoforms, variants, and posttranslational modifications [2, 3]. In this chapter we describe how MS can be combined with the traditional Western blotting method, to provide a selective immuno-proteomic tool for the identification of unknown allergens [2].

Penny Lympany and Meinir G. Jones (eds.), *Allergy: Methods and Protocols*, Methods in Molecular Biology, vol. 2020, https://doi.org/10.1007/978-1-4939-9591-2_17,

1.1 Western Blotting

In western blotting, the proteins (containing unknown or putative allergens) are first separated by gel electrophoresis (either according to molecular weight, isoelectric point, or both). The protein is then transferred onto a membrane made of nitrocellulose or polyvinylidene difluoride (PDVF) and probed with a primary and secondary antibody [4]. The primary antibody binds specifically to the protein of interest. For this, serum from an allergic patient containing specific immunoglobulin E can be used. The secondary antibody binds specifically to the primary antibody, and is also labeled with an enzyme, such as horseradish peroxidase or alkaline phosphatase. The enzyme label reacts with a chemiluminescent substrate, producing light as a by-product, which acts as the detectable protein signal. This technique has often been used in immunological studies to analyze the presence of relevant biological markers [5, 6]. Different western blotting detection methods have varying sensitivities. Chemiluminescence is the most sensitive, where light produced from the enzyme-substrate reaction is captured using charge-coupled device (CCD) cameras [7].

1.2 In-Gel Digestion

Using an optimized in-gel digestion protocol [8], proteins can be excised after gel electrophoresis and prepared for MS analysis. The recipe applies to 1- or 2-dimensional gels stained with Coomassie and comprises four main steps: (1) destaining, (2) reduction and alkylation, (3) proteolytic cleavage, and (4) peptide extraction.

1. To destain the excised gel pieces, a solution of ammonium bicarbonate and acetonitrile is used to break the bonds between the protein and Coomassie dye. For mass spectrometry analysis, Coomassie dye is the more commonly used staining method as glutaraldehyde used in silver staining impairs MS analysis.
2. Reduction of cysteine-disulfide bonds is performed to unfold the tertiary structure of the protein. This allows cleavage sites to be more available for the digestive enzyme. Agents such as tris-2-carboxyethyl phosphine (TCEP) or dithiothreitol (DTT) are used in reduction. Since cysteine-disulfide bonds cannot reform, alkylation is performed in combination with reduction. This is done using iodoacetamide (IAA), which adds an acetamide group to the sulfhydryl groups of cysteine residues, hence blocking bonds from reforming.
3. The unfolded proteins are then cleaved into peptides with a proteolytic enzyme. Trypsin is by far the most widely used enzyme for protein digestion. It is a serine protease that specifically cleaves peptide bonds at the carboxyl-terminal of lysine and arginine residues.
4. After digestion, the peptides generated are extracted from the gel matrix into solution using trifluoroacetic acid (TFA) and

acetonitrile. ZipTip®, a 10 μL pipette tip, is often used in this step as it contains a chromatography media for purifying and concentrating the extracted peptides in solution.

1.3 Nano Liquid Chromatography (LC) Coupled to Tandem Mass Spectrometry (MS/MS)

Prior to MS analysis, peptides will almost certainly be separated by a chromatographic method. The two most commonly used are gas chromatography (GC) for volatile compounds and liquid chromatography (LC) for biological samples. High-performance LC (HPLC) is commonplace in MS-based proteomics and relies on high-pressure pumps to pass the peptide sample in a solvent solution (mobile phase), through a column with an adsorbent material (stationary phase), typically silica particles. It is the interaction between the mobile and stationary phase that determines the pattern of peptide separation.

The coupling of LC with MS was made possible for mainstream clinical research only after the development of electrospray ionization (ESI) and matrix-assisted laser desorption ionization (MALDI). The interfaces between LC and MS available before this were pricey and often unreliable. Developed by Fenn et al. [9], ESI works by pumping liquid samples through a needle to be nebulized at the tip, forming a fine spray of charged droplets. These droplets are rapidly evaporated using heat and dry nitrogen and charged sample ions are released from the droplets that are free from solvent. The ionized sample is then transferred into a high vacuum and then through a small aperture into the mass analyzer. MALDI was developed by Tanaka et al. [10] and is less used in complex proteomics. Briefly, the liquid sample is mixed with organic material (matrix) and applied to a metal plate, positioned in the MS high-vacuum source. A pulsed laser beam irradiates the sample causing desorption from the plate followed by desolvation. The sample is then ionized by protonation/deprotonation and speeds toward the vacuum for entry into the mass analyzer.

A commonly used and trade-marked mass analyzer is the Orbitrap, developed by Hu et al. [11]. An Orbitrap consists of an outer barrel-shaped electrode and an inner spindle-like electrode which together trap ions by "electrodynamic squeezing." The ions oscillate with different rotational frequencies that represent their mass-to-charge (m/z) ratio. After separating ions by their m/z ratio (MS_1), precursor ions can be selected for further fragmentation (MS_2). This is known as tandem mass spectrometry (MS/MS). Collision-induced dissociation (CID) is a popular fragmentation method because of its reproducible fragmentation of the peptide bond. During CID an inert gas (such as helium or argon) is introduced into the ion trap; this induces collision of precursor ions, fragmenting them into n-terminal and c-terminal peptide fragments (termed b and y product ions). This pattern of fragment ions and their mass provides information on the peptide sequence—this is a mass spectrum. The experimental mass spectrum data is then compared against theoretical spectra in protein databases to determine the best match. Software packages are then used to generate reports showing protein matches. The matches will be accompanied by information on the number of peptides/spectra identified, match score, sequence coverage, and other factors that affect the protein identification probability.

1.4 Application of MS to Allergens

It has already been shown that MS can identify and measure specific allergens in addition to assessing variability between allergen extracts. Since allergen proteomics has developed, online directories have become available such as Allergome and WHO/IUIS Allergen nomenclature that contain allergen sequence information. MS has been applied to measure food allergens [3], house dust mite extracts [12], and variability among pollen allergens [13]. The use of MS with other commonly used immunoassays is thought to facilitate allergen standardization and development of new immuno-therapeutics [14].

We provide a protocol to separate, prepare, and identify allergenic proteins by combining western blotting with MS analysis.

2 Materials

2.1 Gel Electrophoresis

2.1.1 Equipment

Vortex mixer.

Glass vial.

Heating block.

NuPAGE™ 4–12% Bis-Tris Protein Gel (manufactured by Invitrogen: Paisley, UK).

Pasteur pipette.

XCell *SureLock*™ Mini-Cell (with gel tension wedge, empty cassette, and gel knife) (manufactured by Invitrogen: Paisley, UK).

PowerEase® 90 W (manufactured by Invitrogen: Paisley, UK).

2.1.2 Reagents

Allergen extract.

Ultrapure water (UPW).

NuPAGE™ LDS sample buffer (4×) (manufactured by Invitrogen: Paisley, UK).

Precision Plus Protein™ Dual Color Standards (manufactured by Bio-Rad Laboratories: Hemel Hempstead, UK).

2.1.3 Running Buffer

Add 50 mL NuPAGE™ MES SDS running buffer (20×) (manufactured by Invitrogen: Paisley, UK) to 950 mL ultrapure water and invert the solution ten times to mix.

2.2 Western Transfer Buffer

2.2.1 Equipment

Gel knife.

Plastic container (at least 1.6 cm length × 11.5 cm width, e.g., Scienceware® antibody saver trays, manufactured by Sigma: Schnelldorf, Germany).

Pasteur pipette.

XCell *SureLock*™ Mini-Cell (with gel tension wedge, empty cassette, and gel knife) (manufactured by Invitrogen: Paisley, UK).

PowerEase® 90 W (manufactured by Invitrogen: Paisley, UK).

XCell II™ Blot Module (with sponge blotting pads and roller) (manufactured by Invitrogen: Paisley, UK).

Nitrocellulose pre-cut blotting membranes, 0.2 µm pore size (manufactured by Invitrogen: Paisley, UK).

Tweezers.

2.2.2 Reagents

Methanol.

Ultrapure water (UPW).

2.2.3 Transfer Buffer

Add 50 mL NuPAGE™ transfer buffer (20×) (manufactured by Invitrogen: Paisley, UK) to 100 mL methanol and 850 mL ultrapure water. Invert the solution ten times to mix.

2.3 Western Blotting

2.3.1 Equipment

Plastic container (at least 1.6 cm length × 11.5 cm width, e.g., Scienceware® antibody saver trays, manufactured by Sigma: Schnelldorf, Germany).

Shaker.

2.3.2 Reagents

Patient serum with positive specific IgE.

Control serum without positive specific IgE.

Goat anti-human IgE secondary antibody, HRP (manufactured by Invitrogen: Paisley, UK).

2.3.3 Blocking Buffer

Phosphate-buffered saline (PBS) pH 7.5, 1% bovine serum albumin, and 0.05% Tween-20.

2.3.4 Wash Buffer

Phosphate buffer pH 7.5 and 0.05% Tween-20.

2.4 Western Detection

2.4.1 Equipment

Tweezers.

Parafilm® M.

ChemiDoc™ Imaging System (incl. UV sample tray) (manufactured by Bio-Rad Laboratories: Hemel Hempstead, UK).

2.4.2 Reagents

Pierce™ ECL Western Blotting Substrate (incl. detections, reagents 1 + 2) (manufactured by Invitrogen: Paisley, UK).

2.5 Coomassie Staining

2.5.1 Reagents

Plastic container (at least 1.6 cm length × 11.5 cm width, e.g., Scienceware® antibody saver trays, manufactured by Sigma: Schnelldorf, Germany).

Ultrapure water.

2.5.2 Equipment

ChemiDoc™ Imaging System (incl. white sample tray for colorimetric imaging) (manufactured by Bio-Rad Laboratories: Hemel Hempstead, UK).

2.5.3 Fixing Solution

Methanol (46%) and acetic acid (7%) mixed in ultrapure water.

2.5.4 Staining Solution

Coomassie® R-250 (0.1%), methanol (46%), and acetic acid (7%) mixed in ultrapure water.

2.5.5 Destaining Solution

Methanol (5%) and acetic acid (7.5%) mixed in ultrapure water.

2.6 Image Laboratory Analysis

2.6.1 Equipment

USB device.

Computer.

2.6.2 Software

ImageLab (Version 5.2.1, manufactured by Bio-Rad Laboratories).

2.7 In-Gel Digestion

2.7.1 Equipment

Scalpel.

Eppendorf.

Centrifuge.

Heating block.

2.7.2 Reagents

ProteoExtract All-in-One Trypsin Digestion Kit (incl. wash buffer, digest buffer, D-buffer reagent, reducing agent, blocking reagent, trypsin) (manufactured by Calbiochem: San Diego, CA).

Trifluoroacetic acid.

Acetonitrile.

Milli-Q-grade water.

2.8 Desalt by ZipTip® and Mass Spectrometry Analysis

2.8.1 Equipment

SpeedVac®.

Eppendorf.

Microcentrifuge.

C18 ZipTip pipette tips (manufactured by Merck: Darmstadt, Germany).

pH paper.

Sonication bath.

Mass spec vial.

Monolithic nano-HPLC column.

Q Exactive Orbitrap mass spectrometer.

2.8.2 Reagents

Trifluoroacetic acid.

Acetonitrile.

2.8.3 Software

Chromeleon.

Xcalibur.

PEAKS Studio 8.

3 Methods

3.1 Gel Electrophoresis

The protein content (μg/μL) in the allergen extract dissolved in ultrapure water (UPW) should be determined prior to electrophoresis using a quantification assay (e.g., *DC*™ Protein Assay Kit (Bio-Rad Laboratories, Hertfordshire, UK)), following the manufacturer's instructions.

1. Calculate the volume needed (up to 22.5 μL) of the allergen solution to run between 2 and 50 μg of protein. (Prior optimization experiments using gel electrophoresis and Coomassie staining may be necessary to determine which protein mass (μg) of the allergen extract is optimal for protein detection.)
2. Pipette this volume in 2.5 μL of NuPAGE™ LDS sample buffer (×4) and make up volume to <25 μL with ultrapure water, in a clean glass vial (*see* **Note 1**).
3. Heat the sample at 70 °C for 10 min in a heat block.
4. Remove the NuPAGE™ protein gel from its pouch and using a Pasteur pipette rinse the gel with prepared running buffer. Peel off the tape at the bottom of the gel and gently pull the comb out of the top of the cassette. Rinse the sample wells three times with prepared running buffer and invert the gel to empty the wells (*see* **Note 2**).
5. Place the gel into the XCell *SureLock*™ Mini-Cell so the taller side of the gel faces outwards and place the empty cassette in the opposite side. Lock the gel into place using the gel tension wedge.
6. Pour prepared running buffer into the inner chamber, ensuring that there is no leak to the outer chambers, and then continue until just exceeding the level of the wells.
7. Using a pipette, load 5–10 μL of the heated sample into a well of the gel and 2 μL of Precision Plus Protein™ Dual Color Standards into another well (*see* **Note 3**).
8. Fill the outer chamber with running buffer to reach the same level as the inner chamber and remove any bubbles with a Pasteur pipette (*see* **Note 4**).

9. Place the lid on the Mini-Cell securely, connect the electrodes to the PowerEase®, and turn on the power supply. Using the keypad on the power supply input a constant voltage of 200 V, current of 80 mA, and time of 35 min.
10. Press start (ensure that bubbles appear at the bottom) and run electrophoresis for at least 35 min, or until the dye front from the sample buffer has reached the bottom of the gel.
11. Once complete, press stop, turn off the power, disconnect electrodes, and remove the lid.
12. Remove the gel from the cell, then separate the three sides of the cassette using a gel knife, and remove the top cassette plate.
13. Proceed to either western transfer or Coomassie staining.

3.2 Western Transfer

1. Take the gel cassette with top plate removed and cut off the wells with gel knife (*see* **Note 5**).
2. Place four sponge blotting pads in a plastic container and submerge in prepared transfer buffer (*see* **Note 6**).
3. Prior to use also place two pieces of filter paper in prepared transfer buffer and in another container using tweezers place the pre-cut nitrocellulose membrane.
4. Place one piece of presoaked filter paper on top of the gel, leaving the gel foot uncovered, and use a roller to remove any trapped air bubbles.
5. Carefully turn over the plate so the gel and filter paper are facing downwards, and then using the gel knife push the gel foot out of the plate slot, so the gel and filter paper fall off the plate.
6. Cut off the gel foot and using a Pasteur pipette wet the gel with transfer buffer.
7. Using tweezers place the presoaked nitrocellulose membrane on top of the gel, and then another piece of presoaked filter paper on top of the membrane. Remove any trapped air bubbles with roller.
8. Place two presoaked sponge blotting pads into the cathode core (−) of the blot module (the larger part of the module). Then pick up the gel-membrane assembly and place on top of the blotting pads. Place another two presoaked sponge blotting pads on top of the assembly.
9. Place the anode core (+) on top, pick up the whole blot module together, and place it into the inner buffer chamber of the Mini-Cell so that the (+) sign is in the upper left-hand corner and the gold post on the right fits into the blot module. Secure the blot module with the gel tension wedge.

10. Fill the blot module with transfer buffer until the blotting sandwich is covered but is not filled to the top of the blot module. Then fill the outer chamber with ultrapure water until it reaches approximately 2 cm from the top and remove any bubbles with a Pasteur pipette (*see* **Note** 7).
11. Place the lid on the Mini-Cell, connect electrodes, and turn on the power supply as before.
12. Input a constant voltage of 30 V, current of 120 mA, and time of 1 h. This will enable the proteins to transfer from the gel to the membrane.

3.3 Western Blotting

1. When the transfer is complete, press stop and turn off the power, disconnect the electrodes, remove the lid, and take out the blot module.
2. Take off the anode core (+), remove the sponge blotting pads, and discard the filter paper.
3. Using tweezers pick up the nitrocellulose membrane and place it into a plastic container with prepared blocking buffer (enough to cover and allow the membrane to freely move). Leave at room temperature shaking at 60 rpm for 90 min (*see* **Note 8**).
4. Prepare the primary antibody solution using patient serum diluted in blocking buffer (recommended dilution is between 1:5 and 1:10, serum:blocking buffer). The total volume will depend on how much is needed to cover the membrane in the container you are using (*see* **Note 9**).
5. Replace the blocking buffer with the 1:5–1:10 diluted primary antibody solution and leave the membrane shaking overnight at 2–8 °C (*see* **Note 10**).
6. Remove the antibody solution and wash the membrane at least five times using wash buffer at room temperature, shaking at 60 rpm.
7. Prepare the secondary antibody solution using goat anti-human IgE secondary antibody, HRP diluted in blocking buffer at a 1:5000 dilution. As before, the total volume will depend on the container you are using. Mix by pipetting the antibody in solution several times to ensure that the antibody is dispersed in the buffer.
8. Replace the wash buffer with the secondary antibody solution and leave the membrane for 30 min shaking at room temperature.
9. Remove the antibody solution and wash the membrane at least five times using wash buffer.

3.4 Western Detection

1. Leaving the membrane in wash buffer, cut out a piece of Parafilm® M slightly larger than the membrane and stick on a lab bench. Using tweezers place the membrane onto the Parafilm® M (*see* **Note 11**).
2. Prepare the substrate working solution immediately before use, by mixing 1 mL each of Pierce™ ECL Western Blotting Substrate detection reagents 1 and 2. Pipette the solution onto the membrane and leave at room temperature for 5 min.
3. During this time, switch on the ChemiDoc™ Imaging System and ensure that the UV sample tray is placed in the imaging stage.
4. Once the substrate incubation is over, immediately place the membrane onto the sample tray, push the transilluminator drawer in, and close the front door of the ChemiDoc.
5. Using the touch screen select "camera view" and specify the image size so the whole membrane is captured on the screen.
6. Press "Application," and then "Blots," and select "Chemiluminescence."
7. Press "Exposure," and then "Manual," and select "Configure Signal Accumulation Mode."
8. For exposure times enter 30 s in the "First Image" box and 300 in the "Last Image" box and in the "Images" box enter 5 as the total number of images. Then tap the Camera icon.
9. Image the dual color standards by selecting "Colorimetric" under "Blots" and "Application." Then tap the Camera icon as before to acquire the image.
10. Once the images are acquired proceed to Image Lab analysis.

3.5 Coomassie Staining

For Coomassie staining all steps should be carried out at room temperature using enough solution to cover the gel.

1. After gel electrophoresis briefly rinse the gel in ultrapure water and place in a plastic container with prepared fixing solution shaking for 1 h.
2. Replace fixing solution with prepared staining solution and leave shaking for 1 h.
3. After staining, briefly rinse the gel with ultrapure water and place in prepared destain solution shaking overnight. Destain solution should be changed at regular intervals to wash off background staining.
4. Once the background is destained, briefly wash the gel in ultrapure water, place the gel onto the white sample tray, and place in the imaging stage of the ChemiDoc Imaging System (*see* **Note 12**).

5. Turn on the imaging system, push in the transilluminator drawer, and close the drawer of the imaging system.
6. Using the touch screen select "camera view" and specify the image size so that all of the gel is captured on the screen.
7. Press "Application," and then "Protein gels," and select "Coomassie."
8. Press "Exposure," and then select "Faint bands."
9. Then tap the Camera icon to acquire the Coomassie-stained gel image.

3.6 Image Laboratory Analysis

1. Export images from the ChemiDoc Imaging System using a USB device.
2. On a computer device open these image files (Type: Image Lab Image Document) on Image Lab (version 5.2.1).
3. Use the left-hand "Analysis Tool Box" to annotate and edit the image in the following ways.
4. For blots, choose the chemiluminescence image with the optimum exposure of the samples and the colorimetric image of the standards. Click on "Image Tools" and select "Merge."
5. For both blots and protein gels, crop the image, so that all the standards and samples are showing.
6. From the "Analysis Tool Box" click on "Lanes and Bands," manually input the number of lanes, and adjust these for your blot. From "Bands," use the "Add" tool to click on the ten dual color standards.
7. Return to the "Analysis Tool Box" and click on "MW Analysis Tools." Select the "Bio-Rad Precision Plus" Standard and tick the standards lane. Select "no" to redetecting the bands.

Using the molecular weights of the standards, determine which bands on the Coomassie gel also appear on the chemiluminescence blot. Use these bands for in-gel digestion.

3.7 In-Gel Digestion

1. Using a clean scalpel excise the bands from the Coomassie-stained gel that match those detected in the chemiluminescence blot (*see* **Note 13**).
2. Cut each band into 2 mm^2 pieces and transfer into an Eppendorf.

   For the following steps use reagents from the ProteoExtract All-in-One Trypsin Digestion Kit, according to the manufacturer's instructions.
3. Wash the gel pieces three times with 80 μL of wash buffer (acetonitrile) at 37 °C in a heating block.
4. Dry the gel pieces by heating to 90 °C for 15 min.

5. Prepare digest buffer by using 0.5 mL of digest buffer solution to dissolve the lyophilized D-buffer reagent.
6. Prepare reducing agent by addition of 120 μL of ultrapure water to make stock solution. Before use, take 1 μL of stock solution and dilute in 9 μL of ultrapure water.
7. Add 20 μL of digest buffer to the gel pieces, mix in 2 μL of diluted reducing agent, and incubate at 37 °C for 10 min. Remove the Eppendorf from the heat block and cool to room temperature.
8. Prepare blocking reagent by addition of 120 μL of ultrapure water to make stock solution. Before use, take 1 μL of stock solution and dilute in 9 μL of ultrapure water.
9. Mix 2 μL of diluted blocking agent into gel pieces and incubate at room temperature for 10 min (*see* **Note 14**).
10. Prepare trypsin by addition of 50 μL of ultrapure water to the lyophilized trypsin to make stock solution. Before use, take 1 μL of stock solution and dilute in 3 μL of ultrapure water.
11. To the gel pieces, add 0.5 μL of diluted trypsin and mix. Incubate in trypsin, shaking for 3–5 h at 37 °C. The gel pieces must be fully submerged (*see* **Note 15**).
12. Centrifuge the sample for 10 min at 10,000 × *g*, and then transfer the supernatant to a new Eppendorf.
13. Add 10 μL of 0.1% trifluoroacetic acid (TFA) to the gel pieces and shake at 37 °C for 10 min. Centrifuge this sample and combine the supernatants.

Proceed with ZIPTIP extraction or samples can be stored at −20 °C.

3.8 Desalt by ZipTip®

1. Dry the gel pieces by placing in a SpeedVac for 10 min.
2. Check the acidity of the sample by addition of 13 μL of 1% TFA and pH paper (should turn red) (*see* **Note 16**).
3. Using a $ZipTip_{C18}$ tip, depress pipette plunger to a dead stop and using a 13 μL volume setting aspirate acetonitrile (100%) into the tip. Dispense, discard, and repeat.
4. Then aspirate 0.1% TFA, dispense, discard, and repeat.
5. Depress pipette plunger to a dead stop, then aspirate, and dispense the peptide sample in 7–10 cycles in the Eppendorf.
6. Aspirate 0.1% TFA, dispense, discard, and repeat.
7. Prepare elution solution as 0.1% TFA and 50% acetonitrile.
8. Dispense 13 μL of elution solution into a clean Eppendorf, then aspirate, and dispense the eluent through the ZipTip pipette three times, without introducing any air bubbles.
9. Dry the sample in a SpeedVac for 10 min.

10. Dissolve the sample in 6 μL of 0.1% TFA and place in a sonication bath for 5 min.
11. Briefly centrifuge the sample and then transfer to a mass spectrometry specialist vial.

The sample is now ready for mass spectrometry analysis. The following is based on using an automated EASY Nano Liquid Chromatograph 1000 coupled to an electrospray ionization Orbitrap mass spectrometer. Chromeleon Chromatography Data System and Xcalibur software should be used to program the instruments. For chromatography, the flow rate should be selected as 200 nL/min over 60 min using a 75 μm column with a linear gradient of acetonitrile in 0.1% formic acid. For mass spectrum scans, a data-dependent switching mode and Top20 collision-induced dissociation fragmentation method should be used.

After samples have been run, the mass spectrum data can be searched against Uniprot protein database. On PEAKS Studio 8 the search should be selected with a fragment ion mass tolerance of 0.80 Da, a parent ion tolerance of 20 ppm, trypsin as the digestion enzyme, and a false discovery rate (FDR) of 1%. These results can then be exported to Excel and scores (−10lgP), coverage (%), signal intensities, and no. of peptides used to determine the most abundant proteins present in your sample.

4 Notes

1. When pipetting the LDS sample buffer and ultrapure water into the allergen solution, use a mix-pipetting technique, to ensure that the final solution is thoroughly mixed.
2. When pulling out the gel comb, hold the gel with both hands and push the comb out using slight pressure upwards with your thumbs.
3. When loading samples and standards with a pipette, do so slowly and continuously, so as not to introduce any air bubbles.
4. To minimize bubbles, pour the running buffer solution slowly.
5. To cut wells, place gel knife directly below them, apply little pressure, and move the gel knife away from the gel.
6. Squeeze the pads while submerged to ensure that any air bubbles are removed.
7. To minimize bubbles, pour the transfer buffer solution and ultrapure water slowly.
8. Prepare blocking buffer prior to use to ensure that solution is dissolved properly.

9. Use a mix-pipetting technique to ensure that the serum is thoroughly mixed into the blocking buffer.
10. Cover the container with parafilm, to avoid any evaporation of solution.
11. Parafilm can be stuck on a lab bench by pushing down the corners with a blunt object such as a pen or pencil.
12. Fixing, staining, and destaining solution can all be prepared before use and kept for further use.
13. To more accurately see the bands which need to be excised, perform this step on a bright surface.
14. Add reducing and blocking reagent by mix-pipetting technique.
15. This can also be left to incubate overnight.
16. If sample is not acidic, continue adding 1% TFA and retesting.

References

1. Schuchardt S, Sickmann A (2007) Protein identification using mass spectrometry: a method overview. EXS 97:141–170
2. Swoboda I, Jilek A, Ferreira F, Engel E, Hoffmann-Sommergruber K, Scheiner O, Kraft D, Breiteneder H, Pittenauer E, Schmid E (1995) Isoforms of Bet v 1, the major birch pollen allergen, analyzed by liquid chromatography, mass spectrometry, and cDNA cloning. J Biol Chem 270(6):2607–2613
3. Koeberl M, Clarke D, Lopata AL (2014a) Next generation of food allergen quantification using mass spectrometric systems. J Proteome Res 13(8):3499–3509. https://doi.org/10.1021/pr500247r
4. Towbin H, Staehelin T, Gordon J (1979) Electrophoretic transfer of proteins from polyacrylamide gels to nitrocellulose sheets: procedure and some applications. Proc Natl Acad Sci U S A 76(9):4350–4354
5. Ebner C, Birkner T, Valenta R, Rumpold H, Breitenbach M, Scheiner O, Kraft D (1991) Common epitopes of birch pollen and apples-studies by western and northern blot. J Allergy Clin Immunol 88(4):588–594
6. Koppelman SJ, Wensing M, Ertmann M, Knulst AC, Knol EF (2004) Relevance of Ara h1, Ara h2 and Ara h3 in peanut-allergic patients, as determined by immunoglobulin E Western blotting, basophil-histamine release and intracutaneous testing: Ara h2 is the most important peanut allergen. Clin Exp Allergy 34(4):583–590. https://doi.org/10.1111/j.1365-2222.2004.1923.x
7. Ghosh R, Gilda JE, Gomes AV (2014) The necessity of and strategies for improving confidence in the accuracy of western blots. Expert Rev Proteomics 11(5):549–560. https://doi.org/10.1586/14789450.2014.939635
8. Shevchenko A, Tomas H, Havlis J, Olsen JV, Mann M (2006) In-gel digestion for mass spectrometric characterization of proteins and proteomes. Nat Protoc 1(6):2856–2860. https://doi.org/10.1038/nprot.2006.468
9. Fenn JB, Mann M, Meng CK, Wong SF, Whitehouse CM (1989) Electrospray ionization for mass spectrometry of large biomolecules. Science (New York, NY) 246(4926):64–71
10. Tanaka K, Waki H, Ido Y, Akita S, Yoshida Y, Yoshida T, Matsuo T (1988) Protein and polymer analyses up to m/z 100 000 by laser ionization time-of-flight mass spectrometry. Rapid Commun Mass Spectrom 2(8):151–153. https://doi.org/10.1002/rcm.1290020802
11. Hu Q, Noll RJ, Li H, Makarov A, Hardman M, Graham Cooks R (2005) The Orbitrap: a new mass spectrometer. J Mass Spectrom 40(4):430–443. https://doi.org/10.1002/jms.856. Accessed 13 Dec 2018
12. Harris J, Mason DE, Li J, Burdick KW, Backes BJ, Chen T, Shipway A, Van Heeke G, Gough L, Ghaemmaghami A, Shakib F, Debaene F, Winssinger N (2004) Activity profile of dust mite allergen extract using substrate libraries

and functional proteomic microarrays. Chem Biol 11(10):1361–1372. https://doi.org/10.1016/j.chembiol.2004.08.008

13. Fenaille F, Nony E, Chabre H, Lautrette A, Couret M, Batard T, Moingeon P, Ezan E (2009) Mass spectrometric investigation of molecular variability of grass pollen group 1 allergens. J Proteome Res 8(8):4014–4027. https://doi.org/10.1021/pr900359p
14. Chapman MD, Briza P (2012) Molecular approaches to allergen standardization. Curr Allergy Asthma Rep 12(5):478–484. https://doi.org/10.1007/s11882-012-0282-3

Index

Penny Lympany and Meinir G. Jones (eds.), *Allergy: Methods and Protocols*, Methods in Molecular Biology, vol. 2020, https://doi.org/10.1007/978-1-4939-9591-2,

MIX
Papier aus verantwortungsvollen Quellen
Paper from responsible sources
FSC® C105338

If you have any concerns about our products,
you can contact us on
ProductSafety@springernature.com

In case Publisher is established outside the EU,
the EU authorized representative is:
Springer Nature Customer Service Center GmbH
Europaplatz 3, 69115 Heidelberg, Germany

Printed by Libri Plureos GmbH
in Hamburg, Germany